STRENGTHENING FAMILY RESILIENCE

Strengthening Family Resilience

SECOND EDITION

FROMA WALSH

THE GUILFORD PRESS
New York   London

© 2006 The Guilford Press
A Division of Guilford Publications, Inc.
72 Spring Street, New York, NY 10012
www.guilford.com

Printed in the United States of America

This book is printed on acid-free paper.

Last digit is print number: 9   8   7   6   5   4   3

Library of Congress Cataloging-in-Publication Data

Walsh, Froma.
    Strengthening Family Resilience / Froma Walsh.—2nd ed.
       p. ; cm.
    Includes bibliographical references and index.
    ISBN-13: 978-1-59385-186-6 (alk. paper)
    ISBN-10: 1-59385-186-3 (alk. paper)
    1. Family—Mental health. 2. Resilience (Personality trait). 3. Problem families.
    4. Family psychotherapy. 5. Family social work.
    [DNLM: 1. Family—psychology. 2. Adaptation, Psychological. 3. Life Change Events.
    4. Mental Health Services. 5. Psychotherapy—methods. 6. Stress, Psychological.
    WA 305 W915s 2006] I. Title.
    RC489.F33W34 2006
       616.89'156—dc22

                                                                    2006004507

About the Author

Froma Walsh, PhD, is the Mose and Sylvia Firestone Professor in the School of Social Service Administration at the University of Chicago. She also has a joint appointment in the Department of Psychiatry, Pritzker School of Medicine, and is Co-Director of the university-affiliated Chicago Center for Family Health. She is a past president of the American Family Therapy Academy and past editor of the *Journal of Marital and Family Therapy*. Dr. Walsh has received awards for her distinguished contributions and leadership in the field of family therapy from the Division of Family Psychology of the American Psychological Association, the American Association for Marriage and Family Therapy, and the American Family Therapy Academy. Her books include *Normal Family Processes: Growing Diversity and Complexity, Third Edition; Living Beyond Loss: Death in the Family, Second Edition; Spiritual Resources in Family Therapy;* and *Women in Families*. She speaks and consults internationally on resilience-oriented research, professional training, and practice.

Acknowledgments

This book is dedicated to the ordinary, everyday families who forge resilience through challenging times. As Studs Terkel, a hero of mine, avows, the real heroes in the world are all around us—parents who work two shifts and still manage to raise their children well; those who sustain an indomitable spirit in the face of illness, disability, or loss; those who rekindle hope and build connection and renewal out of tragedy rather than sink in despair and alienation; those who respond compassionately to the plight of others; those who transcend barriers and show us the value and worth of life.

I am grateful to the many families I've been privileged to know in my professional and personal life who have taught me about resilience through their determination, creative initiative, and perseverance in meeting their life challenges. They inspire my best work and affirm my conviction in the human potential for resilience, healing, and growth. My early Peace Corps experience in Morocco and consultations over the years in many parts of the world have expanded my perspective on resilient families. I've admired strong kinship and community networks that enable families to withstand severe economic hardship, physical suffering, and tragic events. Families with little in material wealth have taught me the immeasurable value of human connections and faith, especially in troubled times. I appreciate the many colleagues and students who have enriched my work immeasurably over the years. It is a joy to teach and learn from the bright and curious students at the University of Chicago and our affiliated family therapy training institute, the Chicago

Center for Family Health. I value my many stimulating contacts and collaborations internationally with colleagues and students on the frontiers of resilience research and innovative practice applications.

I thank the staff at The Guilford Press for their support in the production of this new edition. I'm most grateful for the wise editorial feedback provided by Senior Editor Jim Nageotte. I'd also like to thank all who offered helpful comments on this new edition, particularly John Rolland, Claire Whitney, Michele Scheinkman, Ashley Curry, and Rachel Shapira.

My family and the kinship of close friends have been a wellspring for meaningful connection, joy in good times, and resilience in troubled times. I thank my husband, John, for his steadfast love. I admire my daughter, Claire, for her creative mind, her "can-do" spirit, her compassion, and her deep commitment to international humanitarian work. Above all I want to express my gratitude to my parents for their loving support and encouragement despite their own life struggles. I only wish that while they were alive I had more fully appreciated their courage and resourcefulness in overcoming the many adversities they faced in their lives. I carry their indomitable spirit in my heart.

Preface

Resilience—the ability to rebound from crisis and overcome life challenges—has become an increasingly valuable and timely concept in the field of mental health since the first edition of this volume was published in 1998. Families and societies have been experiencing tumultuous changes and devastating natural and human-caused disasters; the world around us has become more hazardous and the future more uncertain. The media present inspiring accounts of human resilience in courageous responses to crisis situations. Just what is family resilience and why is it so important?

No family is problem free; all face serious challenges over the life course. What processes enable family members to support one another through turbulent times? To cope well with an illness that can't be cured or a problem that can't be solved? To rebuild lives after shattering losses or life-altering transitions? To rise above severe trauma or barriers of poverty and discrimination? It's crucial to understand how families can effectively integrate scarring experiences and go on to live and love well.

This volume presents a research-informed family resilience framework for intervention and prevention to strengthen key family processes in dealing with adversity. This fully updated, revised, and expanded second edition incorporates the latest research and practice advances. Intended to serve both as a clinical resource and course text, it provides practice guidelines and case illustrations to address a wide range of challenges: sudden crisis, trauma, and loss; disruptive transitions, such as job loss, divorce, and migration; persistent multistress conditions of serious

ix

illness or poverty; and barriers to success for at-risk youth. New chapters present resilience-oriented approaches for recovery in the aftermath of major disasters and demonstrate applications of this approach in community-based and international programs.

A family resilience framework is especially relevant to clinical practice and social service delivery because most clients seek help in troubled times. By definition, resilience involves strengths under stress and forged through crisis and prolonged adversity. In contrast to deficit-focused practice models, this resilience-oriented approach draws out family strengths and potential to meet the challenges. Beyond coping or problem solving, resilience involves positive transformation and growth. In building relational resilience, families forge stronger bonds and become more resourceful in meeting future challenges. Thus, every intervention has preventive benefits.

I've long been interested in the concept of resilience. I grew up in a family challenged by many adversities. I was often viewed as hardy, *despite* my family experience. I later came to see that those challenges made me stronger. It took a long time to appreciate my parents' struggles and their remarkable courage, perseverance, and resourcefulness. In my young adulthood, their deficits loomed large. Traditional psychotherapy dredged up all the negative experiences of childhood and elaborated on parental failings. The field of mental health was so heavily skewed toward pathology that it might more aptly have been called the field of mental illness. My clinical training taught me how to diagnose disorders, but gave no attention to healthy functioning or how practitioners might recognize and promote it.

I was drawn to the field of family therapy, which was just flowering in the late 1960s. It was refreshing to cast off deterministic theories of early-childhood, maternal causality for individual problems. The systemic paradigm expanded focus to the multiple influences in functioning through transactional processes in the broad network of relationships. Yet the family field initially overfocused on family deficits, reflecting the broader culture and media views that most families were more or less dysfunctional. As coordinator of the family studies in a schizophrenia research program, when I sought to include a normal control group, my colleagues chided me that I wouldn't find any normal families and they certainly wouldn't recommend their own. Undaunted, I did find them and was impressed by their vitality and diversity. Yet I found that families themselves worried about their adequacy—one mother even asked if her family could receive a "certificate of normality"!

That experience led me to pursue doctoral studies in human development to expand my knowledge about family and social processes that foster healthy functioning, well-being, and growth. My clinical teaching and practice became increasingly strengths-oriented, and I've strived to bridge the divide between the social sciences and the mental health field. I look back on those valuable research and learning experiences as my professional "flight into health."

Two myths about normal families have clouded our understanding. First, the erroneous assumption that healthy families are problem free can overpathologize ordinary families struggling with stressful life challenges or traumatic experiences. Second, the assumption that a single, universal model of the healthy family is essential, fitting an idealized image of families of the past, led to faulty presumptions that varying family values, structures, and gender roles are inherently dysfunctional and damage children. With the growing diversity of families in society, no single model fits all—or even most—families today. In this volume, "family" is defined broadly, to encompass varied family forms, committed couple relationships, and extended formal and informal kin networks. As we will see, research finds that families can thrive and children can be raised well in a variety of kin arrangements: What matters most are effective family processes.

Over the past two decades, family systems research has provided empirical grounding to identify many key processes that support effective family functioning. Drawing together these findings with a growing body of research on resilience, the family resilience framework presented here is flexible for application with a broad diversity of families facing a wide range of stressful challenges. It attends to the interaction of individual, family, and social influences and recognizes that there are many, varied pathways in resilience.

The family resilience practice approach described in this volume builds on recent advances in strengths-based, collaborative, systemic therapies in the field of family therapy. It is distinct in focus on strengthening family functioning in the context of adversity. Incorporating a developmental perspective on stress, coping, and adaptation, this approach links presenting symptoms with disruptive stress events, with ripple effects to all members and relationships. The family response can foster resilience for all members and their relationships.

The framework and practice applications presented in this new edition have been developed, refined, and reformulated over many years of clinical teaching, supervision, and direct practice grounded in a developmental systems orientation. Key processes are identified that enable couples and families facing disruptive crises or persistent stresses to forge stronger bonds, regain functioning, and move forward with their lives. Practical guidelines are offered to assist family members in mastering a wide range of life challenges. Case illustrations draw on many varied examples of family resilience in my professional practice, research, and training of family therapists, as well as in my personal life. Names and details have been carefully altered to protect families' privacy. Throughout this volume, I discuss ways in which couples, families, and helping professionals can identify, affirm, and strengthen ways of turning adversity into opportunities for positive change and growth.

In Part I of the volume, Chapter 1 presents the foundation for a family resilience approach to practice. It clarifies the concept of resilience, surveys what we have learned from studies of individual resilience, and presents a multisystemic view of resilience that integrates ecological and developmental perspectives. Chapter 2 situates family resilience in social context, highlighting trends in the growing diversity and complexity of families and their stressful challenges in our rapidly changing world. This perspective is essential for family assessment and intervention to be attuned to today's families and their varied pathways in coping and resilience.

Part II integrates research findings and practice perspectives to identify key transactional processes that facilitate effective family functioning and resilience. Because practitioners can be overwhelmed by the complexities of family process under stressful conditions, I have found it useful to organize these processes within three domains of family functioning: belief systems, organizational patterns, and communication processes. Chapters 3–5 describe and illustrate key processes for family resilience in each domain.

Part III describes and illustrates practice applications of this family resilience framework. Chapter 6 provides practical guidelines and case examples to foster resilience in work with distressed couples and families. Chapter 7, a new chapter, presents core principles and illustrations of successful family resilience-oriented community-based programs and research both locally, developed at the Chicago Center for Family Health, and internationally, in projects launched in many parts of the world. Helping professionals' own resilience and courageous engagement with families are discussed.

In Part IV, Chapters 8–12 describe and illustrate the application of a family resilience approach to various adverse situations, from crisis events to disruptive transitions to prolonged adversity. Chapter 8 addresses the profound challenges families face with death and dying and key variables in risk and resilience with loss. Chapter 9 tracks the family journey over time with chronic physical and mental illnesses, offering guidelines to reduce stress and enable families to thrive in the face of illness-related demands and uncertainties. Chapter 10 addresses the persistent challenges faced by multistressed, low-income, highly vulnerable families and at-risk youth, presenting principles, guidelines, and case examples of effective strengths-based family and multisystemic interventions. Countering common presumptions that such families are "severely dysfunctional," hopeless, and untreatable, this approach affirms and builds family resources and potential to overcome barriers and thrive in the face of adversity. Chapter 11, new in this edition, focuses on resilience-building approaches for family and community recovery in the wake of major traumatic events, ranging from community violence to large-scale disasters, terrorism, war-related atrocities, and refugee experience. Chapter 12, drawing on my own personal experience as well as many others who have inspired me, encourages possibilities for reconnection, reconciliation, and forgiveness in families, in groups that have suffered oppression, and in parts of our world torn by strife. It challenges common assumptions that those wounded by past trauma and troubled relationships survive best by severing ties to their families and their past, fortifying themselves as rugged individuals.

The family resilience approach presented here is grounded in the firm conviction that we human beings survive and thrive best through deep connections with those around us, those who have come before us, and all who have been, and could be, significant in our lives. Even experiences of severe trauma and very troubled relationships hold potential for healing and transformation across the life cycle and the generations. In facing adversity, resilience is nurtured and sustained through strong family, social, community, and cultural bonds. Caring and committed human connections are "lifelines" for resilience.

This book can serve as a valuable resource for all professionals who are interested in fostering human adaptive capacities, regardless of practice orientation, discipline, or level of experience. A family resilience framework can be applied to a wide range of child and family problems in the fields of mental health, healthcare, human services, child welfare, family life education, juvenile justice, community organization, family law, and pastoral counseling; by practicing professionals, educators, and students; and by marriage and family therapists, social workers, psychologists, psychiatrists, counselors, nurses, and physicians. Although the book is written primarily for helping professionals, it can also be of value for a general readership—especially for family members who have faced stressful life challenges and who are interested in understanding how to build relational resources to strengthen their own individual, couple, and family well-being.

The need to strengthen family resilience has never been more urgent, as families today are buffeted by stresses and uncertainties of economic, social, political, and environmental upheaval. Yet all families have the potential for adaptation, repair, and growth. A family resilience approach provides a positive and pragmatic framework that guides interventions to strengthen family *processes for resilience* as presenting problems are addressed. In this way, families become more resourceful in dealing with unforeseen problems and averting future crises. For helping professionals, the therapeutic process is enriched as we bring out the best in families and practice the art of the possible.

Contents

PART IV
FACILITATING FAMILY RESILIENCE
THROUGH CRISIS AND
PROLONGED CHALLENGES

PART I

Overview

CHAPTER 1

Foundations of a Family Resilience Approach

Come to the edge, life said.
They said: We are afraid.
Come to the edge, life said.
They came. It pushed them . . . and they flew.
—GUILLAUME APOLLINAIRE

We live in turbulent times, on the edge of uncertainty. Family life and the world around us have changed so dramatically in recent years that while we yearn for strong and enduring relationships, we are unsure how to shape and sustain them to weather the storms of life. Although some families are shattered by crisis or persistent stresses, what is remarkable is that others emerge strengthened and more resourceful. With widespread concern about family breakdown, we need more than ever to understand the processes that can foster family resilience—a relational hardiness. In order to support and strengthen couples and families, we need useful conceptual tools as much as techniques. This chapter lays the foundations for a family resilience framework for clinical and community practice, prevention efforts, research, and family policy.

A family resilience approach aims to identify and fortify key interactional processes that enable families to withstand and rebound from disruptive life challenges. A resilience lens shifts perspective from

3

viewing distressed families as damaged to seeing them as challenged, affirming their potential for repair and growth. This approach is based on the conviction that both individual and relational strength can be forged through collaborative efforts to deal with sudden crisis or prolonged adversity.

Resilience has become an important concept in child development and mental health theory and research. Investigators have discovered that many individuals who suffered childhood adversity defied dire expectations of serious and long-lasting damage, instead growing up to lead full, loving, and productive lives. However, the widely held view of resilience as individual hardiness, and the field's skewed focus on family dysfunction, blinded many to the resources that could be found and strengthened in distressed families.

A family resilience framework fundamentally alters traditional deficit-based perspectives. Instead of focusing on how families have failed, we redirect our attention to how they can succeed. Rather than giving up on troubled families and salvaging individual survivors, we can draw out the best in families, building on key processes to encourage both individual and family growth.

This chapter begins by defining and clarifying the concept of resilience. It then surveys what has been learned from studies of resilient individuals, noting the crucial influence of relationships and social support. Next, a systemic view of resilience is advanced: Attention is shifted from individual traits to transactional processes that foster resilience over time. Finally, the concept of family resilience is presented, involving key processes that strengthen resilience in the family as a functional unit.

WHAT IS RESILIENCE?

Resilience can be defined as the capacity to rebound from adversity strengthened and more resourceful. It is an active process of endurance, self-righting, and growth in response to crisis and challenge. The ability to overcome adversity challenges our culture's conventional wisdom: that early or severe trauma can't be undone; that adverse experiences always damage people sooner or later; and that children from troubled or "broken" families are doomed.

Resilience entails more than merely surviving, getting through, or escaping a harrowing ordeal. Survivors are not necessarily resilient; some become trapped in a position as victims, nursing their wounds and blocked from growth by anger and blame (Wolin & Wolin, 1993). In contrast, the qualities of resilience enable people to heal from painful wounds, take charge of their lives, and go on to live fully and love well.

In order to understand resilience, it is important to distinguish it from faulty notions of "invulnerability" and "self-sufficiency." As we will see, resilience is forged through openness to experiences and interdependence with others.

Human Vulnerability, Suffering, and Resilience

The American ethos of the rugged individual (Bellah, Madsen, Sullivan, Swidler, & Tipton, 1985), with its associated images of masculinity and strength, has led many to confuse invulnerability with resilience. The early use of the term "invulnerable child" contributed to an unfortunate image of survivors of destructive environments as impervious to stress because of their own inner fortitude or character armor (Anthony, 1987). These hardy children were likened to steel dolls—so constitutionally sound that, unlike glass or plastic dolls that break under pressure, they could withstand even the most severe stressors.

The danger inherent in the myth of invulnerability and the image of "super-kids" is in equating human vulnerability with weakness and invulnerability with strength. As Felsman and Vaillant (1987) note, "The term 'invulnerability' is antithetical to the human condition. . . . In bearing witness to the resilient behavior of high-risk children everywhere, a truer effort would be to understand, in form and by degree, the shared human qualities at work" (p. 304).

Most studies do not find that resilient individuals maintain a steady state of competence and high functioning through adversity, as some have proposed (Bonanno, 2004). Similarly, the capacity to rebound should not be misconstrued as simply "breezing through" a crisis, unscathed by painful experience, as if fortified with a Teflon ego, troubles bouncing off without causing pain or suffering (Schwartz, 1997). With only two alternatives posed—either to shake off adversity or to "wallow" in it—too many Americans "cut their losses" or simply move on. Our culture breeds intolerance for personal suffering; we avert our gaze from disability, avoid contact with the bereaved, or dispense chirpy advice to "cheer up" and get over it. Well-intentioned loved ones encourage people to get instant closure from personal life crises and to leap into new relationships on the rebound from failed ones. Likewise, we are urged simply to put national crises and past atrocities behind us—whether Vietnam, Abu Ghraib prison abuses, or legacies of slavery—without looking back to draw meaning from them, come to terms with them, and heal as a society. This tendency to cut off from highly stressful and conflict-laden experiences is rooted in our immigrant and pioneer heritage. In order to forge a new life in a strange land, it was more adaptive to focus on meeting new challenges (with a curious blend of stoicism and optimism) than to dwell on the loss of loved ones and communities left behind, or on the extreme conditions many fled as refugees.

This cultural ethos influences us all. At the time of my mother's terminal illness, I was in the midst of a student clinical practicum at Yale; I shuttled back and forth across the country to spend a few days at a time with my parents and still not miss a beat in my demanding schedule. The day after my mother's funeral, I flew right back and hit the ground running. Everyone praised me for being so "resilient." We must be careful not to equate competent functioning with resilience, which involves the whole person, including emotional and relational well-being. It was only much later that I dealt with the full meaning of the loss of my mother and the significance of our relationship.

Unlike the image of the Energizer bunny, or the Timex watch that "takes a licking and keeps on ticking" (Schwartz, 1997), resilience involves "struggling well": experiencing both suffering and courage, effectively working through difficulties both internally and interpersonally (Higgins, 1994). In forging resilience, we strive to integrate the fullness of a crisis experience into the fabric of our individual and collective identity, influencing how we go on to live our lives.

From Rugged Individualism to an Interactional View

Reflecting Western culture's heroic myth of the rugged individual, most interest in resilience has focused on the strengths found within *individuals* who have mastered adversity. Early researchers viewed these qualities in terms of personality traits and coping styles that enable a child or adult to overcome harrowing life experiences. Resilience is commonly seen as inborn, as if resilient persons grew themselves up: They either had the "right stuff" all along—a biological hardiness—or acquired it by pulling themselves up by their bootstraps. This view fosters the expectation that they must become self-reliant and survive through fierce independence. The unfortunate corollary is a contemptuous view of those who don't succeed as deficient, weak, and blameworthy when they can't surmount their problems on their own. In advancing an understanding of personal or family resilience, we must be cautious not to blame those who succumb to adversity for lacking "the right stuff," especially when they are struggling with overwhelming conditions beyond their control.

Led by the work of Sir Michael Rutter (1987, 1999) we've come to understand resilience as an ongoing interaction between nature and nurture, encouraged by supportive relationships. Family and social experiences that open up new opportunities can become beneficial turning points. Recent developments in neurobiology (Siegel, 2005) provide evidence that interpersonal connections play a significant role in shaping neural connections in the emerging mind and that the brain can be rewired through new experiences and altered relationship patterns throughout life. In its recent public education campaign "Road to Resiliency" the American Psychological Association encourages programs to build resilience, much like building muscle, contending that the more we exercise it, the stronger it will get, increasing our ability to handle stress (www.apahelpcenter.org). With supportive relationships, training, and practice, we can strengthen resilience to deal better with traumatic events and life challenges.

Resilience Forged through Adversity

I grew up with a view of myself as resilient. But I believed I was strong *in spite of* my family's deficiencies and the adversities we suffered; it was only in later years that I came to realize that my strengths emerged *because* of those experiences (see Chapter 12). As researchers have discovered, resilience is forged *through* adversity, not despite it. Life crises and hardship can bring out the best in us as we rise to meet the challenges. As Albert Camus wrote, "In the midst of winter I finally learned that there was in me an invincible summer."

Higgins's (1994) study of resilient adults found that they became more substantial because they were sorely tested, endured suffering, and emerged with strengths they might not have developed otherwise. They experienced things more deeply and intensely, and placed a heightened value on life. Often this became a wellspring for social activism, a commitment to helping others overcome their adversities; in turn, they experienced further growth through these efforts. (Of note, half of the resilient individuals studied by Higgins had become mental health professionals!)

Crisis: Threat and Opportunity

The Chinese symbol for the word "crisis" is a composite of two characters: the symbols for "danger" and "opportunity." Although we would not wish for misfortune, the paradox of resilience is that our worst times can also become our best (Wolin & Wolin, 1993). In my experience, many families who have lost a loved one find that the most dreaded and painful end-of-life contacts, when approached caringly, were also their most precious times together. Studies of strong families (Stinnett & DeFrain, 1985) found that at times of crisis, 75% experienced positive occurrences in the midst of hurt or despair, and believed that something good came out of the ordeal. Many families reported that through weathering crises together, their relationships became enriched and more loving than they might otherwise have been. A crisis can be a "wake-up call," heightening our attention to what really matters in our lives. A painful loss may thrust us in new and unforeseen directions. As the Navaho say, the end of a path is the beginning of another. Resilience is about that journey.

STUDIES OF INDIVIDUAL RESILIENCE

In order to understand and foster family resilience, we can learn a great deal from studies of individual resilience conducted over the past three decades. These efforts have countered the predominant view that family and environmental risk factors and negative life events inevitably produce childhood and later adult disorders. As Rutter (1985) noted, no combination of risk factors, regardless of severity, gave rise to significant disorder in more than half of the children exposed. Studies have shown, for instance, that most survivors of childhood abuse do *not* go on to abuse their own children (Kaufman & Zigler, 1987). What accounts for this resilience?

With concern for early intervention and prevention, a number of child development and mental health experts redirected attention toward understanding not only vulnerability or susceptibility to risk and disorder, but even more importantly, the protective factors that fortify children's resources and encourage their resilience (Garmezy, 1974; Luthar & Zigler, 1991; Masten, Best, & Garmezy, 1990; Rutter, 1985, 1987). Most early inquiries sought to understand how some children of mentally ill parents or dysfunctional families are able to overcome early experiences of abuse or neglect to lead productive lives (Anthony, 1987; Cohler, 1987; Garmezy, 1987). Wolin and Wolin (1993) described a cluster of qualities in healthy adults who showed individual resilience despite growing up in dysfunctional, and often abusive, alcoholic families.

Increasingly, studies broadened their focus to include the wider social context, examining individual risk and resilience in the face of devastating social conditions, particularly poverty (Garmezy, 1991) and community violence (Garbarino, 1997). Felsman and Vaillant (1987) followed the lives of 75 high-risk, inner-city males who grew up in poverty-stricken, socially disadvantaged families. Family life was often complicated by substance abuse, mental illness, crime, and violence. Many of these men, although indelibly marked by their past experience, showed courageous lives of mastery and competence. These men took an active initiative in shaping their lives, despite occasional setbacks and multiple factors working against them. As the study concluded, their resilience demonstrated that "the events that go wrong in our lives do not forever damn us" (1987, p. 298). In cross-cultural studies with settings ranging from Brazilian shantytowns and South African migrant camps to U.S. inner cities, Robert Coles (Dugan & Coles, 1989) also found that, contrary to the dire predictions of his mental health colleagues, many children did rise above severe hardship without later "time bomb" effects.

The similar concept of *hardiness* grew out of another line of research on stress and coping (Murphy, 1987). Examining the influence of stressful life events in a range of mental and physical illnesses, a number of investigators sought to identify personality traits that mediate physiological processes and enable some highly stressed individuals to cope adaptively and remain healthy (Antonovsky, 1979; Holmes & Masuda, 1974; Lazarus & Folkman, 1984). Building on earlier theories of competence, Kobasa and her colleagues (Kobasa, Maddi, & Kahn, 1982) proposed that persons who experience high degrees of stress without becoming ill have a personality structure characterized by hardiness (Maddi, 2002).

Grinker and Spiegel's (1945) pioneering study of men under stress in war launched another line of research on the impact of catastrophic events involving trauma and loss (e.g., Figley & McCubbin, 1983; see Chapter 11). That research, too, revealed individual variability in response and in the capacity to recover and move on with life. In *Against All Odds*, Helmreich (1992) found remarkable resilience in the lives forged by many survivors of the Nazi Holocaust. Such accounts attest to the human potential to emerge from a shattering experience scarred yet strengthened.

In one of the most ambitious studies of resilience, Werner (1993; Werner & Smith 1982, 1992, 2001) spent 40 years following the lives of nearly 700 children reared in poverty and hardship on the island of Kauai. Most children were born to sugar plantation workers of mixed ethnic and racial descent. One-third were classified as "at risk" because of exposure before age 2 to at least four additional risk factors, such as serious health problems, and familial alcoholism, violence, divorce, or mental illness. By age 18, about two-thirds of the at-risk children had done as poorly as predicted, with early pregnancy, needs for mental health services, or trouble in school or with the law. However, one-third of those at risk had developed into competent, caring, and confident young adults who were "fine human beings," with the capacity "to work well, play well, and love well," as rated on a variety of measures. In later follow-ups through age 40, all but two of these individuals were still living successful lives. Many had outperformed Kauai children from less harsh backgrounds: More were stably married and fewer were divorced, unemployed, or traumatized by Hurricane Iniki, which destroyed much of the island.

Individual Traits

Most early resilience research focused on individual traits and disposition, such as an easygoing temperament and higher intelligence, which were found to be helpful, although not essential, for resilience. Such qualities tend to elicit more positive responses from others and to facilitate coping strategies and problem-solving skills. More significantly, high self-esteem and self-efficacy, with a sense of hope and personal control, make successful coping more likely, whereas a sense of helplessness increases the probability that one adversity will lead to another (Rutter, 1985). Similar to Antonovsky's (1987, 1998) concept of sense of coherence, studies of hardy individuals found three general characteristics: (1) the belief that they can control or influence events in their experience; (2) an ability to feel deeply involved in or committed to the activities in their lives; and (3) anticipation of change as an exciting challenge to further development (Kobasa et al., 1985). In cross-cultural observations, Coles noted the power of moral and spiritual sources of courage as a life-sustaining force of conviction that lifts individuals above hardship (Dugan & Coles, 1989). Werner (1993) similarly noted that the core component in effective coping is a feeling of confidence that the odds can be surmounted. Even with chaos in their households, by their high school years, resilient youths had developed a sense of coherence, a faith that obstacles could be overcome, and a belief that they were in control of their fate. They were significantly more likely than nonresilient children to have an inner locus of control—an optimistic confidence in their ability to shape events. They developed both competence and hope of a better life through their own efforts and relationships.

Murphy (1987) also described the "optimistic bias" of resilient children. She observed that many latch on to "any excuse for hope and faith in recovery" (pp. 103–104), actively mobilizing all thoughts and resources that could contribute to their success. Based on epidemiological research, Taylor (1989) found that people who hold "positive illusions"— selectively positive biases about such situations as life-threatening illness— tend to do better. Such beliefs allow them to retain hope in the face of a grim situation. Seligman's (1990) research on "learned optimism" also informs our understanding of resilience. His early studies on "learned helplessness" found that people can be conditioned to become passive and give up trying to solve problems when their actions are not predictably linked to rewards. Seligman then found that optimism can be learned through experiences of mastery, as individuals come to believe that their efforts can yield success. (Chapter 3 will examine the power of family belief systems that foster such meaning making, a positive outlook, and transcendence).

Relational Lifelines for Individual Resilience

Increasingly, researchers have linked the emergence of resilience in vulnerable children to key protective influences in the family and social context. Children's resilience to hardship is greater when they have access to at least one caring parent, a caregiver, or another supportive adult in their extended family or social world. Even the emergence of genetically influenced individual traits occurs in relational context (Reiss, Hetherington, Plomin, & Neiderhiser, 2000). As Werner (1993) has emphasized, self-esteem and self-efficacy are promoted, above all else, through supportive relationships. All of the resilient children in the Kauai study had "at least one person in their lives who accepted them unconditionally, regardless of temperamental idiosyncrasies, physical attractiveness, or intelligence" (p. 512). They needed to know that there was someone to whom they could turn, and, at the same time, needed to have their own efforts, sense of competence, and self-worth nurtured and reinforced. Encouraged by their connections with a mentor, many also developed a special interest or skill (e.g., carpentry, art, or creative writing), which enhanced their competence, confidence, and mastery.

Only a few early studies of individual resilience looked for positive family contributions (Hauser, Vierya, Jacobson, & Wertlieb, 1985; Rutter, 1985; Werner & Smith, 1992). They focused on the family organization and emotional climate, noting the importance of warmth, affection, emotional support, and clear-cut, reasonable structure and limits (see Chapter 4). Researchers emphasized that if parents are unable to provide this climate, relationships with other family members, such as older siblings, grandparents, and extended kin, can serve this function. Moreover, shared belief systems transmitted through family interactions are powerful influences in resilience (see Chapter 3). Children's adaptation to crisis events and disruptive transitions is influenced by the meaning of the experience, which is mediated by parental understanding and communication (Kagan, 1984).

Encouragement for individual resilience is also provided by friends, neighbors, teachers, coaches, clergy, and other mentors (Brooks, 1994; Rutter, 1987; Werner, 1993). Resilient children in troubled families often actively recruit and form special attachments with influential adults in their social environment. They learn to choose relationships wisely and tend to select spouses from healthy families. The importance of social support in times of crisis has been amply documented. Although these relationships may sometimes be a source of strain, they can also be a wellspring for positive coping resources (Rutter, 1987).

A SYSTEMIC VIEW OF RESILIENCE

From a Dyadic to a Systemic Perspective

Taken together, the research on individual resilience has increasingly pointed toward the importance of a relational perspective. Worldwide, studies of children of misfortune have found the most significant positive influence to be a close, caring relationship with a significant adult who believed in them and with whom they could identify, who acted as an advocate for them, and from whom they could gather strength to overcome their hardships (Werner, 1993). Yet most resilience theory and research have approached the relational context of resilience narrowly, in terms of the influence of a significant person in a dyadic relationship with an at-risk child. For a fuller understanding of resilience, a complex interactional model is required. Systems theory expands our view of individual adaptation as embedded in broader transactional processes in family and social context. It attends to the mutuality of influences over time.

When we broaden our perspective beyond a dyadic bond and early life determinants, we become aware that resilience is woven in a web of relationships and experiences over the life course and across the generations (Hauser, 1999). Both ecological and developmental perspectives are necessary to understand resilience in social and temporal context.

Ecological Perspective

An ecological perspective takes into account the many spheres of influence in risk and resilience over the life course. The family, peer group, school or work settings, and larger social systems can be seen as nested contexts for social competence (Bronfenbrenner, 1979).

Rutter (1987) also emphasizes that to understand and foster resilience and protective mechanisms, we must attend to the interplay between occurrences within families and the political, economic, social, and racial climates in which individuals and their families perish or thrive. We must be cautious that the concept of resilience is not used in public policy to withhold social supports or to maintain inequities, based on the rationale that success or failure is determined by strengths or deficits within individuals and their families. It is not enough to bolster the resilience of at-risk children and families so that they can "beat the odds"; we must also strive to change the odds against them (Seccombe, 2002).

Developmental Perspective

A developmental perspective is also essential in understanding resilience. Rather than a set of fixed traits, coping and adaptation involve multiple processes that may vary over time. Most forms of stress are not simply a short-term, single stimulus, but a complex set of changing conditions with a past history and a future course (Rutter, 1987). Given this complexity over time, no single coping response is invariably most successful. It is more important to have a variety of coping strategies to meet different challenges as they emerge. The ability to choose viable options is crucial in resilience.

Researchers have explored coping and adaptation under such diverse stress conditions as chronic illness, developmental transitions and role strain, death of a loved one, divorce and stepfamily formation, unemployment and economic insecurity, maltreatment and neglect, war and genocide, and community disasters. Stressful life events are more likely to affect functioning adversely when they are unexpected, when a condition is severe or persistent, or when multiple stressors generate cumulative effects (Boss, 2001). Events that occur "off-time," or out of sync with chronological or social expectations—such as early widowhood—are also more difficult (Neugarten, 1976).

A life cycle perspective on individual and family development is also necessary for an understanding of resilience. Although adaptive functioning in childhood and adolescence serves as a generally good predictor of adult outcomes, the role of early life experience in determining adult capacity to overcome adversity may be less important than was previously assumed (Cohler, 1987; Vaillant, 1995, 2002). Longitudinal studies following individuals through adulthood find that resilience cannot be assessed once and for all on the basis of a quick snapshot of early interactions. If we emphasize continuity and limited short-term perspectives, we may fail to appreciate that people are developing organisms whose life course trajectories are flexible and multidimensional (Falicov, 1988). Moreover, an adaptation that serves well at one point in development may later not be useful in meeting other challenges. Gender differences are also found in vulnerability at different developmental periods (Werner & Smith, 1982). Such variables underscore the dynamic nature of resilience over time.

Werner and Smith's (1982, 1992) longitudinal study of resilient children provides rich evidence for a complex interactional view of resilience, involving multiple internal and external protective influences in lives over time. They concluded that earlier researchers focused too narrowly on maternal influence and the damage of one parent in the nuclear household, and missed the importance of siblings and others in the extended family network. The role of a wide variety of supportive relationships was crucial at every age.

Most children got off to a good start through early bonding with at least one caregiver, often a grandmother, older sister, aunt, or other relative who provided care. Yet even a bad start did not determine a bad outcome. Many overcame early neglect, abandonment, or developmental delays and began to blossom when they benefited from later nurturing care, through adoption or mentoring (e.g., special relationships with teachers). Throughout their school years, the resilient children actively recruited support networks in their extended families and communities. Interestingly, more girls than boys overcame adversity at all age levels. We might postulate the influence of gender-based socialization in seeking out and sustaining supportive relationships: Girls are raised to be both more easygoing and more relationally oriented, whereas boys are taught to be tough and self-reliant through life. Moreover, often *because* of troubled family lives, competencies were built by assuming early responsibilities for household tasks and care of younger siblings.

Werner and Smith found that nothing is "cast in stone" because of early life experiences. A few individuals identified as resilient at 18 had developed significant problems by age 30. However, the most important finding was that resilience could be developed at any point over the life course. Unexpected events and new relationships can disrupt a negative chain and catalyze new growth. Of the two-thirds of at-risk children who were troubled and not resilient as adolescents, fully *one-half* had righted themselves by age 30: Delinquent acts had not led to lives of crime, and many had stable marriages and decent jobs. In these cases, too, most reported that some adult had taken an interest in them when they drifted into trouble. They also credited a major turning point: a good marriage, satisfying work, service in the armed forces, or involvement in a highly structured religious group (Butler, 1997). Such findings support core convictions in a resilience approach to practice: (1) that people with troubled pasts have the potential to turn their lives around throughout adulthood, and (2) that a crisis can become a positive turning point.

Werner and Smith's conclusions are supported by many studies of at-risk children elsewhere (Masten et al., 1990), pointing to the beneficial effects of the web of relationships formed by extended family, friends, and neighbors. Over the years, positive interactions have a mutually reinforcing effect, in positive life trajectories or upward spirals. With multiple pathways in resilience, a downward spiral can be turned around at any time in life.

FAMILY RESILIENCE

The term "family resilience" refers to coping and adaptational processes in the family *as a functional unit*. A systems perspective enables us to understand how family processes mediate stress and can enable families and their members to surmount crises and weather prolonged hardship. Stressors affect children more when they disrupt crucial family processes (Patterson, 1983; Boss, 2001). It is not just the child who is vulnerable or resilient; more importantly, the family system influences eventual adjustment. Even individuals who are not directly touched by a crisis are affected by the family response, with reverberations for all other relationships (Bowen, 1978). How a family confronts and manages a disruptive experience, buffers stress, effectively reorganizes, and moves forward with life will influence immediate and long-term adaptation for every family member *and* for the very survival and well-being of the family unit.

From Family Damage to Family Challenge

In the field of mental health, most clinical theory, training, practice, and research have been overwhelmingly deficit-focused, implicating the family in the cause or maintenance of nearly all problems in individual functioning. Under early psychoanalytic assumptions of destructive maternal bonds, the family came to be seen as a noxious influence. Early family systems formulations, through the 1970s, focused on dysfunctional family processes. Popular movements for so-called "survivors" or "adult children of dysfunctional families" spared almost no family from accusations of failure and blame. With the clinical field so steeped in pathology, the intense scrutiny of family deficits and blindness to family strengths led me to suggest, only half-jokingly, that a "normal" family could be defined as one that has not yet been clinically assessed (Walsh, 2003b).

Beyond the Myths of the "Normal" Family

Views of normality and health are socially constructed, influencing clinical assessment and goals for healthy family functioning (Walsh, 2003a, 2003b). The vision of a so-called "normal" family is largely in the eye of the beholder, filtered by professional values, personal family experience, and cultural standards. Two myths of the "normal" family have perpetuated a grim view of most families.

One myth is the belief that healthy families are problem-free. Based in the medical model, health has been defined clinically as the absence of problems. Unfortunately, this leaves us in the dark about *positive* contributions to healthy functioning. More seriously, it leads to the faulty assumption that any problem is symptomatic of and caused by a dysfunctional family. This belief has tended to pathologize ordinary families struggling to cope with the stresses and disruptive changes that are part of life (Minuchin, 1974). No family is problem-free. Slings and arrows of misfortune strike us all, in varying ways and times over each family's life course. What distinguishes healthy families is not the absence of problems or suffering but rather their coping and problem-solving abilities.

A second myth is the belief that the idealized "traditional family" is essential for healthy child development. In the United States, this conjures up the 1950s image of a white, affluent, nuclear family headed by a breadwinner/father and supported by a full-time homemaker/mother. Early theory and research in the social sciences and psychiatry, seeking to define the "normal" family in terms of a universal set of traits or a singular family form, reified this model of the intact nuclear family with traditional gender roles (Parsons & Bales, 1955). In the wake of massive social and economic upheaval over recent decades, nostalgic images of a simpler past are understandable but are out of touch with the diversity of family structures, values, and challenges in our changing world, as will be seen in Chapter 2. Yet families that don't conform to the "one-norm-fits-all" standard have been stigmatized and pathologized by assumptions that they inherently damage children. Families of varied configurations can be successful. Effective family processes matter most for healthy functioning and resilience.

Strengths in Families Challenged by Adversity

In recent decades, systems-based family therapists have increasingly re-oriented theory and practice from a deficit-based to a strengths-oriented paradigm (Walsh, 2003b). A family resilience framework builds on these developments, shifting our view from seeing distressed families as damaged to understanding how they are challenged by adversity. It also corrects the faulty assumption that family health can only be found in a mythologized ideal model. Instead, this approach seeks to understand how all families, in their diversity, can survive and regenerate even with overwhelming stress. It affirms the family potential for self-repair and growth out of crisis and challenge.

My interest in family resilience was sparked in my early research experience with families of psychiatrically hospitalized and normal young adults (Walsh & Anderson, 1988). The vitality and diversity I observed in families in the normal control group countered the image of normal families as dull and monotone. Most impressive, a number of parents had suffered serious childhood trauma and yet had grown up able to form and sustain healthy families and to raise their children well to adulthood. Along with other emerging research, these cases cast doubt on traditional clinical assumptions that those who have suffered childhood trauma are wounded for life. Particularly striking were the strengths shown by one normal control family, Marcy and Tom and their five children, whose individual and family resilience was interwoven across the generations:

> Marcy, one of three children in her family of origin, told of her father's serious drinking problem, repeated job losses, and family abandonment when she was 7. Despite financial hardship and the social stigma of a "broken home," she emerged quite healthy. She attributed her own resilience to the strong family unit her mother forged with the support of her extended family through troubled times.
>
> Based on her childhood experience, Marcy had developed deep convictions about marriage and raising a healthy family. When she was asked what had attracted her to Tom, her reply was crystal-

clear: "First, I knew I wanted a husband who didn't drink. Second, I wanted my children to have a father who would always be there for them." She consciously sought out and married into the kind of family that she wanted to have. She chose wisely: Tom was the son of a minister, one of six children from a solid, stable family. For his part, he was drawn to her "can do" spirit and admired her family's ability to weather hardship. Together, as they raised their children, they kept close contact and connection with both extended families, which, in different ways, offered strong parenting models and supportive kin networks.

Marcy demonstrated many qualities that other researchers have found to be characteristic of resilient individuals, such as her success in overcoming early life trauma, an ability to learn from traumatic experience to make conscious positive choices, and a determined effort to build a strong marriage and family life. Most striking was the crucial role of her family system in fostering her resilience in the wake of her parents' divorce. Her family's ability to handle crises and persistent challenges over time enabled her to survive and thrive. Moreover, strong sibling bonds through shared adversity provided a lasting mutual resource. As a couple and parental team, Marcy and Tom built a well-functioning family unit, raised their five children successfully, and continued to value and maintain vital extended family connections.

My research also showed that resilience could be brought forth even in the cases categorized as "seriously disturbed." A crisis, such as an emotional breakdown of a family member, can jolt the family into awareness of needed changes. In the following case, a son's psychiatric crisis was precipitated by family reverberations from his father's past trauma at the same age.

While on a summer trip in Europe, 18-year-old Martin had a psychotic episode and was brought home and hospitalized. After a very constrained family interview, his mother asked to meet with me individually. She told of the father's past Holocaust experience as a Jewish refugee from Poland. At the age of 18, he had watched as Nazis shot his brother in the head and took his parents away to their deaths. He survived his own concentration camp experience, came to the United States, and became a physician. On their first date, seeing the camp numbers on his arm, she asked him about his experience. He was so visibly shaken that she never again asked. His past was never mentioned as their children were growing up, even though the tattooed numbers were a visible reminder. An implicit family rule, serving to protect him, rendered the unbearable memories and emotions unspeakable. Then, for Martin's 18th birthday, his father's surprising gift was a trip to Europe. Martin went off, but wrote home revealing that he was unable to enjoy himself, because he was aware that terrible things had happened to his father there. The parents didn't reply. Martin attempted to go to Auschwitz, but broke down en route, becoming incoherent and delusional.

This crisis became a turning point. The family taught me that resilience can emerge even in families that have been rigidly governed by long-standing patterns that have become dysfunctional. What had been unspeakable had gone underground and became expressed in the birthday present when Martin reached the same age as his father's trauma experience. Therapists can help to mobilize new strengths at whatever point they encounter as a family. Family members were commended for their long-standing concern for the father and their wish to spare him pain. At the same time, it was agreed that their silence was no longer needed, since the father was not as vulnerable as he had been years earlier. The "gift" was framed as an opportunity to open up communication and to reintegrate old cutoffs. My follow-up with the family a year later found that the parents had made a trip to the father's family home in Poland, which was immensely healing for him and deepened the couple's relationship. Martin was doing well in college, and, interestingly, was majoring in communications.

My research experience fundamentally altered the direction of my clinical work, shifting my attention from family deficits toward understanding and facilitating the family processes that foster health and growth over the life course and across the generations.

Contributions of Family Process Research

Identifying Core Elements in Healthy Family Functioning

A growing body of systems-based research has advanced our knowledge of the multidimensional processes that distinguish well-functioning from dysfunctional families (Beavers & Hampson, 1990, 2003; Conger & Conger, 2002; Epstein, Ryan, Bishop, Miller, & Keitner, 2003; Ryan, Epstein, Keitner, Miller, & Bishop, 2005; Olson & Gorell, 2003; Schumm, 1985; Walsh, 2003). The family resilience framework presented in this volume draws together the findings of this research to distill core components of effective family functioning, which can usefully inform our efforts to strengthen families in distress.

At the same time, the growing diversity of families and the complexity of contemporary life call for caution in generalizing from normative samples that represent only a narrow band on the wide spectrum of families. Most family process studies have been standardized on white, middle-class, Protestant, intact families that are not under stress. We must be careful not to pathologize families that differ in their cultural values, those that show common reactions to severe stress, or those that have developed their own creative strategies to fit their particular situation. For instance, very high cohesion is too readily labeled as dysfunctional enmeshment; however, togetherness may be highly valued in a family's culture, or needed when family members must pull together to weather a serious crisis. The processes useful for effective functioning may vary, depending on differing sociocultural contexts and life challenges.

Resonant with a family resilience perspective, Falicov's (1995, 1998) multidimensional ecological view recognizes that families combine and overlap features of many cultural contexts based on the unique configurations of variables in their lives, such as ethnicity, social class, religion, family structure, gender roles, sexual orientation, and life stage. Conflict and change are as much a part of family life as are tradition and continuity. For example, the challenges posed by the process of migration involve profound ecological disruption and inevitable uprooting of meanings. We must be careful not to pathologize transitional distress or prolonged strains of adaptation, or to judge families by a single normative standard for family health.

To do justice to these complexities, we must assess family functioning with respect for each family's situation. The concept of family resilience offers a flexible view that can encompass many variables and attend to both continuity and change over time. This volume attempts to strike a balance that allows us to identify core elements in effective family functioning (see Chapters 3–5), while also taking into account the particular strengths called forth to meet varied challenges (see Chapters 8–11). In accord with Falicov's approach to culture, a resilience-based approach views each family in its complex "ecological niche": Each shares some borders and common ground with other families, as well as differences. A holistic assessment includes all contexts the family inhabits, aiming to understand the challenges, constraints, and resources in its position.

A Family Developmental Perspective

An understanding of family resilience must also incorporate a developmental perspective, since varied processes are needed to meet emerging psychosocial challenges over time. We can usefully draw upon the models of vulnerability and protective mechanisms proposed by Garmezy and Rutter to understand individual resilience, as well as a growing body of research on family stress, coping, and adaptation (Boss, 2001; Gilgun, 1999; Hawley & DeHaan, 1996; Lavee, McCubbin, & Olson, 1987; McHenry & Price, 2005; Walsh, 1996).

Models of Vulnerability and Protective Mechanisms. Garmezy (1987) has advocated longitudinal developmental research on high-risk groups to clarify the biological and psychosocial mechanisms in adaptiveness under stress. At each developmental phase, there is a shifting balance between stressful events that heighten vulnerability and protective mechanisms that enhance resilience. Three mechanisms have been proposed through which protective processes may mediate the relationship between stress and competence.

In the *immunity model*, protective factors are thought to serve as reserves against a decline in functioning under stress. The notion of "inoculation" has been expressed often in the resilience literature to describe preventive psychosocial interventions that boost resistance to potentially harmful effects of stressful experiences. For instance, Seligman (1995) has proposed that through a process of "immunization," positive learning experiences can prevent learned helplessness throughout life (see Chapter 3 for discussion).

In the *compensatory model*, personal attributes and environmental resources are thought to counteract the negative effects of stressors. For instance, with aging, the decline in some aspects of mental functioning (e.g., recent memory) can be offset by the gains in wisdom and perspective accrued through life experience.

In the *challenge model*, stressors can become potential enhancers of competence and resilience, provided that the level of stress is not too high. A crisis can challenge us to sharpen our skills and develop new assets. These three mechanisms may operate simultaneously or successively in the adaptive repertoire for resilience, depending on varied coping styles and phases of development (Werner, 1993).

We can apply these protective mechanisms to the family system. Ongoing family processes can boost immunity to stress, preventing or reducing harmful impact. Family processes can be rallied as resources to compensate for negative stress effects. Family processes can even be strengthened through shared coping efforts. Let's consider the crisis and challenges when a mother is hospitalized with a serious illness. If ongoing family interaction is generally strong in communication and problem-solving skills, these processes can serve as psychosocial inoculation to bolster immunity to the negative stress effects (reducing its impact from severe to moderate or mild) and to sustain competence during the crisis period. To compensate for the mother's lost role functioning, the family may reorganize its daily routines and reallocate responsibilities to ensure that the children's needs are met, with the father flexibly altering his work schedule, older children helping out more, and extended family members pitching in. As they rally together to meet this challenge, family members' bonds are strengthened, and individuals may develop new competencies and perspectives on their lives. For instance, the father's previously untapped potential to nurture his children may be developed as he is thrust into new responsibilities.

This transactional perspective and the contextual nature of resilience fit well with Sir Michael Rutter's (1987) model of risk and protection, which emphasizes resilience processes and intervention possibilities (see Chapter 6). Resilience is fostered in family interactions through a chain of indirect influences that ameliorate the direct effects of a stressful event. Strains can be compounded by ineffective family coping efforts and heighten the risk for further complications. Positive coping strategies can buffer or reduce stress and restore well-being.

Family Stress, Coping, and Adaptation. McCubbin and Patterson (1983) developed a family crisis framework, grounded in Hill's (1949) pioneering work on family coping in wartime stress. They examined family vulnerability and regenerative power to understand how some families are able to withstand stress and recover from crisis when others are not. They have emphasized the importance of "fit" and "balance" to the development of both the family unit and its individual members. Families need to achieve a functional fit between their challenges and resources and between different dimensions of family life. A fit at one system level may precipitate strains elsewhere, as in dual-earner families when efforts to manage job and childrearing demands deplete the energy available for couple intimacy. With many adaptational pathways possible, family members need to weigh and balance costs and benefits in their options. Promising research on family resilience has begun to emerge (McCubbin, Thompson, Thompson, & Futrell, 1998; McCubbin, Thompson, Thompson, & Fromer, 1998a, 1998b; Patterson, 2002).

Family Resilience as Interactive Processes over Time. Family resilience cannot be captured in a snapshot at a single moment in time. More than immediate crisis response or adjustment, resilience involves many interactive processes over time—from a family's approach to a threatening situation, through its ability to manage disruptive transitions, to varied strategies for coping with emerging challenges in the immediate and long-term aftermath. For instance, postdivorce functioning and well-being of family members, especially children, are influenced not simply by the "event" of divorce, but even more by the family processes involved in dealing with the many unfolding stressful challenges and in making meaning of the experience (Hetherington & Kelly, 2002; see Chapter 2, this volume).

Shared beliefs shape and reinforce interactional patterns governing how a family approaches and responds to adversity (Reiss, 1981). A critical event or disruptive transition can catalyze a major shift in a family belief system, with reverberations for both immediate reorganization and long-term adaptation. Moreover, a family's perceptions of a stressful situation intersect with legacies of previous experience in the multigenerational system to influence the meaning the family makes of a challenge and its response (Carter & McGoldrick, 2004).

A cluster of stressors complicates adaptation as family members struggle with competing demands, and emotions can easily spill over into conflict (Walsh, 1983). One family was able to cope with the challenges of their small child's severe developmental disabilities until the father's job loss and accompanying loss of medical benefits multiplied the strains. Over time, a pileup of stressors, losses, and dislocations can overwhelm a family's coping efforts, contributing to family strife, substance abuse, and emotional or behavioral symptoms of distress (often expressed by children in the family).

Psychosocial challenges of stress events vary with their circumstances, timing, and meaning. Catastrophic events that occur suddenly and without warning can be especially traumatic (Figley & McCubbin, 1983; see Chapter 11, this volume). Reverberations, like a shock wave, can extend throughout family networks and communities. In their wake, some families are devastated but most are able to pull together, right themselves, and move on. Recurrent stressors, such as family or community violence, may well strike again at any time, fueling anticipatory anxiety. The sudden, unpredictable, life-threatening nature of such events is especially unsettling. Acute posttraumatic complications are common.

A persistent challenge requires tenacity over the long haul; it poses very different demands from those of a sudden crisis, when families must mobilize quickly but can then return to regular daily life. Some families face episodic stress alternating with periods of calm, as in the case of migrant workers: With temporary employment and repeated job layoffs, families must repeatedly switch gears and get by as best they can. Prolonged challenges face families when a member's permanent disability irrevocably alters lives. In most cases, psychosocial demands on the family change over time, with subsequent phases in the adaptation process, as in the variable course of a serious illness; at each transition, the family must readjust and recalibrate (Rolland, 1994). Therapeutic responses must be attuned to these varied and changing demands and tap into family resources to meet them. When a crisis looms, and in its immediate and long-term aftermath, a systemic approach to intervention strengthens key interactional processes that foster healing, recovery, and resilience, enabling the family and its members to integrate the experience and move forward with life.

Future Research Priorities

A redirection of research focus and funding priorities is needed, from studies of dysfunctional families and how they fail, to studies of well-functioning families and what enables them to succeed, particularly in the face of adversity. As an analogy, after a devastating earthquake, we need to study not only the buildings that crumbled; more importantly, we need to examine those structures that withstood the crisis and aftershocks, in order to identify the essential elements and construct more resilient structures. Rather than proposing a blueprint for any singular model of "the resilient family," this volume offers a flexible family resilience framework, identifying key processes that can strengthen each family's ability to overcome the challenges they face.

A FAMILY RESILIENCE APPROACH: LOOKING AHEAD

A family resilience framework can serve as a valuable conceptual map in orienting a wide range of human services. A systemic view of resilience is important in all efforts to help individuals, couples, and families to cope and adapt through crisis and adversity. The family has been a neglected resource in interventions aiming to foster resilience in children and adults. A narrow focus on individual resilience has led clinicians to attempt to salvage individual "survivors" without exploring their families' potential, and even to write off many families as hopeless. A family resilience approach fosters a compassionate understanding of parental life challenges, encourages reconciliation, and searches for unrecognized strengths in the network of family relationships (see Chapter 12).

In the field of family therapy, we have come to realize that successful interventions depend as much on tapping the resources of the family as on the techniques of the therapist (Karpel, 1986). What we need most are strength-oriented conceptual tools that guide intervention. A family resilience framework offers such tools, and is distinct in its focus on surmounting crisis and challenge. Symptoms are assessed in the context of past, ongoing, and threatened crisis events, their meanings, and family coping responses. Therapeutic efforts are attuned to each family's particular challenges and family resources are mobilized to meet them.

A resilience-based stance in family therapy is founded on a set of convictions about family potential that shapes all intervention, even with highly vulnerable families whose lives are saturated with crisis situations. Collaboration among family members is encouraged, enabling them to build new and renewed competence, mutual support, and shared confidence that they can prevail under duress. This approach fosters an empowering family climate: Members gain ability to overcome crises and challenges by working together, and they experience success as largely due to their shared efforts and resources. Experiences of shared success enhance a family's pride and sense of efficacy, enabling more effective coping with subsequent life adaptations.

A family resilience approach provides a positive and pragmatic framework that guides interventions to strengthen the family as presenting problems are resolved. This approach goes beyond problem solving to problem prevention; it not only repairs families, but also prepares them to meet future challenges. A particular solution to a presenting problem may not be relevant to future problems, but in building *processes for resilience*, families become more resourceful in dealing with unforeseen problems and averting crises. Thus, in strengthening family resilience, every intervention is also a preventive measure.

The growing body of resilience studies and systems-based research on healthy family processes can inform our efforts to identify strengths and vulnerabilities and target interventions to strengthen core processes for family resilience. Part II of this volume (Chapters 3–5) presents and integrates our knowledge and perspectives on these elements. I have found it useful to organize these findings into a conceptual framework comprising three domains: belief systems, organizational patterns, and communication processes. In Chapters 3–5, key processes in family resilience are identified in each domain (see Table 1.1): These processes may be expressed in different ways and to varying degrees by families to fit their values, structures, resources, and life challenges.

To summarize, several basic principles grounded in systems theory serve as the foundations for a family resilience approach:

- Individual resilience is best understood and fostered in the context of the family and larger social world, as a mutual interaction of individual, family, sociocultural, and institutional influences.
- Crisis events and persistent stresses affect the entire family and all its members, posing risks not only for individual dysfunction, but also for relational conflict and family breakdown.
- Family processes mediate the impact of stress for all members and their relationships and can influence the course of many crisis events.
- Protective processes foster resilience by buffering stress and facilitating adaptation.
- Maladaptive responses heighten vulnerability and risks for individual and relationship distress.
- All individuals and families have the potential for greater resilience; we can maximize that potential by encouraging their best efforts and strengthening key processes.

TABLE 1.1. Keys to Family Resilience

Family belief systems
- Making meaning of adversity
- Positive outlook
- Transcendence and spirituality

Organizational patterns
- Flexibility
- Connectedness
- Social and economic resources

Communication processes
- Clarity
- Open emotional expression
- Collaborative problem solving

CHAPTER 2

The Growing Diversity and Complexity of Families in a Changing World

> If we are to achieve a richer culture . . . we must recognize
> the whole gamut of human potentialities, and so weave a less
> arbitrary social fabric, one in which each diverse human gift
> will find a fitting place.
> —MARGARET MEAD, *Blackberry Winter*

The concept of family resilience is especially timely as our world grows increasingly unpredictable and as families face unprecedented challenges. With profound social, economic, and political upheavals over recent decades, families and the societies around them are changing at an accelerated pace. It is useful to highlight four major trends and to view them in sociohistorical context:

- Varied family structures
- Changing gender roles
- Growing cultural diversity and socioeconomic disparity
- Varying, expanded family life course

In this chapter, we consider the implications of these trends for our understanding of family challenges and resources. Our efforts to strengthen

27

family resilience must be relevant to this growing diversity and complexity in family life.

VARIED FAMILY STRUCTURES

Family structures have become increasingly varied over recent decades. The very survival of the family has been called into question with this reconfiguration of human relationships. Popular images of the typical "normal family" and the ideal "healthy family" both shape and reflect dominant social norms and values for how families are supposed to be (Walsh, 2003a). Fears of the demise of the family have escalated in periods of social turbulence, as in our times. Yet controversy and change have surrounded the definition of the family for well over a century (Coontz, 1997). In the United States, two eras have become mythologized: the traditional family of the preindustrial, rural past and the modern nuclear family of the 1950s.

Many people hold an idealized image of intact, multigenerational family households in the distant past (Walsh, 2003a). Actually, family patterns were no more orderly and stable than today's complex and varied family structures and roles. Family transitions were more unpredictable due to many life uncertainties, particularly unplanned pregnancies and untimely deaths. Family units were frequently disrupted by early parental death, which led to remarriage and stepfamilies, or to placements of children with extended kin, foster care, or orphanages. Today, we have greater control over the options and timing of marriage and parenting, largely due to birth control and to medical advances that have increased fertility and childbearing options and have lengthened life expectancy.

Family households before the mid-20th century were quite diverse and complex, as they continue to be in most parts of the world. Flexible structures and fluid boundaries with extended kin and communities enabled resilience in weathering harsh and unstable life conditions. Households commonly included non-kin boarders, providing surrogate families for individuals on their own and facilitating the adaptation of new immigrants, as well as furnishing income and companionship for widows and the elderly.

The nuclear family structure, which arose with industrialization and urbanization, peaked in the United States in the 1950s. The household comprised an intact, two-parent family unit headed by a breadwinner husband and a full-time homemaker wife who devoted herself to household management, raising children, and elder care. Many mistake this model as an essential, and now endangered, institution when it was actually unique to its times (Skolnick & Skolnick, 2001). Following the Great Depression and World War II, U.S. prosperity—fueled by a strong postwar economy and government benefits—provided for education, jobs, and home ownership, enabling most families to live comfortably on one income. After a steady decline in the birth rate, couples married younger and in greater numbers, producing the "baby boom."

In earlier eras, the family fulfilled a broad array of economic, educational, social, and religious functions intertwined with the larger community. Relationships were valued for a variety of contributions to the collective family unit. The modern nuclear family household, fitting the resurgent ethos of the rugged individual, was expected to be self-reliant within the borders of its white picket fence. Too often, it became a rigid, closed system, isolated from extended kin and community connections—relational sources of well-being and resilience. It also lost the flexibility and diversity that had enabled households to reconfigure according to need. Unrealistically high expectations for marital relationships to fulfill all needs for intimacy, support, and companionship contributed to the fragility of marriage (Coontz, 2005). Yet, nostalgia for the stability, security, and prosperity of those times is understandable.

Today, the idealized 1950s model of the white middle-class, intact nuclear family, with a breadwinner father and a homemaker mother, is only a narrow band on the wide spectrum of families (Coontz, 1997). A diverse reshaping of contemporary family life encompasses multiple, evolving family cultures and structures: working mothers and two-earner households; divorced and single-parent families and stepfamilies; and domestic partners, both gay and straight.

Dual-earner families now comprise over two-thirds of all two-parent households (Fraenkel, 2003). Most families need two paychecks to maintain even a modest standard of living. Traditional gender role divisions are no longer typical, as women's career aspirations, economic pressures, and divorce have brought over 70% of all mothers into the workforce. By choice, and even more by necessity, most mothers (both married and single-parent) are currently in the workforce.

Marriage and birth rates have declined. More people are living on their own: The number of single adults has more than doubled over the past two decades. At the same time, more young adults are living with their parents, usually for financial reasons. First marriage is occurring at a later age (on average, at 27 for men and 25 for women). Childbearing is increasingly delayed, with employed women often waiting until their

30s or even later. Many couples choose not to have children, defining their relationship as family.

The number of unmarried couples living together has risen dramatically. Nearly half of all adults live in a cohabiting relationship at some time. Although most go on to marry, many break up within a few years. When there are children, studies suggest that high instability in partnerships increases the risk of adjustment problems.

Single-parent households, headed either by an unmarried or a divorced parent, have become increasingly common, accounting for over 25% of all households. Nearly half of all children, and over 60% of poor, ethnic minority children, are expected to live for at least part of their childhoods in one-parent households (Anderson, 2003). Nearly 90% of primary residences are headed by mothers. The lack of financial support and low involvement with their children by over half of nonresidential fathers have been the largest factors in child maladjustment. Growing numbers of older, single women and men are choosing to parent on their own if they haven't found a good partner with whom to share parenting. Children generally fare well in financially secure single-parent homes where there is strong parental functioning, especially when extended family and informal kin networks are involved. There has been a welcome decline in unwed teen pregnancy, which holds high risk for long-term poverty, poor-quality parenting, and a cluster of health and psychosocial problems for mothers and their children (McLanahan et al., 2003). At the same time, there's been an increase in families headed by grandparents, especially grandmothers, who assume primary caregiving roles for their grandchildren, in most cases when parents are unable to provide care (Ehrle & Green, 2002).

Divorce rates, after climbing rapidly in recent decades, have leveled off at around 45% for first marriages. The vast majority of divorced individuals go on to remarry, making stepfamilies increasingly common (Visher, Visher, & Pasley, 2003). Yet the complexity of stepfamily integration contributes to the risk of divorce, at nearly 60% of remarriages (Fine & Harvey, 2004).

Adoptive families have also been increasing, for single parents as well as for couples (Rampage, Eovaldi, Ma, & Weigel-Foy, 2003). Most adoptions are now open, based on findings that children benefit developmentally if they know who their birth families are, have the option for contact, and especially in biracial and international adoptions, are encouraged to connect with cultural traditions (Pertman, 2000). In foster care families, permanency in placement is seen as optimal, with extended

kin wherever possible, keeping siblings together, and avoiding the instability and losses of multiple placements (Ehrle & Green, 2002).

The social movement for gay and lesbian rights has brought increasing normalization and legalization of same-sex domestic partnerships,
although stigma and controversy persist over legal and religious marriage rights. Growing numbers of gay and lesbian single parents and
couples are raising children through adoption and varied reproductive
strategies. Research finds that their children grow up healthy, but do
face challenges of social stigma (Green, 2004; Laird, 2003; Sanders &
Krall, 2000). In a landmark decision in 2002, the American Pediatric
Association endorsed the rights of gay and lesbian parents to adopt children, citing the large body of research finding that children in these families fare as well psychologically and socially as those raised by hetero-
sexual parents.

Although family structures are changing dramatically, the vast majority of people still view loving, committed relationships as the most
important source of happiness in life. Many will marry more than once
or form committed partnerships without legal marriage, often in later
life. The varied family forms have different structural constraints and
resources for functioning. With changing role relations, two-earner families must organize their households and family lives quite differently
from the traditional breadwinner–homemaker model.

Myths of the ideal family compound a sense of deficiency and failure for families in transition. Our language and preconceptions about
"the normal family" can pathologize or stigmatize relationship patterns
that don't conform to the intact nuclear family model. The term "single-
parent family" can blind us to the important role of a noncustodial
parent or a caregiving grandparent and kin network. A stepparent or
adoptive parent is viewed as inherently deficient when seen as not the
"real" or "natural" parent. With the death of a biological parent or with
divorce, the former spouse can be legally disenfranchised from rights to
continuing contact with children he or she has been raising. However,
gains are being made in broadening the definition of family. In one landmark court decision supporting gay parental rights, the judge concluded:
"It is the totality of the relationship, as evidenced by the dedication, caring, and self-sacrifice of the parties which should, in the final analysis,
control the definition of family" (quoted in Stacey, 1990, p. 4).

It is unfortunate when public discourse frames as "profamily" those
who adhere to the 1950s nuclear family as the sole standard for healthy
families while denouncing as "antifamily" those who hold a pluralistic

view. Abundant research evidence shows that children can be raised well in a variety of family arrangements (Walsh, 2003a). We need to be mindful that families in the distant past and in cultures worldwide have had multiple, varied structures and that effective family processes and the quality of relationships matter most for the well-being of children (Amato & Fowler, 2002).

CHANGING GENDER ROLES AND RELATIONS

Over the centuries—and still today in many traditional cultures—marriage has been viewed in functional terms: matches made by families on the basis of economic and social position (Coontz, 2005). In traditional patriarchal cultures, wives and children have been regarded as the property of their husbands and fathers, who held authority and controlled all major decisions and resources. For a husband to be certain of his (male) heirs, the honor of the family has required the absolute fidelity of the wife and the chastity of marriageable daughters. These values have often been enforced in traditional Arab societies, for instance, through the veiling and cloistering of women in the household (Walsh, 1985). In many patriarchal cultures, polygamy has been considered the normal family arrangement. The husband, his co-wives, and their many children often live together in one household, and a man's social status is enhanced with each wife, whose status in turn increases with the birth of each son. In other cultures, men commonly have kept a mistress and their children apart from the primary family unit.

Although families had many more children in the past, women invested relatively less time in parenting, contributing to the shared family economy in varied ways, from fieldwork to bookkeeping. Fathers, older children, extended kin, and neighbors all participated actively in child rearing. The integration of family and work life facilitated intensive sharing of labor among all family members. With industrialization and urbanization, family work and paid work became segregated into separate gendered spheres of home and workplace. Women were assigned exclusively the roles of custodian of the hearth, nurturer of the young, and caretaker of the old. In North American and British societies, strongly influenced by psychoanalytic movements, mothers came to be regarded as the primary, essential, and irreplaceable caregivers for children and blamed for all child and family problems (Braverman, 1989).

The belief that "proper gender roles" are essential for healthy family functioning and child development dominated sociological conceptualizations of the normal American family, based on Talcott Parsons's observations of white, middle-class, suburban U.S. families in the 1950s (Parsons & Bales, 1955). In that view, the nuclear family structure provided for a healthy complementarity in the division of roles into male instrumental leadership and female socioemotional support. The fields of social psychiatry, and child development adhered to this family model and to its corollary: that the failure to uphold proper gender roles would damage children (Lidz, 1963).

The breadwinner–homemaker model was highly adaptive to the demands of the industrial economy, and men with wives covering the home front were most successful. However, rigid role expectations came at great personal and family cost. Job demands limited men's involvement in family life and women carried a disproportionate burden in caring for others, while denying their own needs and identities (McGoldrick, Anderson, & Walsh, 1989). Unpaid domestic work was devalued and rendered invisible, with women and children dependent financially on male breadwinners. The loss of community further isolated men and women from companionship and support.

In the 1960s, the feminist movement grew in reaction to the exploitive and stultifying effects of the modern family model. With reproductive choice and family planning, women turned to the work sphere, seeking personal growth, greater financial autonomy, and equal status. However, women found that their wages and job status were lower than men's, and they remained bound to their primary family obligations—a dual disparity that widely persists. The belief that women's full-time homemaking role was essential for the well-being of all family members fueled the persistent myth (together with maternal blame and guilt) that outside work was harmful to their children's healthy development. Research has not supported that contention.

In combining jobs and child rearing, women found that they were adding a "second shift" as most men were not making reciprocal changes in sharing family responsibilities. The women's movement refocused on efforts to redefine and rebalance gendered role relations, so that both men and women could share equitably in the joys and obligations of family life, be gainfully employed, and seek personal fulfillment (McGoldrick et al., 1989). Men's movements have encouraged more active involvement in parenting and deeper connections with their own fathers. Most men today are doing substantially more in home life than their own fathers, yet shouldering far less than employed wives' share of household, childcare, and elder care burdens (Barnett & Hyde, 2001; Hochschild, 1997; Lamb, 2004). Although some advocate a return to

34   OVERVIEW

the traditional patriarchal model, most men today share with women the desire for a full and equal partnership and involvement in family life (Haddock, Zimmerman, & Lyness, 2003). Living out this aim is still a work in progress.

CULTURAL DIVERSITY AND SOCIOECONOMIC DISPARITY

One of the most striking features of North American families today is the rapid increase in cultural diversity. The foreign-born population in the United States has more than tripled since 1970, with most coming from Latin America and Asia (McGoldrick, Giordano, & Garcia-Preto, 2005). Currently, over one in five persons is either foreign-born or a first-generation resident. Through immigration and higher birth rates, the proportion of Latino, Asian, and African American families has risen to nearly half of the U.S. population and is expected to increase further in coming decades. Growing numbers of children and families are multiethnic and bi- or multiracial (Root, 2001).

Contrary to the myth of the melting pot, American families, with a long tradition of immigration, have always been diverse. In earlier periods, strong pressure for assimilation into mainstream society led many immigrants to cut off from their extended family ties and ethnic traditions left behind. More recently, experts working with immigrant families find that they are more resilient in navigating the challenges of adaptation when they maintain continuities with their past alongside the changes they must make, essentially becoming bicultural (Falicov, 1998, 2003). Parents are encouraged to raise their children with knowledge of and pride in their kin and community roots, language, ethnic heritage and religious values. Cultural pluralism can be seen as a source of strength that vitalizes a society. Sadly, recent economic insecurities and fears of terrorism have aggravated racial discrimination and intolerance toward non-European immigrants and minorities, complicating adaptive challenges for those families.

Socioeconomic influences must be taken into account in appraising family functioning and resilience. Social scientists have too often generalized to all families on the basis of white middle-class experience. With the intact, self-sufficient nuclear family model taken as the norm, there has been insufficient appreciation of the strong extended family bonds that foster resilience in low-income families, especially in African American and immigrant families who have had to struggle to overcome conditions of poverty and discrimination (Boyd-Franklin, 2004). Over recent decades, due to economic and political forces, the broad middle class has been shrinking, and the gap of inequality between the rich and poor has widened. The financial prospects of most young families today are lower than those of their parents, with a decline in median income and more families living in poverty. Most families require two incomes to support even a modest standard of living, health care expenses, and their children's education. Many are struggling anxiously through uncertain times as businesses downsize and workers are let go despite loyal service. As the economy has shifted from industrial manufacturing to services and computer-based technology, working-class and poor families with limited education, job skills, and employment opportunities have been hit hardest.

Declining economic conditions and job dislocation can have a devastating impact on family stability and well-being (McLanahan et al., 2003). Persistent unemployment or recurring job transitions can fuel substance abuse, family conflict and violence, marital dissolution, homelessness, and an increase in poor single-parent households. Studies have found that young inner-city fathers are less likely to marry or maintain financial support of their children when they lack job opportunities and face bleak earning prospects, reinforced by racism (Wilson, 1996).

The economic and social conditions of women and children have worsened disproportionately (Barnett & Hyde, 2001). In the workplace, the earnings gap between men and women, although improving somewhat over the past decade (due in part to a drop in male earnings), still leaves women currently earning about 78 cents to each dollar earned by men. The number of children in poverty has increased over 40% since 1970. Their life chances are worsened by persistent conditions of discrimination, neighborhood decay, poor schools, crime, violence, and lack of opportunity.

Harry Aponte (1994) stresses that the emotional and relational problems of poor ethnic minority families must be understood within their socioeconomic and political contexts: They are dependent on and vulnerable to the overreaching power of society and cannot insulate themselves. They can't afford private schooling for their children when their public school fails or move into an upscale neighborhood when their housing project becomes too dangerous. Such immense structural disparities perpetuate a vast chasm between the rich and the poor, increasing the vulnerability of the growing numbers of families struggling to make ends meet. Structural changes in the larger society are necessary to support and sustain family vitality and resilience.

VARYING AND EXTENDED FAMILY LIFE COURSE

Families and societies worldwide are rapidly aging. In the United States, life expectancy has increased from 47 years in 1900 to over 75 years currently. By 2030, the over-65 age group will exceed 20% of the population. This trend makes possible—and more challenging—long-lasting couple and intergenerational relations (Walsh, 1999a). Four- and five-generation families are increasingly common. Sibling relationships assume growing significance as people age (McGoldrick & Watson, 1999). Yet, in later life, chronic illness and disability also pose stressful family caregiving challenges (see Chapter 9). Adults over 85 are the fastest-growing and most vulnerable age group; nearly half are likely to suffer with dementia. Adult children past retirement, and with limited resources, are increasingly called upon to care for their aged parents. Adult children at midlife have been dubbed "the sandwich generation" with childrearing and college expenses on one side and caregiving for parents, grandparents, and extended kin on the other side. With fewer young people in families to support the growing number of elders, threats to Social Security and health care benefits are likely to fuel growing insecurity and intergenerational tensions.

Marriage vows "till death do us part" are harder to keep over a lengthening life course. It's difficult for one relationship to weather the storms and to meet changing needs and priorities, as Margaret Mead (1972) noted. In youth, romance and passion stand out in choosing a partner. In rearing children, relationship satisfaction is linked more to the sharing of family joys and responsibilities. In later life, needs for companionship and caregiving come to the fore. In view of these developmental shifts, Mead predicted that time-limited, renegotiable contracts and serial monogamy would become more common and might better fit contemporary life. Despite today's high divorce rate, most people remain optimistic; they long for a romantic, committed relationship, and if their attempt fails or their needs change, they try again. Two or three committed relationships in a (long) lifetime, along with periods of cohabitation and single living, are becoming increasingly common. Thus, most adults and their children will move in and out of a variety of family structures as they come together, separate, and recombine. For resilience, we will need to learn how to navigate these transitions and how to live successfully in complex kin arrangements.

Our view of the family must also be expanded to the varied course of the life cycle, to a wider range of life phases and transitions fitting the diverse preferences and challenges that make each family unique. Some become first-time parents at the age when others become grandparents. Others start second families at midlife. Some who remarry have children as young as their own grandchildren. Single adults (Anderson & Stewart, 1994) and couples without children forge a variety of intimate relationships and significant kin and friendship bonds, such as the close-knit networks of gays and lesbians termed "families of choice" (Weston, 1991).

Reproductive technologies and the increase in surrogate pregnancies offer new opportunities to individuals and couples yearning to become parents, often at a later age. Medical technologies prolonging life and the dying process pose unprecedented family challenges. Yet, in impoverished communities, the lack of adequate health care and the risks of toxic environmental conditions, neighborhood violence, drug abuse, and HIV/AIDS drastically foreshorten life expectancy.

NAVIGATING FAMILY TRANSITIONS: RISK AND RESILIENCE

As we've seen, today's families are increasingly diverse and complex. Adults and their children are likely to transition in and out of several household and kinship arrangements over the life course. Research finds that no family form is essential for healthy child development; children can fare well in a variety of family arrangements. Nevertheless, family transitions are disruptive and upsetting. Highly unstable households and relationships increase the risk for children's maladaptation. Therefore, it's crucial to identify risk variables and facilitate family processes that foster resilience through stressful transitions.

The family transitions with divorce, for instance, pose a series of challenges over time. Claims that divorce inevitably damages children have not been substantiated by carefully controlled, longitudinal research (Greene, Anderson, Hetherington, Forgatch, & DeGarmo, 2003; Hetherington & Kelly, 2002). Although some studies have found a higher risk of problems for children in divorced families than those in intact families, it should be noted that most intact families are happily married and that fewer than one in four children from divorced families show serious or lasting difficulties. The vast majority of children do reasonably well after divorce, and many do remarkably well. In high-conflict and abusive families, children tend to do better after divorce than those in families that remain intact. Moreover, other factors, particularly economic strain and a cutoff of contact and support by the nonresidential parent, are critical variables that heighten risk for children's maladjustment. If parents live far apart or differ greatly in their lifestyles and expectations, children have a burden of reconciling their place in two worlds when they navigate between households. As children grow up, many do have painful memories of the divorce or its aftermath, but most are not seriously impaired psychologically or socially and have no greater difficulty developing committed intimate relationships than those whose parents remain unhappily married. Above all else, the healthy adaptation of children is influenced by the quality of relationships with parents and between the parents before and after the divorce (Ahrons, 2004).

Thus, divorce entails a complex set of changing conditions over time. Studies have tracked family processes associated with successful adaptation versus dysfunction, from an escalation of tensions in the predivorce climate, through separation, legal divorce processes, and subsequent reorganization of households, roles, and relationships. Most undergo further transition with remarriage and stepfamily integration (Hetherington & Kelly, 2002). Give this complexity, different strategies may prove useful in meeting new challenges that emerge (Greef & Van der Merwe, 2004). Family resilience thus involves varied adaptational pathways over time, from a threatening event on the horizon, through disruptive transitions, and subsequent shockwaves in the immediate aftermath and beyond.

Because separation, divorce, and remarriage are evolving processes over time, clinicians need to inquire about previous relationships and family units, the timing and nature of transitions, and future anticipated changes, in order to understand a problem in family developmental context. In particular, recent or impending changes in membership or household composition should be noted, as these changes may precipitate a crisis related to presenting problems. Focusing only on the present family household can result in tunnel vision, as the following example illustrates:

A single-parent father with custody of his two children, Matt, age 14, and Maggie, age 12, sought help for Maggie's stormy behavior with him. In presenting the case for supervision, the therapist diagrammed the family structure as follows:

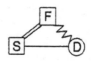

The therapist had assessed the problem as a triangle in which the father's strong bond with Matt excluded Maggie, who then sought attention through misbehavior. Interventions had focused on rebalancing this triangle, with no progress. Outside the household and the frame of assessment and intervention, however, were critical relationship complications in this system (as illustrated in this diagram):

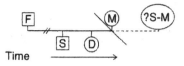

Time

The father had divorced the mother 3 years earlier after learning she had carried on an affair with his best friend in the family home. He fought and won a bitter custody battle and continued to demonize the mother to the children, severely restricting their contact with her. In the midst of the divorce, he plunged into a serious relationship with a new partner, a divorced woman with custody of her two children, who was now pressuring him to get married. Maggie was angry at having been being turned against her mother by her father, saddened by her loss of contact, and resentful of the new "replacement" mom in the wings. The father, in an individual session, then revealed his own catastrophic fears of remarriage, rooted in his shattered trust and sense of betrayal by his ex-wife. Therapy focused on dealing with these issues and facilitating positive connections between the children and their mother before moving on to possible remarriage and the complications of new stepparenting relationships. (See Chapter 12 for discussion of post-divorce reconciliation).

FAMILY TRANSFORMATIONS: FORGING RESILIENCE

Families today are in transformation, with growing diversity and complexity in structure, gender roles and sexual orientation, cultural and class differences, and life cycle patterns. Debates about the future of the family have touched a vulnerable core of anxiety about contemporary life (Gergen, 1991). Families are struggling with actual and symbolic losses as they alter family arrangements and as their world changes around them. Many feel adrift on their own fragile life rafts in a turbulent sea (Lifton, 1993). Disoriented and uncertain, many struggle to hold on to familiar patterns and yet question idealized family models from the past that don't fit their current situation, resources, and challenges. There is widespread confusion about the very structure and meaning of family relationships—about what is "normal" (i.e., typical and expectable) in family life and how to construct "healthy" families that function well and are resilient under stress.

Yet most families are showing remarkable resilience, making the best of their situations and inventing new models of human connectedness. As sociologist Judith Stacey (1990) has observed, these "brave new families" are creatively reworking family life in a variety of household and kinship arrangements, drawing on a wide array of resources, and devising new gender and relationship strategies to cope with new challenges. In her ethnographic study of working-class families, she found men and women sharing housework and child care, unmarried working women choosing to have children on their own, strong extended family connections sustained across serial marriages, and longtime close friends claiming kinship. She also found same-sex couples exchanging marital vows, sharing childrearing commitments, and more openly seeking community and spirituality outside mainstream institutional forms. Particularly impressive were bold and creative initiatives to reshape the experience of divorce from a painful, bitter schism and loss of resources into a viable kin network involving new and former partners, multiple sets of children, step-kin, and friends—into households and support systems collaborating to survive and flourish. It is ironic that such families are termed "nontraditional" as their flexibility, diversity, and community recall the resilience found in the varied households and loosely knit kinship of the past.

Because today's world is marked by tumultuous changes, our lives can seem utterly unpredictable, with few certainties. The rise in religious fundamentalism may be seen in part as a reaction. The loss of bearings can be overwhelming and alarming. Yet rather than collapsing under these pressures and threats, Robert Lifton (1993) contends that we humans are surprisingly resilient. He compares our predicament and response to those of the Greek god Proteus: Just as Proteus was able to change shape in response to crisis, we create new psychological, social, and familial configurations, exploring new options and transforming our lives many times over the life course. Similarly, Mary Catherine Bateson (1994) contends that adaptation "comes out of encounters with novelty that may seem chaotic" (p. 8). An intense multiplicity of vision, enhancing insight and creativity, is necessary. Although we can never be fully prepared for the demands of the moment, Bateson argues that we can be strengthened to meet uncertainty:

> The quality of improvisation characterizes more and more lives today, lived in uncertainty, full of the inklings of alternatives. In a rapidly changing and interdependent world, single models are less likely to be viable and plans are more likely to go awry. The effort to combine multiple models risks the disasters of conflict and runaway misunderstanding, but the effort to adhere blindly to some traditional model for a life risks disaster not only for the person who follows it but for the entire system in which he or she is embedded, indeed for all other living systems with which that life is linked. (1994, p. 8)

If we knew the future of a particular family, therapists and other helping professionals might be able to prepare that family with all the necessary skills and attitudes. But such stability or certainty has never existed. Instead, ambiguity is the essence of life; it cannot be eliminated. We must help families to find coherence within complexity. In Bateson's apt metaphor, "We are called to join in a dance whose steps must be learned along the way. Even in uncertainty we are responsible for our steps" (1994, p. 10).

Gergen (1991) observes that when we become aware of the multiplicity in diverse human experience, we begin to see that each ethnic community, political group, and economic class has its own limited, partial perspective and frames the world in its own terms. We may lose the safe and sure claims to truth, objectivity, and authority—and the idea of self as the center of meaning. Yet, he contends, we may gain something scarcely known in Western culture: the reality, the centrality, and the fundamental necessity of relatedness.

Amid the swirling confusion and upheaval, we can help families to prevail by sustaining continuities along with change and by gaining coherence in the midst of complexity and uncertainty. In the process of small victories, families build competence and confidence. Also, as Bateson (1994) urges, families must be encouraged to carry on the process of learning throughout life in all they do—"like a mother balancing her child on her hip as she goes about her work with the other hand and uses it to open the doors of the unknown" (p. 9). The ability to combine multiple roles and to embrace new challenges can be learned. A family resilience approach to practice encourages such vision and skills.

Clinician and Family Views of Family Normality and Health

With the many changes in family life, what is a normal family in our times? Our views of normality and health are socially constructed (Walsh, 2003a). Widely held cultural ideals of the "normal" family become standards by which families are judged—and judge themselves—to be healthy and successful. When families that don't conform are viewed as pathological and are stigmatized, it makes their adaptations more difficult. In these uncertain times, families worry about their own normality and deficiency if they don't fit the socially desirable standard. In my research experience with nonclinical families, many sought confirmation that they were, indeed, normal. One family even asked if they would receive a certificate of normality! Some families who declined to participate feared that under scrutiny they would be found abnormal. This gave me perspective on what is commonly labeled as "resistance" in clinical practice. Families often don't come for help because they fear being judged dysfunctional or deficient. They may have had such blaming or shaming experiences in the past. Too often their reluctance is misconstrued as a further sign of pathology.

As helping professionals, we also need to be aware of implicit assumptions about family normality, health, and dysfunction we bring to our work from our own world views, based in our cultural standards, personal experience, and clinical theories (Walsh, 2003b). Through these filtered lenses, we and our clients, together, construct the problems and deficits we "discover" in families, and set therapeutic goals tied to preconceptions about healthy functioning. This makes it imperative to examine our own views of family normality and to explore those brought by our clients to the therapeutic encounter. These beliefs influence how we define and explain problem situations, success or failure, and therapeutic goals.

The definition of "family" has broadened to encompass a wide spectrum of relationship options. It is important to explore each family's own identity and notions of normality. We might ask members such questions as: How do view your family? How do you believe others see your family? How do you compare your actual family to perceived cultural ideals? Beliefs of deficiency can fuel feelings of failure and misguided efforts to fit inappropriate standards. For instance, the belief that stepfamilies are inherently deficient often leads them to emulate intact nuclear families—sealing their borders, cutting off ties with nonresidential parents, and feeling they have failed when they don't immediately blend. As family therapy pioneer Carl Whitaker noted, the very attempts to fit the social mold of a normal family are often sources of problems and deep pain.

Assessing Families: A Broad, Inclusive Perspective

A family resilience framework for practice searches for strengths and potential alongside family problems and limitations. In all assessments, it's important to gain a holistic view of the family system and its community linkages. This includes all members of current households, the extended kin network, and key relationships that are—or have been—significant in the functioning of the family and its members. A genogram (McGoldrick, Gerson, & Shellenberger, 1999) is essential to construct as a systemic diagram, enabling both clinicians and family members to visualize the network of relationships and significant patterns. While the genogram is a useful tool in exploring past family-of-origin patterns, it also has immense value in showing the current configuration of the family system; demarcating living arrangements in various households; noting patterns of alliance, conflict, and cutoff; and identifying existing and potential resources in kin and social networks.

We must look beyond the household unit, particularly with single-parent families and stepfamilies, and with individuals living on their own. Clients who presume that "family" is equated with "household" may not mention an intimate partner or other kin who are, or could become, important resources, such as grandparents, aunts and uncles, and godparents. The potential contribution of a nonresidential parent may be overlooked if focus on a single-parent household renders him (or her) invisible or if the primary parent has written the ex-spouse off as hopeless. An elderly woman living alone may say that she has no family, meaning that her husband has died or that her children have little contact with her. A genogram can help to identify significant losses and potential resources.

It is important to ask who family members include in defining their own kinship: who is significant and what roles they play. Legal and blood definitions of "family" and social norms of the idealized nuclear family may constrain clients from disclosing important relationships, such as a gay or lesbian partner, or a live-in boyfriend of a single parent. It's important to clarify their roles and involvement with children.

We should also note the relational significance of companion and assistance animals, which are often vital supports in resilience (Walsh, 2006). Studies have found that pet owners enjoy better health, and that simply stroking a dog or cat can lower stress effects, heart rate, and blood pressure—in both the person and the animal! Our dog was a constant companion for our daughter through disruptive family transitions and our move into a new community. Targa was featured prominently on the multigenerational genogram she constructed for her stepgrandfather's 90th birthday.

A developmental perspective is needed to track significant events and transitions in families. A family timeline, accompanying the genogram, is extremely helpful in noting a pile-up of stressors and the confluence of stressful events and symptoms of distress. One family, who came for therapy after their 17-year-old son's drug overdose, did not initially mention an older son, who had died two years earlier at age 17. In another family, a child's school grades plummeted just after his father's job loss.

Clinicians can usefully draw on research to inform families that a variety of family structures can function well; none is inherently healthy or pathological. Research also sheds light on the processes families can strengthen for resilience, as we will see in the following chapters. Too often, problems of a child living in a single-parent household are reflexively attributed to "a broken home" or the absence of a father in the house. Key issues are whether the child feels abandoned or cared for by those who are important in his life, and how positive bonds can be strengthened. A resilience-based approach taps into each family's resources and builds on their potential.

Helping Families Meet the Challenges of Our Times

In the public rhetoric on "family values" we need to keep in mind that despite cultural and structural differences, the vast majority of families hold strong traditional values of commitment, responsibility, and mutual support. Yet today's families are struggling in the face of overwhelming challenges, such as time pressures in meeting job and homefront demands, as well as economic dislocations affecting job security, medical coverage, and retirement benefits. Parents worry about the impact of larger forces on their children, from war and terrorism to the cultural transmission of violence, sexism, and racism (Pipher, 1997). For individual and family well-being, quality-of-life issues are at the fore, including a desire for more community involvement, spiritual meaning, social justice, and a concern for the environment.

As we create more viable approaches to family life in our times, our families and society can experience new growth and transformation for greater individual and family well-being. Such attempts must overcome tremendous institutional resistance. To support family resilience, we must press for larger systemic changes and creative strategies for workplace security and flexibility; adequate, affordable health care; and quality day care for children and frail elders. Our challenge is to craft social and economic policies as well as clinical and community services that are responsive to the new family realities and challenges.

Crisis and challenge are inherent in the human condition. The concept of family resilience affirms the potential for survival, repair, and growth in all families, and offers a valuable framework for strength-oriented approaches to practice. Because families have varied resources, challenges, and adaptive strategies, there are many pathways in family resilience. Clinicians and community-based professionals equipped with an understanding of key processes can mobilize resilience-building resources in distressed families, and those at risk. Chapters 3–5 describe and illustrate these keys to resilience.

PART II

Key Family Processes in Resilience

CHAPTER 3

Belief Systems
The Heart and Soul of Resilience

Deep in my heart I do believe
We shall overcome someday!
—GOSPEL SONG, CHARLES TINLEY, 1900

Belief systems are at the core of all family functioning and are powerful forces in resilience. We cope with crisis and adversity by making meaning of our experience: linking it to our social world, to our cultural and spiritual beliefs, to our multigenerational past, and to our hopes and dreams for the future. How families view their problems and their options can make all the difference between coping and mastery or dysfunction and despair. This chapter draws on research and practice knowledge to identify key beliefs that facilitate resilience in families facing serious life challenges.

In the empirically based Western world, it is often said that "seeing is believing." Native Americans would say, "It may have to be believed to be seen" (Deloria, 1994). Beliefs are the lenses through which we view the world as we move through life, influencing what we see or do not see and what we make of our perceptions (Wright, Watson, & Bell, 1996). Beliefs are at the very heart of who we are and how we understand and make sense of our experience. Our core beliefs, whether secular or sacred, anchor us "in the dizzying vastness of the great unknown we call reality" (Taggart, 1994, p. 20). In this way, beliefs come to define our reality.

Belief systems broadly encompass values, convictions, attitudes, biases, and assumptions, which coalesce to form a set of basic premises that trigger emotional responses, inform decisions, and guide actions. Facilitative beliefs increase options for problem resolution, healing, and growth, whereas constraining beliefs perpetuate problems and restrict options (Wright et al., 1996). Affirming beliefs—that we are valued and have potential to succeed—can help us to rally in times of crisis. Beliefs that our own needs are "selfish" or unimportant can lead to selfless caregiving or relentless accommodation, leaving us depleted, guilty, or resentful. Some beliefs are more useful than others, depending on our situation. Some are more acceptable within a particular culture. Beliefs and actions are intertwined: our actions and their consequences can reinforce or alter our beliefs.

In this chapter, we first examine the ways in which shared belief systems evolve in families over time, and the importance of storytelling and narrative coherence. Key beliefs that facilitate family resilience are then identified and discussed. Professional belief systems regarding treatment and healing are also considered.

SHARED BELIEF SYSTEMS

Our beliefs are socially constructed, evolving in a continuous process through transactions with significant others and the larger world (Gergen, 1989; Hoffman, 1990). We experience commonalities not only because of similar events, but also when we construe and interpret the implications of events in a similar way (Wright et al., 1996). In living and being together we influence each other's beliefs. We develop our identities within our families, professions, and communities by the belief systems that we share. We live our lives only slightly aware of many beliefs that powerfully influence us.

Each family's shared beliefs are anchored in cultural values and influenced by their position and experiences in the social world over time (Falicov, 1995; Hess & Handel, 1959; McGoldrick et al., 2005). Family belief systems provide coherence and organize experience to enable family members to make sense of crisis situations. David Reiss (1981) demonstrated that families construct shared beliefs about how the world operates and their own place in it. These paradigms influence how family members view and interpret events and behavior. They provide a meaningful orientation for understanding one another and for approaching new challenges. Shared beliefs develop and are reaffirmed or altered over the course of the family life cycle and across the multi-generational network of relationships.

While sharing a congruent mythology, members of well-functioning families maintain openness to many differing viewpoints, lifestyles, and perceptions. Truth is seen as relative rather than absolute; this permits family members to approach human experience as subjective and unique for each person and situation. Because the family and its environment vary over time and for each individual, not all beliefs in a family will be shared. Different perspectives among siblings, for example, may arise out of non-shared experiences from their unique positions, influenced by genetic predisposition, birth order, gender, family roles, relationship dynamics, and the timing of critical events (Reiss et al., 2000). Nevertheless, the dominant beliefs in a family system—and its culture—most strongly influence how the family, as a functional unit, will deal with adversity.

Family Norms, Identity, Rituals

These shared beliefs shape family norms, expressed through patterned and predictable rules governing family life. Relationship rules, both explicit and implicit, provide expectations about roles, actions, and consequences that guide family life. Beginning in courtship, every couple makes a relational bargain, or "quid pro quo" (Jackson, 1977; Walsh, 1989)—a largely unspoken contract defining what the partners expect of each other and the relationship. In well-functioning families, relationship rules organize interaction and maintain system integration by regulating members' behavior. Core beliefs are fundamental to family identity and coping strategies, expressed in such rules as: "We never give up when the going gets rough," or "Men don't cry." Over time, mutual expectations need to be reappraised and rules altered in light of changing needs and constraints, such as when a father's disability disrupts assumptions about his role as breadwinner.

Family rituals store and convey each family's identity and beliefs in the celebration of holidays, rites of passage (e.g., weddings, bar/bat mitzvahs, graduations, and funerals), and family traditions (e.g., anniversaries, reunions), as well as routine family interactions (e.g., dinnertime). Rituals also facilitate life cycle transitions and transformations of beliefs. Rituals are encouraged in family therapy to mark important milestones, restore continuities with a family's heritage, create new patterns, and foster healing from trauma and loss (Imber-Black, Roberts, & Whiting, 2003).

The deep social and cultural roots of our beliefs often make it difficult to step outside our own context to notice and comment on them.
My experiences while living and working in Morocco as a Peace Corps
volunteer, and later serving as a consultant, not only immersed me in a
culture quite different from my own; they also brought new perspectives
on my social world upon reentry. I began to notice and question patterns
of family organization and gender roles that I had always taken for
granted as normal and ideal. As Mary Catherine Bateson has observed,
"Seen from a contrasting point of view or seen suddenly through the
eyes of an outsider, one's own familiar patterns can become accessible to
choice and criticism" (1994, p. 31).

Organizing Belief Systems: Storytelling and Narrative Coherence

Meanings and beliefs are expressed in the narratives we construct together to make sense of our world and our position in it. Storytelling has
served in every time and place to transmit cultural and family beliefs that
guide personal expectations and actions. For centuries, Moroccans have
gathered around storytellers in the lively marketplace of Marrakech, the
J'maa el F'na, to hear tales of life and love, of tragic plights and comic
relief, of human foibles and heroism. These stories are often dramatically acted out in costume and mime, with the perils and triumphs ac-
centuated by Berber drumming. Like storytelling and theatre in cultures
the world over, they convey personal mores, family values, and adaptive
strategies for mastering life's challenges.

Cultural changes, disrupting traditional modes of understanding the
self and others, generate heightened concern for coherence and integrity
in life stories (Geertz, 1986). In today's technological societies, culture
stories are transmitted through the mass media, in images that both por-
tray and saturate family life. Films and television powerfully shape and
reflect the values and concerns of our times: what it means to be a family, a husband and father, or a wife and mother; to be successful or to
fail. These images reach around the world, via satellite TV and the internet, where they are often strangely incongruent with local life. I've sat
bemused among remote villagers who are shocked and fascinated by
images from programs such as *Desperate Housewives*. Not surprisingly,
cultural anthropologists find multiple, conflicting identities in the life
narratives of young people worldwide who are challenged by shifting
norms and incongruities in our rapidly changing world.

Our need for enduring values and traditions, for stability and continuity admist rapid change can be seen in the multigenerational family transmission of myths and legends. Stories and rituals that preserve links to a family's cultural heritage are especially valuable for recent immigrant families, whose members can too easily lose their sense of identity, community, and pride in pressures for assimilation to the dominant culture (Falicov, 1998, 2003). It's important to ask about their families' migration experiences, attending to the traumas and losses they suffered and to the sources of resilience that enabled them to survive, regenerate, and make their way in a new world. Recovering stories, when lost, can restore a vital sense of connection and meaning (see Chapters 11, 12).

Researcher Elizabeth Stone views family stories as the DNA of family life (Stone, Gomez, Hotzoglou, & Lipnitsky, 2005). She found that family stories told by new immigrants in the United States and their American-born children help retain affiliation with their country of origin, reinforcing a dual identity and affiliation. Across cultures, the stories' motifs celebrate and idealize the country of origin/ethnic group, denigrate their past and present enemies, and share detailed knowledge of the country. American-born children of immigrant families in the past have tended to stress assimilation, and their family stories often reflected the ideology of "the Melting Pot." American-born children of recent immigrants are more transnational, more likely to be proudly bilingual, and more likely to maintain ties with the family's country of origin themselves.

In sharing stories we come to know ourselves, and we build coherent identities to make sense of the larger social context and our place in it. Susan Griffin (1993) asserts that we all have a deep need to be connected to the larger society and to our own history. She contends that all history is a part of us, such that when stories are told and secrets revealed—whether about our own family members or about tragic events or heroic deeds long ago or far away—our lives are made clearer to us.

Stories have particular significance in response to crisis and adversity. In his memoirs of the Holocaust experience, Elie Wiesel (1995) attests to the importance of memory and storytelling: "Memory is a passion no less powerful or pervasive than love. . . . What does it mean to remember? It is to live in more than one world, to prevent the past from fading, and to call upon the future to illuminate it." Wiesel continues, "Survivors have only words, poor, ineffectual words, with which to defend the dead. So some of us weave these words into tales, stories, and pleas for memory and decency. It is all we can do, for the living and for the dead."

Adversity and the accompanying distress become tensions and organizing principles for coherent life stories and belief systems (Bruner,
1986). Whether a widespread catastrophe, a personal tragedy, or persistent hardship, adversity generates a crisis of meaning and a potential disruption of personal integration. This tension prompts the construction
or reorganization of our life story and beliefs. Over time, we revise our
stories of adversity and resilience to gain narrative coherence and integrity (Cohler, 1991). A major therapeutic task involves the effort to reorganize a life story that presents past or ongoing misfortune as an impedi-
ment to the ability to move forward.

Psychotherapy can offer a healing context for dialogue and storytelling. Kleinman (1988) has found that individuals and family members
who have experienced serious illnesses benefit greatly from the opportunity to tell their stories of suffering. Yet professionals need to be attuned
to cultural differences. For instance, counselors for Cambodian refugees
who fled widespread massacres in the 1970s found that many families
told their stories of the terror and atrocities just once, and then preferred
to go on with their lives and speak of it no more (Mollica, 2004). Community-based, resilience-oriented approaches elicit stories of courage,
perseverance, and mastery alongside suffering with those who have experienced extreme trauma (see Chapter 11).

Family therapists can help clients to recover important stories from
the past that have become fragmented or lost in family processes of
secrecy, denial, distortion, and relationship cutoff (Byng-Hall, 1995a;
Imber-Black, 1995; McGoldrick, 1995). Such stories may concern stigmatized situations, such as gay relationships, or involve blame-, shame-,
or guilt-laden incidents involving substance abuse; violence or sexual
abuse; suicide; or accusations of unethical, scandalous, or illegal conduct. In narrative therapy approaches (Anderson, 1997; Freedman &
Combs, 1996; White & Epston, 1990), the therapist and family collaborate in developing alternative meanings and new, more hopeful, affirming stories in place of problem-saturated narratives.

Key beliefs in family resilience can be organized into three areas, as
outlined in Table 3.1. These beliefs involve efforts to make meaning of
adversity, a positive outlook, and transcendent or spiritual beliefs.

MAKING MEANING OF ADVERSITY

The meaning of adversity is filtered through family transactions. How
families make sense of a crisis situation and endow it with meaning is

TABLE 3.1. Belief Systems: Keys in Family Resilience

1. Making meaning of adversity
   • Viewing resilience as relationally based
     • "Lifelines" versus "rugged individual"
     • Viewing crisis as shared challenge
   • Normalizing and contextualizing experience
     • Family life cycle orientation
     • Viewing vulnerability as human; distress as understandable, common in situation
   • Gaining a sense of coherence
     • Viewing crisis as a challenge: comprehensible, manageable, meaningful
   • Appraisal of adverse situation: issues of control/responsibility/blame
     • Causal, explanatory attributions: How could this happen?
     • Future expectations/catastrophic fears: What will happen? What can be done?

2. Positive outlook
   • Hope: optimistic bias
     • Confidence in overcoming odds/barriers
   • Affirming strengths; building on potential
   • Seizing opportunities: active initiative and perseverance
   • Courage—En*courage*ment
   • Mastering the possible; accepting what can't be changed

3. Transcendence and spirituality
   • Larger values, purpose
   • Spirituality: faith, rituals, congregational support
   • Inspiration: envisioning new possibilities
     • Role models, life dreams
     • Innovative solutions
     • Creative expression (e.g., art, music, writing)
   • Transformation: learning, change, and growth out of crisis
     • Crisis is both threat and opportunity; holds gifts, potential
     • Reassess, reaffirm, or redirect life priorities
     • Concern and action to benefit others; social responsibility

most crucial for resilience (Antonovsky, 1998; Patterson & Garwick, 1994). As Kagan (1984) found, for instance, families have a positive mediating influence in children's adjustment to an emotionally stressful experience, such as a father's prolonged absence or parental divorce, by sharing helpful perceptions and an understanding of what is happening and what will happen to them. The ability to clarify and give meaning to a precarious situation makes it easier to bear.

As Reiss (1981) observed, an enduring set of beliefs about the social world is forged through pivotal family experiences and, in turn, shapes and reinforces interactional patterns. This shared world view influences how family members approach a stressful new situation and the meanings they attach to life challenges. A critical event or disruptive transition can catalyze a major shift in a family belief system, with reverberations for immediate reorganization and long-term adaptation.

Relational View of Resilience

The gospel song "We Shall Overcome" became the clarion cry of the 1960s civil rights movement and has inspired hope and creative action in many parts of the world. This simple yet profound phrase expresses the core conviction in relational resilience: In joining together, we strengthen our ability to overcome adversity.

The individualistic ethos underlying the myth of the rugged individual denies the critical importance of the communal and the interpersonal. Although the definition of the family is fluid and diverse, at the core is a value of kinship and pride in family identity. This strong affiliative value has been found to be vital for optimal family functioning (Beavers & Hampson, 2003). Genuine caring proves effective even in families where parenting skills are more modest. An expectation of satisfaction from relationships, in turn, reinforces involvement and mutual investment.

Like Dorothy in *The Wizard of Oz*, we find in life's journeys that there's no place like home. The poet Maya Angelou has remarked on this powerful yearning for "home": "The ache for home lives in all of us." In our turbulent times, our challenge is to expand the relational meaning of "home" and construct new maps to find our way home. The idea of home also extends to a sense of community beyond immediate family and intertwined in meaning and experience (Carter & McGoldrick, 2004). All concepts of the self and constructions of the world are fundamentally products of relationships, and it is through our interdependence that meaningful lives are best sustained (Bellah et al., 1985). Mary Catherine Bateson avows, "Community, like the sacred, is an idea that becomes reality because we believe in it" (1994, p. 42). We must then act on this belief, reaffirming it by putting it into practice.

Crisis as a Shared Challenge: Lifelines in Distress

Meaningful kin and community connections are lifelines in times of distress. Investment in affiliation and collaboration increases our potential to surmount overwhelming challenges. Stinnett and DeFrain's (1985) research on strong families found that pulling together was one of the most important processes in weathering crises.

As we will see in Chapters 4 and 5, a relational view is expressed in a family's organizational connectedness and communication processes. For instance, a shared commitment to the marital vow "in sickness and in health" can bolster actions to support optimal recovery and to sustain the relationship through an illness ordeal. A relationship is strengthened when a crisis is viewed as a shared challenge, to be tackled together. One husband conveyed this relational view in recounting how he and his wife approached her diagnosis of breast cancer as partners. He realized not only that her life was at risk and that she needed his support, but also that their *relationship* was endangered by the illness and required their mutual support in facing the challenges. In striking contrast, in the film *The Doctor*, a hotshot surgeon is thrown into a life crisis when he is diagnosed with cancer. Framing it as his individual crisis, he shuts out his wife and seeks comfort in an affair. Throughout his treatment ordeal, he distances from his wife, refusing to let her into his emotional turmoil, and preventing them from comforting each other. He recovers, but the damage to the marriage is irreparable.

Optimally, when families hold a positive view of human nature as essentially good, or at least as not malign in intent it enables them to relate with trust, without erecting stultifying interpersonal defenses (Beavers & Hampson, 2003). However, the ability to be trustful of the world and to view others as caring or benign can be impaired by repeated experiences of discrimination, exploitation, or abuse. And yet family members must at least be able to assume benign intentions in their own significant relationships rather than believe that one another's actions are fundamentally hostile or destructive in intent. We can encourage mutuality by affirming the belief that family members are all struggling to do as well as they can under their particular constraints. Confidence in one another's basic goodwill is essential to achieve closeness and collaboration, and to support trust, joy, and comfort in relating. In times of trouble, family members do best when they believe they can turn to one another as trusted partners and true kin.

Families are best able to weather adversity when members have an abiding loyalty and faith in one another, rooted in a strong sense of trust (Beavers & Hampson, 2003). They share confidence that home is a safe and welcoming place and that they can count on one another. Here again, beliefs and actions are intertwined. When members are trustworthy they stand by their word and stand by each other. Relationships are strengthened by actions toward trustworthiness, based on consideration

of one another's welfare. Trust is essential for open communication, mutual understanding, and problem solving, as pioneer family therapists
observed. Boszormenyi-Nagy (1987) has emphasized this ethical dimension of family relationships in multigenerational legacies of parental accountability and filial loyalty, which guide members over the life course.
His concept of "merited trust" dovetails with Whitaker's view (Whitaker
& Keith, 1981) of the importance of loyalty, accountability, and mutual
commitment in sustaining a strong relational foundation and buffering
periods of stress and disorganization.

Normalizing and Contextualizing Adverse Experience

Resilience is fostered when family members are able to view their crisis
situation or prolonged adversity in context. In the midst of crisis or facing overwhelming challenges, people commonly feel overwhelmed and
out of control of events impinging on their lives. We can foster their
resilience by *normalizing* and *contextualizing* distress, so that family
members can enlarge their perspective to see their reactions and difficulties as understandable in light of their particular situation, such as a
painful loss or daunting obstacles. The tendency for blame, shame, and
pathologizing is reduced in viewing their complicated feelings and dilemmas as "normal," in other words, common and expectable among families facing similar predicaments.

Family Life Cycle Orientation

Well-functioning families have an evolutionary sense of time and of
becoming—a continual process of growth and change across the life
course and the generations. Members experience strong transgenerational
connections, with internal images updated and modified as a guiding
mythology evolves over time. This family life cycle orientation (Beavers
& Hampson, 2003) helps members to accept the rhythms and flow of
family life as children grow up and parents grow old; new members are
born and loved ones die.

   Family resilience is strengthened through acceptance of the passage
of time and the need for change with new developmental challenges. Life
cycle transitions, while disruptive, are also seen as milestones that can be
an impetus for reevaluation of assumptions about one's place in the
world. In this way, painful transitions can catalyze growth and transformation. In contrast, risk of dysfunction is heightened when members
can't accept the passage of time and the continuities between past, pres-

ent, and future (Carter & McGoldrick, 2004). Symptoms commonly occur at times of disruptive transition. Family members may seem frozen in time. Some are terrified to move forward into the unknown. Many live only in the present moment, without a sense of past connection or future direction. Some become preoccupied with the past or so focused on future goals that they are unable to live fully in the present. Some attempt to escape the past through detachment from painful relationships and aspects of their history. Some reject their past by making reactive, oppositional choices in their lives.

Traumatic past experiences become encoded into family scripts that are often out of awareness, providing a blueprint for meaning and behavior when a family is facing a dilemma or crisis (Byng-Hall, 1995a). Unresolved conflicts, secrets, and losses can reverberate underground, erupting in painful symptoms or destructive behavior, or enacted in family dramas at the next generation, as we saw in Martin's family in Chapter 1. Family myths can be either empowering or debilitating, depending on their underlying themes and their fit with new challenges. Clinicians who are trained to search for negative family-of-origin influences need to seek out positive multigenerational stories, heroes, and legacies, which can inspire hope and courageous action in the face of adversity.

For some, positive family ties may be overshadowed by past disappointment, conflict, or loss. Yet resilience and growth involve family members' coming to terms with their past, and integrating that meaningful understanding into their current lives and their future hopes and dreams. As Bateson (1989) has observed, "Composing a life involves a continual re-imagining of the future and reinterpretation of the past to give meaning to the present" (pp. 29–30).

Sense of Coherence

The concept of *sense of coherence* was developed by Aaron Antonovsky (1987, 1993, 1998) as a model for understanding the emergence of health—a "salutogenic" orientation in contrast to the dominant "pathogenic" paradigm in biomedical and social science research (Cederblad & Hansson, 1996). Antonovsky remarked that, given the stress-producing nature of the human condition, the miracle and mystery are that any organism ever survived for any length of time. The important question then is, what resources promote stability and health in the face of disruption and change?

A sense of coherence is defined as a global orientation to life as comprehensible, manageable, and meaningful. A strong sense of coherence involves confidence in the ability to clarify the nature of problems so that they seem ordered, predictable, and explicable. Demands are believed to be manageable by mobilizing useful resources, including relational resources. Stressors are viewed as challenges that we are motivated to deal with successfully. The construct addresses meaningfulness, including existential feelings of social integration and purpose in life, as opposed to a sense of alienation, drifting, or stuckness.

A sense of coherence has been found to contribute significantly to health, mental well-being, and quality of life, and to be more influential than such individual traits as temperament or intelligence (Cederblad & Hansson, 1996). This concept taps into important elements missing in such concepts as *locus of control* and *mastery*, which focus more narrowly on self-reliance and specific coping strategies. The concept of sense of coherence (SOC) cuts across such influences as culture, class, and gender, emphasizing flexibility in selecting varied strategies that are useful and preferred to deal with diverse challenges.

Antonovsky and Sourani (1988) attempted to measure *family sense of coherence*, the perceived coherence of family life in coping with a specific crisis. They studied working-class couples faced with the husband's disability and subsequent pileup of stresses. They found that a high sense of family coherence predicted better coping and adaptation, with greater satisfaction within the family and in terms of its fit with the community.

Appraisal of Crisis, Distress, and Recovery

Our appraisal of stress events and our resources to deal with them will strongly influence our response (Lazarus & Folkman, 1984). The same event may be perceived as burdensome, threatening, harmful, benign, or irrelevant. Stressful life events are most distressing when we feel little control over them or when they pose a major threat to our lives, our loved ones, and our understanding of ourselves and the meaning of life (Cohler, 1987).

The meaning of adversity varies across cultures. Whether an event is viewed as a problem and how distress is handled vary with different family and cultural norms. Epidemiologists find that at any given time, 75% of all Americans are "symptomatic," experiencing physical or psychological distress. Yet most don't seek treatment, instead defining their distress as part of normal life (Kleinman, 1988). A troubled family may not seek professional help or may attempt to deal with problems in other ways. Conversely, as mental health professionals are the first to avow, seeking help can be a sign of strength. In fact, studies have found that highly resilient people do reach out for help when needed, turning to kin, social, and religious support systems—most often before going to professionals.

Causal and Explanatory Beliefs

When adversity strikes, we attempt to make sense of how things have happened through causal and explanatory attributions (Kleinman, 1988). Some families hold a core belief that misfortune is a sign that they are sinful and deserve to suffer or be punished. Some blame others, or view themselves as victims in a dangerous and hostile world beyond their control. Many believe that adversity is simply a matter of bad luck. It's important to explore the family, cultural, and religious roots of such beliefs and their implications.

Western culture emphasizes personal responsibility, in the belief that we are masters of our fate. In U.S. society, we hold a curious split of individual and family responsibility: We tend to credit individuals for their success but blame their families for any problems. A Moroccan Muslim friend once told me of his father's drinking and abandonment of the family, and of his mother's retreat into her own sorrows. When, from my American perspective, I was puzzled that he harbored no anger or blame toward them for his own life difficulties, he replied, "But you don't understand. I'll always be grateful to them: my parents gave me life."

In many cultures and religions, adversity is ascribed to fate, destiny, or God's will, and regarded as beyond human comprehension. Hindus believe that misfortune may be the result of bad karma, due to one's conduct or circumstances in a previous life. In many indigenous traditions, when things go wrong in a family, people externalize blame in the belief that others who are envious, spiteful, or wish them harm may have brought about their plight; they turn to highly respected shamans or faith healers to restore health or good fortune (Falicov, 2003; Wright et al., 1996).

Studies of families in mainstream U.S. culture find that high-functioning families tend to view problems as resulting from many contributing variables rather than from one cause—essentially holding a systemic orientation, although they never heard of systems theory (Beavers & Hampson, 2003). Their responses vary with the situation in a pragmatic fashion. For example, they see that attempts at autocratic control can trigger reactions of angry defiance, just as uncooperative defiance invites tyrannical control. Realizing mutual influences, family members avoid blaming or typecasting others as villains or victims. In contrast, poorly functioning families tend to adhere fanatically to one explanation, get locked into a belief in a single cause, or personal failing, and are prone to blaming and scapegoating. Families whose members repeatedly blame one another tend to have more conflict and less solidarity than families who unite by attributing blame beyond their borders (Wright et al., 1996). However, a united front mobilized by the belief "Us against the world" can have a cost in social isolation, alienation, and mistrust.

How family members define and frame a problem situation will influence how they attempt to deal with it. A family's general worldview may not fit well with a particular challenge (Rolland, 1994). For instance, a family that believes that no effort should be spared until a solution is found may have difficulty accepting and living with a problem that can't be solved, such as an illness that cannot be cured.

In all family assessments, it is useful to explore patterns of problem explanation and attribution. Preoccupation with causal questions and accusations—"Who is at fault?"—invites blaming and scapegoating. Even in well-functioning families, parents (especially mothers) are particularly vulnerable to blame and guilt when something happens to a child, because of expectations of responsibility for their children's wellbeing. When adversity strikes, issues of blame, shame, and guilt can loom large, becoming as problematic as the crisis event.

> In one clinical case, Jean and Jerry were on the brink of divorce several months after their 3-year-old son had drowned in the lake behind their vacation cabin. Each blamed the other for not watching the boy, who waded into water to retrieve a ball and dropped from sight. They fought bitterly, faulting each other for negligence. It was crucial to explore and acknowledge each parent's own painful self-doubts and self-blame under the surface of their mutual attacks. Eventually, they both owned partial responsibility for the ambiguity in their communication about who was "on duty" at the time of the accident. Other contributing factors were also acknowledged, such as the rocky shoreline, which increased the risk of a fall. In shifting from blame to a fuller appreciation of many variables, Jean and Jerry became better able to share their sorrow, to consider what might be learned from the tragedy, and to begin a healing process together.

When people who are locked into a particular explanation of their experience are invited to reflect on their beliefs, they become freer to consider other possibilities. The following questions can be useful in guiding inquiry with families in crisis: How do family members make sense of the problem or crisis? How do they think it occurred? Do they fault themselves or anyone else? Do they believe it was accidental or intentional? Are family members overly preoccupied with blame, shame, or guilt? How do they agree or disagree in their views? What connections do they make to other adversities that have occurred in their lives and in their family's past history? How do cultural beliefs influence their views? Often this is the first time members have shared their private beliefs with one another. They may be surprised to learn that, deep down, each person blames himself or herself in some way, or that they've been fighting over assignment of blame in order to deflect unbearable pain, which can be eased through more empathic interaction.

Future Expectations and Catastrophic Fears

In troubled times, we look to the future with anticipation or dread, and at times, some of both. We ask: What will happen to us? What can be done to improve our situation? Our expectations, both conscious and out of awareness, are validated or disconfirmed in our daily lives and transactions. Assumptions that we will succeed or fail may lead us to take actions that fulfill our prophecies. Aaron Beck (Beck, Rush, Shaw, & Emery, 1987) identified three self-defeating cognitive distortions, or types of faulty thinking, that increase human vulnerability: (1) minimizing or underestimating strengths; (2) magnifying or exaggerating the seriousness of each mistake; and (3) "catastrophizing," that is, expecting disaster. These beliefs can be a major source of depression.

Catastrophic fears are paralyzing assumptions that block constructive action and fuel self-defeating behavior. For instance, the catastrophic fear of loss, through rejection or abandonment, can lead us to behave in ways that bring about loss. Fear of abandonment may also propel a partner to leave before being left. James, happily remarried after the death of his first wife from breast cancer, left his second wife abruptly within weeks of her diagnosis of breast cancer. She recovered; their relationship did not. The realization that there is no love without loss—that loss is inevitable in any relationship—can be a facilitating belief, enabling us to love more fully and to appreciate the time we do have together (see Chapter 8).

Perceptions of a current event intersect with legacies of previous multigenerational family experiences in making meaning of their challenge (Carter & McGoldrick, 1999). Traumatic past experiences—particularly a similar situation, a crisis, or a bad outcome, at the same nodal point in the life cycle a generation earlier—load apprehension onto the present situation (Walsh, 1983). If a family experienced courage and success in mastering similar crises in the past, its members will approach the new situation with greater confidence. It is important to search for such stories in dealing with past adversity—they offer positive models that can be transposed to new challenges.

People offer a variety of explanations for their success or failure in a challenging situation. In our mastery-oriented culture, resilient children tend to perceive success as largely due to their own efforts, resources, and abilities (Brooks, 1994). They assume realistic ownership for their achievements and possess a sense of some personal control over what happens in their lives, which enhances self-esteem. In contrast, children with low resilience more often believe that success and failure are matters of chance or luck, forces beyond their control. Such perceptions lower their confidence of future success.

When mistakes or failure occur, highly resilient children view them as experiences from which to learn, rather than as occasions of defeat. They are more likely to attribute mistakes to factors they can change, such as insufficient effort or an unrealistic goal. In contrast, children with low resilience and self-esteem are prone to believe that their mistakes are due to their own deficits (e.g., "I'm just stupid") and that these deficiencies can't be modified. The senses of competence and control are intertwined.

Severe and persistent adverse conditions with forces largely beyond personal control, such as chronic poverty, breed helplessness and hopelessness. For poor minority youth, especially young African American men, both self-esteem and resilience erode when job opportunities and encouragement for success are lacking (Wilson, 1996). Future success becomes less likely as individuals and their families expect to fail and retreat from demands, or resort to self-defeating coping strategies that worsen their situation.

High-functioning families recognize that success in human endeavors depends, in part, on variables beyond their control; yet they share the conviction that with goals and purpose, they can make a difference in their lives (Beavers & Hampson, 2003). They accept human limitations, believing that no one is completely helpless or all-powerful in any situation. Self-esteem comes from achieving relative competence, rather than absolute control, in dealing with a challenging situation. It's important for clinicians to explore beliefs about personal agency, power, and control. Who and what could be helpful in making things better? Can their efforts make a difference? We can help families find ways for each member to contribute in some valuable way.

POSITIVE OUTLOOK
IN OVERCOMING ADVERSITY

A positive outlook has been found to be vitally important for resilience. Key elements involve hope and optimism; focus on strengths and potential; initiative and perseverance; courage and en-*courage*-ment; and active mastery and acceptance. All are essential in forging the strength needed to withstand and rebound from adversity.

Hope: An Optimistic Bias

"What oxygen is to the lungs, such is hope to the meaning of life" (Brunner, 1984, p. 9). Sustaining hope in the face of overwhelming odds enables us to carry on our best efforts. The word "hope," originating in Old English, has a similar connotation in many languages: "to leap with expectation." Hope combines an internal decision—a leap of faith—with an external event we strongly desire to happen.

Hope is essential in repairing troubled relationships. Too often, partners give up on a marriage when they have lost hope that change can occur. Research-based couple interventions find that in many seemingly hopeless relationships, "reservoirs of hope" can be found and strengthened (Markman & Notarius, 1994).

In the wake of devastating loss or trauma, we need to help families regain hope to invest in rebuilding their lives and revising lost hopes and dreams. Hope is a future-oriented belief; no matter how bleak the present, we can envision a better future. Hope for a better life for their children keeps beleaguered parents in impoverished communities from being defeated by their immediate circumstances (Hines, 1998). The words of Martin Luther King inspire this hope: "We must accept finite disappointment but we must never lose infinite hope."

Learned Optimism

Although the "power of positive thinking" has become a cliche, considerable research evidence documents the strong effects of an optimistic orientation in dealing with stress and overcoming adversity (Seligman & Csikszentmihalyi, 2000). High-functioning families have been found to hold a more optimistic rather than a pessimistic view of life (Beavers & Hampson, 1990).

The concept of *learned optimism*, introduced by Martin Seligman (1990), has relevance for fostering resilience. Seligman's earlier studies on "learned helplessness" found that people can be conditioned to become helpless and to give up on trying to solve problems, particularly when rewards and punishments are unpredictable or random, regardless of their behavior. When people learn that their actions are futile and that nothing they do matters, they no longer initiate action and become passive, dependent, and hopeless. Qualities of permanence, pervasiveness, and personalization contribute to learned helplessness in such beliefs as "Things like this always happen to me." There is evidence that depression and pessimism are mutually reinforcing and can deplete the immune system, impair physical health, and even hasten death.

Interestingly, Seligman's own family experience heightened his interest in beliefs and explanatory styles. When he was 13, his father was paralyzed by a series of strokes that left him "physically and emotionally helpless." It was a foundation-shaking event that first depressed Seligman, but then lit a fire in him to do something to overcome passivity. The question that intrigued him was: Why did it spark that fire and not render *him* helpless, too? He became convinced that the difference had to do with dogged determination, persistence, and competitiveness: "I don't lie down and die." Family therapists will find it interesting that Seligman shifted his research attention from learned helplessness to learned optimism when he reached the age that his father had been at his paralysis.

An encounter with Jonas Salk, at a conference on psychoneuroimmunology, also redirected Seligman's focus to preventive work: Salk told him that if he himself were a young scientist today, he would focus on *psychological* immunization, not simply biological. Seligman contends that if helplessness can be learned, then it can be unlearned by experiences of mastery, in which people come to believe that their efforts and actions can work. He has theorized that through a process of "immunization," early learning that responsiveness matters can prevent learned helplessness throughout life. His research team developed approaches to "vaccinate" 10- to 12-year-olds at risk for depression, working with suburban children, inner-city youths, children and their parents, and teachers who train children in cognitive-behavioral techniques (Seligman, 1995). He found that children who learn such skills as challenging their negative thoughts and negotiating with peers showed less depression than control children, with effects increasing over time. Such findings point to the importance of strengthening family communication skills for problem solving and success (see Chapter 5).

Not everyone can change in every way, yet Seligman is convinced that a pessimistic orientation can be altered. Although research suggests that pessimists may see the world more clearly (and are more likely to be depressed), he believes that we must be able to use pessimism's keen sense of reality when needed, but without dwelling in its dark shadows. Yet a cheerful mindset is not sufficient; conditions must offer predictable and achievable rewards. Positive thinking is reinforced by successful experiences and a nurturing context.

Positive Illusions

In epidemiological research, Shelley Taylor (1989) found that people who hold selective positive biases about stressful situations tend to do better than those who have a hard grasp of a reality that may be depressing, such as life-threatening illness. These "positive illusions" sustain hope in the face of crisis, enabling individuals to carry on their best efforts to overcome the odds. Taylor also found that most people tend to see themselves as less vulnerable than others to a wide variety of risks. Among normal college students, individuals facing traumatic events, cancer and heart disease patients, and men at risk for AIDS, 85–90% of all subjects held such biases.

Taylor emphasizes that positive illusions are distinct from defensive denial or repression of distress, in that information about a stressful event or a threat is incorporated and its implications are absorbed (Taylor, Kemeny, Reed, Bower, & Gruenwald, 2000). Whereas defense mechanisms become more exaggerated in response to anxiety and break down under extreme stress, positive illusions function as a buffer against extreme stress and promote strong mental health. They are associated with a wide variety of indices of adaptive coping, such as persistence at tasks, willingness to help others, and high functioning.

Such positive illusions are also common in couple and family relationships. Despite the high divorce rate, just under 50%, few people believe that they will be among the divorce statistics. Fowers found that married couples, on average, thought their own chance of divorce was only 10%. Over 75% of the couples did not even acknowledge divorce as a remote possibility (Fowers, Lyons, & Montel, 1996). Fowers then looked more closely at "marital illusions"—fantasies and unrealistic ideas people hold about marriage in general and their own relationship in particular. He found that happy couples were more likely than unhappy ones to hold unrealistically rosy images of their relationships. They idealized their spouses, attributing more positive qualities to them and crediting them for the positive aspects of their marriage. However, extremely unrealistic expectations that a partner can meet all needs placed an undue burden on the relationship.

Resilience is not fostered by simply looking at "the sunny side" without acknowledging painful realities and giving voice to concerns. Each family's suffering is unique, and attempts to have members "cheer up" or "count their blessings" can unintentionally trivialize their experience. Reassuring platitudes such as "It'll all work out," or "Life could be worse," though meant to offer comfort and solace, are usually felt to be unempathic and unhelpful when the pain and heartache experienced in the particular crisis situation are not heard and acknowledged.

Shared Confidence in Overcoming Challenges

Science has begun to understand the chemistry of the will to live and dogged efforts to recover as fully as possible. Norman Cousins (1979) has written of his success in beating the odds when informed that he had a progressive and incurable collagen disease. Told to expect only months to live, he refused to accept the verdict. He was not in denial, because he was fully mindful of the seriousness of his condition. Yet deep down he believed he had a good chance to survive for much longer, and he relished the idea of bucking the odds. As Cousins observed, "I have learned never to underestimate the capacity of the human mind and body to regenerate—even when the prospects seem most wretched." The conviction that his own total involvement was necessary in achieving his aim was a major factor. Yet he didn't do it alone; he was selective in finding a physician with whom he could collaborate to fully mobilize all his resources in that endeavor.

Similarly, resilient families show unwavering confidence through an ordeal: "We always believed we would find a way out." This conviction and the relentless search for solutions fuel optimism and make family members active participants in the problem-solving process. Confidence in one another—a belief that each member will do his or her best—builds relational resilience as it reinforces individual efforts.

Affirming Strengths; Building on Potential

When families are dealing with a major crisis or pileup of stresses, they can easily lose sight of their strengths and resources. Therapy too, can become problem-saturated, attending to all that has gone wrong or bogging down with recurrent crises. By noticing, affirming, and commending family members for their strengths and potential in the midst of difficulties we help them to counter a sense of helplessness, failure, or blame. Seeing potential in everyone reinforces a sense of pride, confidence, and a "can do" spirit.

Initiative and Perseverance

For resilience, a positive outlook must be acted upon in personal initiative, rather than waiting passively for things to work out. Clinicians can help families to see and seize opportunities. Beliefs that their efforts and actions can make a difference fuel this initiative.

Perseverance—the ability to "struggle well" and persist in the face of overwhelming adversity—is a key element in resilience. What may be taken for rigidity or stubbornness may also be seen as tenacity, a strong determination to persevere. At times, this requires bouncing back from failure to try and try again—or try a new way—until we succeed. As Lillian Rubin (1996) put it, "We must be able to fall down seven times and get up eight."

At times, we must make the best of a grim situation and stand firm, holding on with resolve. The endurance and survival of harrowing life experiences can themselves be a source of pride. In studying resilience in African American men born into poverty and racism in rural Mississippi, Franklin (in Butler, 1997) was struck by their sheer capacity to survive to the age of 70 in those harsh circumstances. Elie Wiesel (1995), in describing the dehumanizing effects of the Nazi concentration camps, said that to survive Auschwitz while remaining a human being was itself heroic.

In Memory's Kitchen (DeSilva, 1996), a poignant collection of recipes, poems, and stories was written by the women starving in a Nazi concentration camp at Terezin in Czechoslovakia. In an effort to endure the hunger, cold, and terror at the camp, the women met secretly to share and gather together memories of their family life to which they might never return. They believed that they needed imagination and a link to their traditions to survive and preserve their identity and heritage. Their way of coping was to think of wonderful food—to transport themselves back into their kitchens and dining rooms, filled with joyous gatherings, loving husbands, and lively children. The recipes evoked memories of feasts and celebrations, such as the blue plum strudel served at Rosh Hashanah, the Jewish New Year, and "Mrs. Pachter's *Gesundheit*

Kuchen," "good health" cakes traditionally taken to the mothers of newborn babies. Their positive remembrances were written on scraps of paper, stitched together by hand and hidden, to be retrieved after the war as a legacy of their lives. Although the women did not survive the camp, their endurance and their collected memories attest to the survival of the spirit.

Courage and En-*courage*-ment

The word "courage" is embedded in the word "encouragement." Personal courage is strengthened by the encouragement of family, friends, and community. One woman, abandoned by her husband, dreaded her divorce hearing and the difficulties that lay ahead. Her brother accompanied her to the hearing, saying simply, "I came to sit at your side to give you courage." In the gay community, supportive social networks have been vital in sustaining the courage of persons dealing with HIV/ AIDS (Weston, 1991).

The courage shown in the everyday life of ordinary families often goes unnoticed. In the housing projects in Chicago, parents and their children must pass through gang- and drug-infested courtyards daily to go to work and school; returning at night from a late shift is always hazardous (Kotlowitz, 1991). Mothers show enormous courage in steeling themselves each morning to get their families through another harrowing day, and to encourage their children to strive and overcome barriers, for a better life.

The extraordinary courage shown by an ordinary person can also inspire others. Rosa Parks is well remembered as the African American woman whose refusal to sit in the back of the bus became a defining moment at the start of the civil rights movement. Her courage emboldened others and shaped the spirit of the times. As Goethe wrote: "What people call the spirit of the times is mostly their own spirit in which the times mirror themselves."

The Art of Mastering the Possible

For resilience, we need to take stock of our situation—our challenges, constraints, and resources—and then focus on making the most of our options. Both active mastery and acceptance are required, akin to the Serenity Prayer at the heart of recovery movements. In Higgins's (1994) study, resilient adults reported that they had overcome childhood adversity by channeling energy and efforts to master what they could control and accepting what couldn't be changed. Higgins aptly termed them masters of the art of the possible.

Remarkable mastery is often brought forth in the experience of immigration, which poses the challenges of loss and adaptation; strengths are forged through interweaving the old with the new for continuity and change. Immigrant women have often found cooking to be both a source of livelihood in the new land and a cherished link to the families and homelands they had to abandon. My great-grandmother Frimid came to Milwaukee from Budapest to escape pogroms against the Jews in the late 1880s. She used her cooking skills to start a catering business while her husband, who had been a Talmudic scholar, learned a trade. One year, the strange weather reminded her of a certain season in Hungary when all the onion crops had failed. With her husband's encouragement, she withdrew all their savings from the bank and invested them in onions. Sure enough, the crop failed, and, having cornered the market, they became rich. Her picture on the front page of the newspaper was captioned, "Frimid: The Onion Queen." Family stories of her bold resilience have been a source of inspiration for me, as her namesake. (However, I have yet to realize any financial windfall!)

Beliefs concerning mastery and acceptance must be counterbalanced. Resilience requires acceptance of the limits of our power—appraising and acknowledging what we can influence and what we can't control, and then putting our best efforts into what is possible. A philosophical acceptance is more common among older people, and is an important source of wisdom with aging (Walsh, 1999a). Those of Eastern and Native American traditions are less focused on mastery and more attuned to living in harmony with nature. Those of us with a European American mindset are often uncomfortable in situations beyond our control. Striving to "beat the odds" fits our competitive culture. The practice of Western medicine provides an illusion of control over life and death. Seeking comfort in that illusion is one way to deal with our fear of mortality. But each time a patient dies or "fails" to recover, doctors—and family members—must confront the fact we live in an uncertain universe and can't "master" death. Still, we do have the ability to heal psychosocially and spiritually from an illness or traumatic experience, even when we can't control or reverse it.

Family members may not be able to control the *outcome* of events, but they can make choices and find meaningful ways to participate actively in the *process* of unfolding events, influencing the quality of life and relationships. In situations beyond their control, or those with a good deal of uncertainty, they can be encouraged to carve out aspects they can influence. For instance, when an illness is terminal, and no treatment options remain, family members can actively choose ways to participate in caregiving, the relief of suffering, and preparation for death. In such ways, they make the most of the time they have together and find comfort in loving one another well in the face of loss.

TRANSCENDENCE AND SPIRITUALITY

Transcendent beliefs provide meaning, purpose, and connection beyond ourselves, our families, and our troubles. They provide continuity with the past and into the future, with generations before us and those that will come after us. The need to find greater meaning in our lives is most commonly met through spiritual faith and cultural heritage. It may also be expressed through deep philosophical, ideological, or political convictions. Transcendent beliefs offer clarity about our lives and solace in distress; they render unexpected events less threatening and foster acceptance of situations that cannot be changed.

Values and Purpose: A Moral Compass

A transcendent value system, whether conventional or unique, enables us to define our lives and our relationships to others as meaningful and significant. Just as individuals prosper within significant relationships, families thrive when connected to larger communities and value systems (Beavers & Hampson, 2003; Doherty, 1996). To accept the inevitable risks and losses in loving and being close, families need a value system that transcend the limits of their experience and knowledge. It enables family members to view their particular reality, which may be painful, uncertain, and frightening, from a perspective that makes some sense of events and allows for hope. Without this larger view, or moral compass, we are more vulnerable to hopelessness and despair.

Most families uphold values and commitments that maintain continuity with their past. In recent surveys (Gallup & Lindsey, 1999), most Americans ranked "family ties, loyalty, and traditions," and secondly, "moral and spiritual values," as the main factors thought to strengthen the family. In clinical practice, it's important to explore each family's values and how they may have been strengthened or shaken by crisis events. Persistent adversity may prevent families from fully living out their best values. Family members can be encouraged to get in touch with their deepest values and to commit themselves to live in ways that support their best aspirations.

Spirituality

Many of our most fundamental beliefs are founded in religion and spirituality. Religions are organized belief systems, including shared and institutionalized moral values, beliefs about a higher power, and involvement in a faith community (Wright et al., 1996). Religions, through their teachings, rituals, and ceremonies, provide guidelines for the living out of core beliefs and scripted ways to mark major life transitions, as well as congregational support in times of need.

"Spirituality," a broader and more personal overarching construct, can be defined as "that which connects one to all there is" (Griffith & Griffith, 2002). Spirituality involves an active investment in internalized beliefs that bring a sense of meaning, wholeness, and connection with others. It may involve belief in an ultimate human condition or set of values toward which we strive; belief in a supreme power or an inner light; or belief in a holistic oneness with the human community, nature, and the universe. It may also include holy or mystical experiences, which are difficult to explain in ordinary language and imagery. Spirituality invites an expansion of awareness, and with it personal responsibility for and beyond oneself, from local to universal concerns.

Spirituality can be experienced either within or outside formal religious structures. A discontinuity can exist between religious and spiritual domains in a person's life (Walsh, 1999b). Some may adhere to religious rituals and practices and yet not find spiritual meaning in them. Others may disavow formal religion, while finding and expressing spirituality in daily life. Congruence between religious and spiritual beliefs and practices yields a general sense of well-being and wholeness.

Universally, the spirit is seen as our vital essence, the source of life and power. In many languages the word for "spirit" and "breath" are the same: Greek, *pneuma*; Hebrew, *reach*; Latin, *spiritus*; Sanskrit, *prana* (Weil, 1994). In contrast to the emphasis on the individual in many Western cultures, most spiritual orientations in the world see human experience as sociocentric, embedded within the family and larger community. In Chinese culture, for instance, the centrality and continuity of family relations remain very important after death through spiritual connections (McGoldrick et al., 2005). Prayers may be said daily in front of portraits of ancestors in the belief that their spirits can be communicated with directly and, if honored appropriately, will confer their blessings and protect their progeny from harm.

Spiritual beliefs and practices have been found to foster strong family functioning, especially in times of crisis (Beavers & Hampson, 2003; Stinnett & DeFrain, 1985). In Gallup surveys, nearly 75% of Americans report their family relationships have been strengthened by religion in the home (Gallup & Lindsey, 1999).

Suffering invites us into the spiritual domain (Wright et al., 1996). Religion and spirituality offer comfort and meaning beyond comprehension in the face of adversity. Personal faith gives people strength to endure hardships, overcome challenges, or turn their lives around (Werner & Smith, 2001). In the Bible, the book of Job is a story of resilience in which persistent adversity holds meaning beyond comprehension, testing both faith and endurance.

Yet, spiritual distress can impede coping and mastery and may render us unable to invest life with meaning. Religious beliefs may become harmful if they are held too narrowly, rigidly, or punitively. One mother's self-destructive drinking was fueled by the belief, rooted in her childhood Catholic upbringing, that the death of her son was God's punishment for not having baptized him. Although she had not practiced her religion in years, this conviction seized her mind in her tragic loss. She had not shared her belief and guilt with her husband, who was not religious but was raised Jewish and was very close to his family. In other cases, a crisis may precipitate a questioning of long-held spiritual beliefs or it may launch a quest for a new form or dimension of faith that can be sustaining.

Numerous studies of resilience have noted the importance of spiritual faith and involvement in a religious community (e.g., Werner, 1993). In the African American community, religion has been a wellspring for resilience, countering despair (Boyd-Franklin, 2004). The Reverend Martin Luther King, Jr., has been a guiding spirit to many oppressed people through his abiding faith that social justice would prevail. Yet his was not a passive faith to wait for God's deliverance. Rather, his dream became a rallying call to collective action to bring about change, with an emphasis on personal responsibility and initiative.

Surveys find that those who are deeply religious cope better with stress, have fewer alcohol or drug problems, less depression, and lower rates of suicide than those who are not religious (Gallup & Lindsey, 1999). What matters most is drawing on the power of faith to give meaning to a precarious situation and find hope, comfort, and solace.

Medical studies find abundant evidence that faith, prayer, and meditation can actually promote health and healing, reducing stress by strengthening the immune and cardiovascular systems (Dossey, 1993; Kabat-Zinn, 2003; Koenig, McCullough, & Larson, 2001). Brain research finds that meditation activates the region of the brain associated with well-being. With quiet contemplation or memories of being in a favorite place or with a comforting person, chemical activity in the pain area of the brain is drained away to other areas.

Spiritual connectedness and renewal can be found in communion with nature—in mountain vistas, a walk through the woods, a sunset, or the rhythm of waves on the shore. Many are drawn to places with high spiritual energy, such as cathedrals, healing waters, and pilgrimages to sacred shrines and temples. Beauty in many forms can have spiritual, healing effects. We can be inspired by great art, music, literature, or drama that communicates our common humanity. Music offers a powerful transcending experience in many cultures, from African American gospel singing, blues, and jazz to the ecstatic drumming rhythms of Gnawa tribes of the Sahara. As the Hopi Indians say, "To watch us dance is to hear our hearts speak."

For me, music has a deep spiritual resonance as well as a bond with both my mother and my daughter. Throughout my childhood, my mother was a concert pianist, a music teacher, and the organist at our Jewish temple. With an ecumenical command of the great spiritual music, she also served as organist on occasion for various Christian congregations in our town. Whenever she played music, from Chopin to Gershwin, I could see that the weariness and sorrow she carried from the hardships and losses she had suffered in life were released and she was transported to another realm by the music she loved. Music has been that spiritual wellspring for me, as well, especially through times of illness and loss. Although I don't quite share my daughter's taste in hip-hop, I love her passion for music and dance. When stressed out, we both feel inspired and revitalized by music from around the world.

The linchpins of resilience, faith, and intimacy are linked (Higgins, 1994). Faith is inherently relational, from early in life to the end of life, when fundamental convictions about life and death are shaped and nourished within caregiving bonds. Loving relationships with partners, family members, and close friends—our soul mates and kindred spirits— infuse our lives with meaning. Viktor Frankl (1946/1984) recounted how in Nazi prison camps he was sustained by his deep spiritual connection with his wife, visualizing her image: "I didn't even know if she were still alive. I knew only one thing—which I have learned well by now:

Love goes very far beyond the physical person of the beloved. It finds its deepest meaning in the spiritual being, the inner self" (pp. 59–60).

Over past decades, the mental health field considered spirituality not the province of secular or scientific therapies, but rather as a matter best left for clergy to address (Walsh, 1999b). Clinicians shouldn't presume spiritual matters to be unimportant if not voiced. Over 75% of Americans surveyed want to be able to express spiritual concerns to their physicians and other helping professionals (Gallop & Lindsey, 1999). When clients are not asked about their spiritual beliefs and practices, they are likely to edit out the spiritual dimension of their lives. Just as we would inquire about ethnic or cultural belief systems, we need to show comfort and respect in exploring the spiritual aspect of experience. It is useful to draw out multiple stories, deconstructing harmful aspects while encouraging more healing possibilities. For instance, some family members may hold an old childhood image of an all-powerful God as harsh and punitive, often connected to experiences of shame and helplessness. We can invite stories of other spiritual experiences that have been positive, or moments of inner peace, communion, and nurturance that can be drawn upon to meet current challenges.

As we expand our vision of psychotherapy as both a science and a healing art, we approach researcher Martin Seligman's belief that the soul, which is deep within the personality, is the key to change, and that our change efforts must take the human spirit into account. Wright and her colleagues (1996) urge systems-oriented professionals to conceptualize human experience as bio-psycho-social–spiritual. To be most helpful to families, we must acknowledge that suffering, and often the injustice or senselessness of it, are spiritual concerns and that religion and spirituality can be powerful resources for recovery, healing, and resilience.

Inspiration, Innovation, Creativity

The struggle to overcome adversity can bring new vision to one's life. As Eleanor Roosevelt once said, "The future belongs to those who believe in the beauty of their dreams." Creativity is often born of adversity. Our imaginations can transport us beyond our crisis situation and can enable us to envision new possibilities and illuminate pathways out of our dilemmas.

Art and education can empower and transform lives. The film *Born into Brothels* (Kauffman & Briski, 2004) documented the resilience of children and the restorative power of art. A New York–based photographer, living in the brothels of Calcutta to document life there, became interested in the prostitutes' children, who are not recognized by society. She decided to teach them photography, assuming a valuable mentoring role in their lives. As they began to observe and record their world through the lens of the camera, they awakened to their own talents, sense of worth, and future possibilities.

Resilient persons—and communities—often draw something positive out of a tragic situation by finding something to salvage and seeing new possibilities in the midst of the wreckage. We are all enriched when such creativity adds something valuable to culture and society (Csikszentmihalyi, 1996). Through their own creative processes, such writers as Ralph Ellison and Toni Morrison have drawn upon and transformed the brutalizing elements of the African American experience into art. Similarly, jazz and blues powerfully express and transcend the painful life conditions and oppression of that experience.

Families must also be inventive to weather and rebound from adversity. A well-functioning family draws on a wide variety of inspirations to solve its problems, including past experience, family myths and stories, creative fantasy, and new and untried solutions. Bateson (1994) has underscored the need for an attitude of improvisation: "In trying to adapt, we may need to deviate from cherished values, behaving in ways we have barely glimpsed, seizing on fragmentary clues" (p. 8). With life-altering transitions, families often need to envision new models of human interaction.

Role Models and Heroes

We can transcend the constraints of our own particular situations through the positive examples of others who model resilience and inspire our strength and success. Beyond the borders of our everyday world, we can be inspired by the life stories of great men and women of courage and high attainment who have overcome adversity.

Michael Jordan, the basketball giant who was a sports hero to so many youths, embodied many of the best qualities of resilience throughout his career. Not resting on the laurels of his extraordinary talents, he worked out many hours daily—honing his skills, pushing his limits, always striving for excellence, and developing new ways to compensate for injuries and aging. He maintained a tenacious will to win, to persevere even when injured, and to rebound from failure and loss, which he viewed as challenges sparking him to try even harder. Although Jordan was seen as simply innately gifted, his many qualities of resilience were relationally honed in his strong family upbringing (D. Jordan, 1996).

His own heroes were his parents—his nurturing and spiritually devout mother, who instilled strong values, and his father, who was his mainstay and closest companion. In a life that seemed charmed, however, even Michael Jordan was not spared tragedy when his father was brutally murdered. In shock and grief, he left basketball, losing passion for the sport with the loss of his father. After turning to baseball (an earlier life connection with his father), he returned to basketball to lead a remarkable team in winning a fourth NBA title for the Chicago Bulls—on Father's Day. Hugging the trophy, he wept openly and dedicated the victory to the memory of his father.

Great literature opens up the world, enabling us to envision possibilities beyond our immediate circumstances and inspiring us to reach for them. Henry David Thoreau's famous essay on civil disobedience—speaking out against slavery and advocating for the weakest in society—was a source of inspiration to both Martin Luther King, Jr., and Mahatma Gandhi in their leadership of peaceful protests against injustices.

Parents can open windows to many realms and possibilities by reading together with their children from infancy. I grew up in a poor, working-class neighborhood, where most of my peers married and got factory jobs after high school. My own world and aspirations were enlarged through stories and reading. Some were constraining: such classic fables as "Cinderella" and "Snow White" were stifling in their gendered expectations that if I was sweet, compliant, and uncomplaining, I would be rescued by a prince and live happily ever after. Fortunately, in reading the life stories of Jane Addams, who founded Hull House, and the scientist Marie Curie, I could imagine possibilities for my own life dreams beyond the limitations of my immediate surroundings. Although I didn't consciously plan to follow those particular pathways, curiously enough, I later found myself drawn to social change and research. The book I remember most vividly from early childhood was *The Little Engine That Could*, which is a wonderful story of resilience. When tempted to think of my own resilience as self-made, I need only remember that it was my parents who read that story to me at so many bedtimes.

With the complexities and ambiguities of life today, families need a variety of models to inspire a wide range of strategies for meeting life challenges. Yet, in seeking models, we often fail to see the many examples of heroism in our own families and communities. We attribute neglect to single mothers working out of the home when we need to appreciate the heroic feat of an undersupported parent who must juggle job, parenting, and household demands. Stories of uncommon courage and triumph over tragic events are valuable, but so too are stories of the remarkable strengths and vitality of ordinary families in weathering the storms of life. In *Hope Dies Last*, Studs Terkel (2004) documents the courage and comebacks everyday people make every day—the heroic feats that don't get media fanfare. For helping professionals, seeing the ways ordinary families draw on the capacity for resilience can inspire us to see and affirm the unrecognized strengths in every family we work with.

Transformation: Learning, Change, and Growth from Adversity

Resilience is promoted when hardship, tragedy, failure, or disappointment can also be seen as instructive and can serve as an impetus for change and growth. Resilient persons believe that it's a waste of time and energy to be preoccupied with regret or bound up in retribution or nursing old wounds. Instead, they survey their experience and attempt to draw lessons from it that can be valuable in guiding their future course. In accepting what has happened and any persisting scars, they try to incorporate what they have learned into attempts to live better lives, and strive so that others can gain from their experience. A prominent African American judge, the son of a sharecropper, told how he transcended early life trauma: "I've learned to use the hardships that I endured from that time to become my source of strength. I converted the energy and, to some extent, the anger that the system caused within me, into motivation." He dedicated his life to a career in justice based on fairness and what he believed to be right.

   In such ways, families, too, forge new meaning and growth out of the cauldron of adversity. Learning from adversity, resilient families believe that their trials have made them more than what they might have been otherwise. One couple nearly lost a son in a freak accident that shook the very foundation of the family. They share the belief that this crisis was like an epiphany, crystallizing a deeper appreciation of their family bonds, a stronger sense of purpose in life, and a dedication to practice their values more fully. In the uncertainty and pain wrought by a life crisis, core beliefs come to the fore. As events are assimilated, they may come to be seen as a gift that opens a new phase of life or new opportunities.

   The paradox of resilience is that the worst of times can also bring out our best. A crisis can yield transformation and growth in unforeseen directions. It can awaken family members to the importance of loved ones or jolt them into healing old wounds and reordering priorities for more meaningful relationships and life pursuits. Resilient individuals and families commonly emerge from shattering crises with a heightened moral compass and sense of purpose in their lives, gaining compassion for the plight of others. The experience of adversity and suffering may spark community action on behalf of others, as in Mothers Against Drunk Driving, formed by parents so that other families could be spared the tragedy they had experienced. Many express their spirituality through working passionately for social justice (Perry & Rolland, 1999).

It's most important for families in problem-saturated situations to envision a better future through their efforts, and for those whose hopes and dreams have been shattered to imagine new possibilities, seizing opportunities for invention, transformation, and growth. We might best view resilience as the ability to do the best of things in the worst of times, seizing every opportunity.

TREATMENT AND HEALING PARADIGMS

For helping professionals, our understanding of healing is important in fostering resilience. Distinct from curing or problem resolution, healing is a natural process in response to injury or trauma. Sometimes people heal physically but don't heal emotionally or spiritually; wounded relationships may remain unhealed. Some may survive an illness, trauma, or loss but may not regain the spirit to live and love fully. Yet we are able to heal psychosocially and spiritually even when we do not heal physically, or when a traumatic event cannot be changed. Similarly, resilience can be fostered even when problems cannot be solved or when they may recur. The literal meaning of healing is becoming whole—and, when necessary, adapting and compensating for losses of structure or function.

Treatment and healing are quite different concepts. Treatment is externally administered; healing comes from within the person, the family, and the community. In the West, scientific medicine has focused on identifying external agents of disease and developing technological weapons against them. Metaphors of war are prominent: "fighting" and "combating" illness; developing "aggressive" treatments to "destroy" disease. The "battle against" each new disease requires a new "weapon." An unbalanced focus on disease rather than health, and many patients' skewed clinical experience with serious and chronic illness, all contribute to fear and pessimism (Weil, 1994). Even the word "remission" refers to a temporary abatement of disease processes that may recur.

In contrast, Eastern medicine is based on a different philosophy—
a set of beliefs about healing processes and the importance of mind–
body interactions (Kabat-Zinn, 2003). The healing system is a functional system, not an assemblage of structures. Chinese medicine, for
example, explores ways to increase internal resilience as resistance to
disease, so that whatever harmful influences people are exposed to,
they can remain healthy. This belief in strengthening protective processes assumes that the body has a natural ability to heal and grow
stronger. Mechanisms of diagnosis, self-repair, and regeneration exist
in all of us and can be activated as the need arises. Knowledge about
the healing system enables practitioners to enhance those processes at
every level of biological, social, and health care organization, as the
best hope for recovery and wellbeing. Interventions to promote these
healing mechanisms are more effective than those that simply treat or
suppress symptoms.

In the field of family therapy, the treatment paradigms of medical
and psychoanalytic models influenced early formulations of family pathology and strategies to reduce it. The more recent shift to strength-
based approaches is based on the recognition and activation of a family's
own healing resources. Healing approaches to practice put faith in our
clients' potential to reduce their vulnerability and increase their resilience. If we believe in and encourage this potential, chances are greater
for success. Resilience-oriented practice approaches inspire people to believe in their own possibilities for regeneration to facilitate healing and
healthy growth. Therapeutic work best fosters healing when it is collaborative, activating a family's own resources. Interventions draw on kin
and social networks to become a healing environment for the relief of
suffering and renewal of life passage. This approach helps family members to shift from helplessness and despair to believe in their potential to
make things better.

We must be cautious, however, not to attribute inability to overcome the odds or recover from illness or adversity to insufficient positive
beliefs, willpower, or spiritual purity. In middle age, Helen Keller (1929/
1968) wrote:

> I had once believed that we were all masters of our fates—that we could
> mold our lives into any form we pleased. . . . I had overcome deafness
> and blindness and I supposed that anyone could come out victorious if
> he threw himself valiantly into life's struggle. But as I went more and
> more about the country . . . I learned that the power to rise in the world
> is not within the reach of everyone.

Our conviction in the potential for human resilience must be joined with compassion for those who have not been able to overcome their challenges. In addition, as helping professionals encourage families to alter constraining beliefs and overcome the odds against them, we must also strive to change the odds against them. For sustained commitment and success, an empowering belief system must be validated by experience and reinforced by larger social structures. Therefore, we must work with larger systems to transform policies and practices to better enable families to bring their dreams to fruition. Families want to be healthy; as practitioners, we can encourage their best efforts through genuine faith in each family's potential for healing and resilience.

CHAPTER 4

Organizational Patterns
Family Shock Absorbers

The road to success is always under construction.
—ANONYMOUS

Families, with varied forms and relationship networks, need to provide structure to support the integration and adaptation of the family unit and its members (Watzlawick, Beavin, & Jackson, 1967; Minuchin, 1974). Family organizational patterns are maintained by external and internal norms, influenced by cultural and family belief systems. Patterns are also based on mutual expectations in particular families and persist out of habit, mutual accommodation, or functional effectiveness. To deal effectively with crises or persistent adversity, families must mobilize and organize their resources, buffer stresses, and reorganize to fit changing conditions. This chapter identifies the organizational elements in effective family functioning, highlighting key processes for relational resilience: flexibility, connectedness, and social and economic resources (see Table 4.1).

FLEXIBILITY

Families need to develop a flexible structure for optimal functioning in the face of adversity. Families, like all human systems, tend to resist

83

TABLE 4.1. Structural/Organizational Patterns: Crisis Shock Absorbers

Flexibility

- Adaptive change: "bouncing forward"
  - Rebounding, reorganizing, adapting to fit new challenges
- Stability through disruption:
  - Continuity, dependability, rituals, routines
- Strong authoritative leadership: nurturing, guiding, and protecting children and vulnerable family members
  - Varied family forms: cooperative parenting/caregiving teams within/across households
  - Couple relationship: equal partners; mutual respect

Connectedness

- Mutual support, collaboration, and commitment
- Respecting individual needs, differences, and boundaries
- Seeking reconnection, reconciliation of wounded relationships
  - Forgiving and remembering

Social and economic resources

- Mobilizing extended kin, social, community support networks
- Recruiting mentoring relationships
- Building financial security; balancing work–family strains
- Larger systems: institutional/structural supports

---

change beyond a certain familiar or acceptable range. Yet, change is an inevitable part of the human condition. Families must be able to adapt to changing developmental and environmental demands—both normative (expectable, predictable) and nonnormative (uncommon, untimely, or unexpected). A dynamic balance between stability ("homeostasis") and change ("morphogenesis") enables a stable family structure while also allowing for change in response to life challenges (Olson & Gorall, 2003; Beavers & Hampson, 2003).

Bouncing Forward: Capacity for Adaptive Change

Leading family therapists and researchers have found that the capacity to change is essential for high functioning in couples and families, especially under stress. As Virginia Satir (1988) observed in healthy families, the rules for members are flexible, appropriate, and alterable. Similarly, studies find that the capacity for adaptability, flexibility, and change predict the long-term success of a couple relationship (Holtzworth-Monroe & Jacobson, 1991). Partners must be able to evolve together and cope with the multitude of internal challenges and external forces in their lives. When people a hold rigid conception of marriage as an institution with unchanging rules and roles, they are more wary of long-term commitment. As the fabled Hollywood film star Mae West once put it, "It's not that I'm opposed to the institution of marriage; I'm just not ready for an institution." Instead, couples and families do best when they construct relationships with a flexible structure that they can mold and reshape to fit their needs and challenges over time.

Resilience is commonly thought of as "bouncing back," like a spring, to our precrisis shape or norm. A more apt metaphor for resilience might be "bouncing forward," rebounding and reorganizing adaptively to fit new challenges or changed conditions. A serious crisis can be so disruptive that there's no going back. For instance, with a major loss—a job, a home, or a life partner—we must forge a new pathway. When events of great magnitude occur, such as a natural disaster like a hurricane, we may not be able to return to "normal" life as we knew it. In rebuilding our lives, we must construct new patterns and recalibrate "normal" settings to meet unanticipated challenges. With major catastrophic events, we may have to question old assumptions and grapple with a fundamentally altered conception of ourselves in relation to others in our shared world (see Chapter 11).

Stability through Disruption

When families are overwhelmed by a crisis or a pileup of stressors, members yearn for calm and order. In times of upheaval, families commonly lose structure, daily routines fall by the wayside, and established patterns become disorganized. We can foster resilience by helping members regain stability and restore predictable, consistent rules, roles, and patterns of interaction. Members need to know what is expected of them and what they can expect of each other. Reliability is crucial: family members need assurance that they can depend on one another to follow through with commitments they've made.

Rituals and routines maintain a sense of continuity over time, linking past, present, and future through shared traditions and expectations (Imber-Black et al., 2003). Routines of daily life, such as family dinner or bedtime stories, provide regular contact and order in a hectic family schedule. In family assessment, we can learn about structure by asking what a typical day and week are like, and how family life has changed with a crisis or transition experienced by the family. Some families become too overloaded and fragmented even to have dinner together; parents may work on different shifts, with precious little time together at home. Seemingly small routines can make a big difference. Often children with school or behavior problems have no set bedtime, or it is a nightly hassle, with overtired children becoming more wound up and exhausted parents' tempers likely to flare. Setting a reasonable bedtime is assisted by a nightly routine with pleasurable contact, such as reading, a bedside chat, and "tucking in." Enlisting older children to assist with younger ones builds their competencies as it allows adults much-needed quiet time for respite.

In times of crisis and major transitions, disruption in family structure and daily routines compounds upset and confusion, especially for children. In one family, when a single parent's illness required several hospitalizations, extended family members took turns moving in to stay with the children, enabling them to sleep in their own beds, have their belongings at hand, and keep up daily routines and friendships, rather than experience further dislocation by moving to stay with various relatives. When family life is reorganized, as with divorce, it is important for families to create new routines that provide continuity of significant bonds, such as Sunday brunch at Dad's house. After a divorce, the predictability and reliability of contact with a nonresidential parent are very important for children's adjustment (Hetherington & Kelly, 2002). Children are more likely to feel abandoned or uncared for when a parent drops in and out of their lives without clear expectations about the next visit, or when promises to call are vague and plans repeatedly fall through.

Strong Leadership: Nurturance, Guidance, and Protection

Parents (and their elders) are the architects of a family, laying the foundation for healthy family life in the structural arrangements, roles, and rules they construct. Strong leadership is crucial for nurturance, protection, and guidance of children, as well as caring for elders and family members with special needs. Leadership is also needed to provide basic resources (e.g., money, food, clothing, health care, and shelter) and to manage the many pressures and demands of everyday life (Epstein et al., 2003).

In well-functioning families, leadership is strong and clear; adults in charge do not abdicate their authority or responsibilities. At the same time, they are careful not to abuse their relative power over children. Children's choices and responsibilities increase with developing maturity. Frustrating, self-defeating power struggles occur infrequently.

Moderately structured relationships have somewhat democratic leadership, with some negotiations including the children. Roles are stable, with some role sharing. Rules are firmly enforced with few changes. Moderately flexible relationships have more egalitarian leadership, with a democratic approach to decision making. Negotiations are open and actively include the children. Roles may be shared, and change is fluid when necessary. Rules are age-appropriate and can be modified over time (Olson & Gurell, 2003).

In contrast, families at dysfunctional extremes tend to be either overly rigid or chaotic, with too much or too little structure. At the chaotic extreme, disorganization prevails. Leadership is limited or erratic, with roles unclear and shifting. Decisions tend to be impulsive and not well considered. Parents vacillate between overindulgence and neglect. Family members have difficulty following through with plans and promises. This sets up repeated disappointments in expectations. Similarly, limit setting and discipline may swing between extremes of laxness and overly harsh crackdown. In rigid systems, one person tends to dominate through autocratic, highly controlling leadership. Most decisions are imposed, with limited negotiations. Roles are narrowly defined, and rules are inflexible. Under stress, families low in structure tend to become more chaotic and out of control, whereas rigid systems tend to become even more inflexible and their behavioral repertoire still more tightly constricted. As Satir (1988) observed, when families are rigid, rules become nonnegotiable and everlasting.

Families are critical social learning contexts, created and responded to by all members. They function best when the exchange of benefits is far more frequent than punishments or mutual coercion (Patterson, 1983; Sexton & Alexander, 2003). Parents encourage children's success and reward adaptive behavior through attention, acknowledgment, and approval. They try not to reinforce maladaptive behavior. In less functional families, parents use more coercion and focus on misbehavior, failure, control, and punishment. Positive efforts and successes go unnoticed and unrewarded. Therapists can serve as models, helping families to affirm the positive behaviors and to encourage interests and talents. We can help distressed families find opportunities for rewarding exchanges that enhance the relationship along with individual competence and self-esteem.

Families need effective methods of control to keep behavior within bounds and neither dangerous nor destructive. It's important to assess the rules and standards a family sets and the latitude allowed. Authoritative yet flexible behavior control has been found to be the most effective style (Olson & Gorell, 2003; Steinberg, Lamborn, Dornbusch, & Darling, 1992). Standards are reasonable, with opportunity for negotiation and change. Parents/caregivers are in accord when setting and enforcing rules. They are clear about what behavior is unacceptable, and intervene consistently when infractions occur. They make allowances when a situation calls for it, yet still maintain consistent expectations.

Less functional is rigid behavior control, with narrow standards and minimal negotiation or variation across situations, or laissez-faire behavior control, with few standards and total latitude allowed. Most dysfunctional is chaotic structure, out of control with unpredictable and random shifts. Parents may swing from one extreme to the other, letting children run wild without rules or limits and then suddenly becoming rigid, overly harsh, and punitive. Children then don't know what standards apply in any situation or how much leeway is possible.

In highly disruptive crisis situations, very strong leadership is essential to maintain or restore order and direction in the midst of chaos or overwhelming stress. More authoritarian leadership is needed in families where community structures have broken down. Above all, caring discipline with firmness *and* warmth is most effective.

The resilience literature underscores the vital importance of mentoring: guiding and inspiring children in positive directions. In the clinical field's focus on behavior control, we've given insufficient attention to the ways that parents, older siblings, extended family members, and community elders can all play a part in providing values, motivation, and active mentoring to children. Unlike lecturing youth about what they should and shouldn't do, a mentoring relationship makes active investment in each child's interests and talents and nourishes hopes and dreams. This positive involvement is especially important in the resilience of high-risk adolescents (Ungar, 2004a, 2004b). This neglected dimension in clinical practice can be usefully approached by identifying and encouraging mentoring opportunities within the family network, supplemented by community resources.

Varied Family Forms: Cooperative Teams

In today's diverse family forms, leadership is increasingly varied, from an intact two-parent family to single-parent and binuclear households, stepfamilies, and extended kinship care. Families function best and children thrive when parents and other involved kin work collaboratively, with mutual respect and accommodation within and across households. Clarity and consistency in expectations and consequences for children are crucial. Parenting arrangements that involve a grandparent or span separate households can function well as long as lines of authority and responsibility are clearly drawn and maintain mutual respect. With divorce and remarriage, children and their families do best when the adults are able to form cooperative parenting teams across households, involving both biological parents and stepparents (Ahrons, 2004). Rather than fight over custody, parents can be encouraged to focus on how they can make the most workable parenting plan. Families may need help for former spouses to put aside past grievances and for both old and new partners to overcome feelings of rivalry in order to work together for the sake of the children (see Chapter 12).

Couple Relationships: Equal Partners

Couple relationships function best when each partner supports the better characteristics and creative aspects of the other in a mutual, equitable way. Family process research has shown the importance of role flexibility and balance to promote adult growth and development for both partners, with rigid, skewed relationships contributing to distress and divorce. Children are also affected by how parents treat each other, not only how each parent relates to the child.

Gender, like generation, is a basic structural axis in families (Goldner, 1988), differentiating husband and wife, father and mother, son and daughter. Issues concerning gendered roles and relations concern two distinct yet overlapping aspects of the traditional (and persisting) gender gap: assumptions of innate *differences* between men and women, and the *differential* in their power and privilege. Although some differences arise from biologically influenced predispositions, research finds broad overlap in individual traits, abilities, and preferences that have been culturally defined as "masculine" or "feminine" (McGoldrick et al., 1989). Most gender differences in family role expectations, relational styles, and constraints are shaped and reinforced by cultural norms through socialization from early childhood on.

As we've seen in Chapter 2, in the traditional gender role split, women (as wives, mothers, daughters, and daughters-in-law) have been held responsible for the well-being of all family members and expected to tend to the needs of their spouse, children, and elders. Men, defined by job success, have been expected to be breadwinners and instrumental problem solvers, and have been constrained from intimate involvement in family life. This gender gap is being bridged as women and men increasingly challenge gender-linked role constraints and seek more equitable partnership in couple and family relationships. Studies have found that optimally functioning couples and families show less gender stereo-typing, both in couple relationships and in child rearing (Beavers & Hampson, 2003; Haddock et al., 2003).

In clinical practice, we can invite families to deconstruct the subtle yet powerful cultural messages and constraining stereotypes that are played out in actual family life (Silverman & Goodrich, 2003). We can explore preferential treatment of sons over daughters. We can question constraining assumptions such as: "Housework is women's work," "Women are naturally more nurturant," "Men are better with money," or "It's not manly to cry." Labeling *human* qualities as either "mascu-line" or "feminine" casts them as "proper" and "natural" for only one sex. We are all capable of a wide range of human functioning, and our resilience as individuals, couples, and families is strengthened as we de-velop our full potential.

The balance of power is also a fundamental issue in couple relation-ships. Equal sharing of power has been found to contribute to relation-ship success, intimacy, stability, and satisfaction for married men and women, and for gay and lesbian couples (Gottman & Silver, 1999; Kurdek, 2002). In high-functioning families, partners are able to work out strong egalitarian leadership and authority (Beavers & Hampson, 2003). Power is experienced through close, loving bonds, not through coercion. Control is expressed through self-control rather than control over others. Midrange and more dysfunctional families show more skewed power differentials, and wives, typically in a "one-down" posi-tion, are more likely to report being overburdened and depressed. The greater the power imbalance—in both gay and straight relationships—the more unsatisfying is the relationship and the greater is the risk for conflict and dissolution.

In well-functioning families, both partners' contributions are equally valued and neither carries disproportionate burden or privilege. Couples are more prone to power imbalances in traditional family structures, given the different status of paid work versus unpaid housework and child care. Dual-earner couples, today's norm, with more symmetrical relationships, face different challenges (Risman, 1999; Schwartz, 1994). Family and work life, to a large extent, remain organized around gendered structural patterns, which operate on "automatic pilot." Most men are more involved than their fathers were on the home front but still carry far less household responsibility than their wives. When both partners hold jobs and share child care and housework, a division of la-bor needs to be worked out for their particular situation, with demands, skills, preferences, and fairness taken into account. Bombarded by multiple, conflicting job and family pressures and by changes in role expectations, dual earners need to establish a very clear structure and yet to be highly flexible to shift gears and cover for each other as needs arise.

When couples have difficulties related to skews in power and privilege, therapists can encourage partners to explore these dilemmas. We can notice gendered role assumptions and bring biases or disproportionate burdens into greater awareness for discussion and change. For instance, we might ask: "Since both of you work full-time, how was it decided that one of you would do all the housework?" It can be an eye-opener to review the management of a typical week in family life. For instance, we can actively encourage fathers to become more directly involved and build competencies in child care, elder care, and housework, as well as in the coordination of home/family demands. Tasks and directives can be useful—for instance, asking a father take to charge of all housework and parenting responsibilities for a week without help (or criticism) from the mother.

Reciprocity is essential for a fair and equal partnership. A good relationship requires continuous balancing in terms of partners' priorities and responsiveness so that each carries a fair share of responsibilities and enjoys equal privileges. This give-and-take is based on trustworthiness and follow-through—mutual assurance that each member's needs will be honored and that the exchange will balance out over time. We can help partners negotiate to rebalance power and entitlement, to share burdens more equitably, and to appreciate each other's contributions (Knudson-Martin & Mahoney, 2005).

Family therapists have become aware that a therapeutic stance of neutrality tacitly reinforces cultural biases and ignores harmful power skews in families and society. Ethically, we must foster equal respect and challenge beliefs and practices—in families and larger systems—that perpetuate abuses of power, particularly in demeaning treatment and in violence or sexual assault. Change is also needed in societal, institutional, and workplace structures for equal opportunities, status, and pay and for more flexible work and child care arrangements. Relational resilience is strengthened when men and women can share fully and equally in the responsibilities and joys of family and work life.

Navigating Stressful Life Challenges: Counterbalancing Stability and Change

Family resilience requires the ability to counterbalance stability and change as family members deal with adversity. Skiing provides a useful metaphor to visualize the dynamic balance needed to navigate life challenges. Going down the mountainside, good skiers maintain stability while shifting position fluidly to meet the changing demands of the terrain. When a skier stiffens up out of fear of losing control, the rigid stance heightens risks of falling and of serious injury.

My personal experience with skiing held valuable lessons for my practice as a therapist. As a novice, with a catastrophic fear of speeding out of control and tumbling all the way to the bottom of the mountain, I once sat down at the top of a slope and refused to budge from terra firma. Lessons with a pro not only enabled me to overcome my fear and enjoy skiing, but furnished useful clinical insights. A good ski instructor first teaches novices how to stop (control over runaway processes) and how to fall and minimize injury. Next, skiers learn how to sustain that dynamic balance of steadiness and flexibility, which requires repeated adjustments, shifting positions while moving forward through changing conditions. Although my internal cues signaling fear (e.g., pounding heart) protested that I wasn't ready, my instructor calmly yet firmly encouraged me to try short runs on a gentle slope (behavior change preceding and facilitating internal change). He provided a secure mentoring relationship by demonstrating skills and going just ahead of me, assuring me that he would catch me (quite literally a "holding environment") if I went too fast and lost control. Each small success, along with his praise, increased my competence and confidence.

Applying this analogy to work with families helps me understand much of what is commonly labeled as "resistance" to change and how to work with it. Change is frightening largely because family members fear losing control of their lives in a runaway process that might leave them even worse off than in their present predicament. Fear of the unknown can outweigh current distress, which is painful yet familiar. Those who have been in crisis and have experienced a terrifying and overwhelming state of chaos quite understandably hold catastrophic expectations about change; they may feel an acute sense of helplessness as they fear that their lives will spiral out of control yet again. This apprehension is especially intense in the aftermath of major traumatic events (see Chapter 11) and for multistressed families (see Chapter 10). Therapy may seem particularly threatening, because its objective and methods promote change. Therapists, indeed, are often thought of as change agents.

Helping professionals need to respect clients' hesitation to engage in a change process when they are already in crisis or a precarious situation, or when they are struggling with an overwhelming pileup of stressors. We need to better appreciate their yearnings for less change and

more stability, and strive to achieve a flexible balance. Like the ski instructor, we can encourage a collaborative process in which we actively
structure the therapy and contribute our expertise and support, yet help
clients to feel in control of the therapy process and more in charge of
their lives. An initial priority is to help them learn how to prevent runaway change by building skills and confidence in small, manageable in-
crements. We can also help them maintain continuities and build new
structures as they undergo disruptive transitions and must reorganize
(e.g., after the loss of a parent). In exploring what clients need and
value—what family members *don't* want to change or lose—we can then
help them find ways to conserve those elements, or to transform or
replace them. For instance, with separations, children lose their intact
family structure but parents can be helped to establish new role relations, routines, and rituals that preserve parent–child connectedness
(Ahrons, 2004). Tasks and directives are valuable in building new skills
and confidence, as well as in learning how to fail (fall) safely, try again,
and succeed.

These insights have particular relevance for helping families withstand and rebound from crisis. Families in crisis experience an immediate period of rapid disorganization, which is disorienting and chaotic. A
fear of runaway change and a sense of being out of control are common
at such times. It can be reassuring to normalize this experience, to slow
down change processes, and to provide strong structure to contain reactions and support the ability to tolerate uncertainty as families gradually
attain a new, more functional equilibrium.

Crisis events often require a family to reorganize. With a major disruption or turning point in the family life cycle, such as stepfamily formation, a basic shift of rules and roles (second-order change) may be
needed. Significant losses stress the family even further and require major adaptational shifts of family rules to ensure both the transformation
and continuity of family life.

Rituals are valuable in marking important events and promoting
both continuity and change. Celebrations of holidays, birthdays, rites of
passage, weddings, anniversaries, and funeral rites are important in all
cultures, although they have varied forms and symbolic meanings
(Imber-Black et al., 2003). Whether secular or sacred, rituals and ceremonies offer both transcendence and connection. They assist in facilitating life transitions as they strengthen family and community ties. Wedding rituals are as important in remarriage as in a first marriage,
signifying the formation of a new family unit. Involving children from
previous marriages in the joyous occasion fosters the process of integra-

tion. Ceremonies celebrating commitment vows are especially important for gay and lesbian couples who are denied legal or religious sanction of their union. For partners who wish to repair a rupture in their relationship, the renewal of vows can serve as a healing recommitment (see Chapter 12).

CONNECTEDNESS

A second core element of family organization involves *connectedness*, or *cohesion*, the emotional and structural bonding among family members. Olson has assessed cohesion in terms of structural variables such as boundaries and coalitions; time and space together or apart; and involvement with friends and interests (Olson & Gorrell, 2003). Similarly, Beavers and Hampson (1990, 2003) find that families with a highly connected (centripetal) style orient their lives inward. Members seek satisfaction and connection primarily within the family. In more disengaged (centrifugal) families, members turn more outside the family for satisfaction and often leave home early. Families tend to do best when they balance closeness, mutual support, and commitment with tolerance for separateness and individual needs and differences.

Mutual Support and Commitment; Respect for Differences

In surmounting adversity, family members need to be able to turn to one another and at the same time have own efforts, sense of competence, and self-worth valued. A well-functioning family provides what attachment theorists describe as a "holding environment" for its members: a context of security, trust, and nurturance to support individual development (Bowlby, 1988; Byng-Hall, 1995b). Family members take an active interest in what is important to each other, even when interests vary, and can respond empathically to others' distress.

In times of crisis, families function best when members rally together and know they can count on each other. Pulling together is one of the most important processes in weathering crises (Stinnett & DeFrain, 1985). Every member—even a small child, a disabled parent, or a frail grandparent—can have a part to play in easing family burdens or providing comfort, and each is helped by being included in some way. In assigning tasks or solving problems in family therapy, it's important to help the family find ways for every member to participate actively. The comfort and security provided by warm, caring relationships is especially critical in withstanding catastrophic events, such as natural disasters (see Chapter 11). In adoption and foster care, there is increasing recognition of the value of kinship care and placement of siblings together (Minuchin, Colapinto, & Minuchin, 1998) (see Chapter 10).

At times of crisis, intense upset can precipitate conflict and cutoffs. Alliances and splits may fluctuate erratically or rigidify. In one case, two adult sisters, distraught over their mother's death, fought over her jewelry. They refused to speak to each other for many years, although they continued to live next door to each other.

Well-functioning families enable individuals to be both differentiated and connected. In highly connected families, emotional closeness and loyalty are strong. Time spent together is highly valued, and many interests, activities, and friends are shared. However, mutuality is best achieved when individuals possess a clear sense of themselves. In less connected yet supportive families, there may be considerable emotional separateness and time spent apart; yet members still share some time together, make some joint decisions, and support one another.

Although cultural norms and family organizational styles vary considerably, extreme patterns of *enmeshment* and *disengagement* tend to be dysfunctional, especially under stress. In enmeshed families, diffuse boundaries, blurred differentiation, and strong pressure for togetherness block autonomy and competence. Individual differences, privacy, or independence are seen as threats to group survival and are sacrificed for the sake of unity and loyalty. Pressures for consensus can interfere with communication and problem solving. Enmeshed families may have a large network proffering support; however, in crisis they can readily become overloaded and overreactive and have difficulty managing stress. In disengaged families, distance or rigid boundaries leave family members emotionally cut off, lacking caring or commitment. With little involvement or synergy in the family, the whole becomes less than the sum of its parts. Members drift off—or are cast off—on their own, unable to turn to each other for the mutual support and problem solving that are so necessary in times of crisis. Instead, individuals are isolated and left to fend for themselves, as depicted in a cartoon captioned "The Dysfunctional Family Robinson": family members are each huddled alone on separate small islands.

Also, for resilience as families and their members move through the life cycle, they need to alter their functional balance of connectedness and separateness to meet changing developmental needs (Carter & McGoldrick, 2003; Olson & Gorell, 2003). For instance, with the birth of the first child, a couple must reorganize from dyad to triad, assuming new parental roles and responsibilities as nurturance and protection of the newborn become primary concerns (Cowen & Cowen, 2003). Adolescent children and their parents must renegotiate patterns of connectedness, allowing for increasing separateness and autonomy. When the children are launched, parents refocus to personal or couple priorities and reorganize the household. When aging elders—or any family members—become ill or disabled, families need to shift attention and resources to provide needed caregiving.

A family's *style* should not be equated with its *level* of functioning. Family and cultural norms vary widely in preferences for closeness and separateness. In ethnic groups that value solidarity and community, families expect individual needs to be deferred to the common good. They live by the motto "All for one and one for all."

In clinical practice, the terms "enmeshment" and "disengagement" have tended to be overused, erroneously pathologizing patterns of high connectedness or separateness that may be normal (typical) and functional in different contexts (Green & Werner, 1996). In most cases, "high cohesion" or "strong connection" would be preferable descriptions. In many ethnic groups, such as Middle Eastern families, respectful deference to elders and high concern and involvement in one another's lives may mistakenly be labeled as "enmeshment." In traditional Latino families, adult children are expected to sideline their own pursuits to care for parents with serious illness, even if it means leaving jobs or relocating their own families (Falicov, 1999). The emphasis on independence and self-reliance in the dominant U.S. culture can lead to faulty assumptions of dysfunction and inappropriate therapeutic goals. Most other cultures are more sociocentric, valuing mutual dependency and placing family and community commitments above individual preferences.

Another error is to presume that a family is pathologically enmeshed when high cohesion may be functional and even necessary, to pull together to deal with a crisis or pileup of stressors. High cohesion in lesbian couples has mistakenly been labeled as fusion (Laird, 2003), when it may be mutually satisfying and functional in dealing with a homophobic social context.

Family Boundaries, Subsystems, and Individual Differences

Connectedness can be assessed more specifically in terms of proximity and hierarchy (Wood, 1985). Family boundaries—rules defining who participates how—function to clarify and reinforce roles and to protect the differentiation of the system (Minuchin, 1974). Boundaries must be firm, yet also be flexible enough for both autonomy and interdependence for the psychosocial growth of members, for maintaining the family unit, and for restructuring in response to stress. The *clarity* of boundaries and subsystems, particularly between adult caregivers and children, is especially important. Ambiguity in boundaries, roles, and membership can complicate adaptation, as in families with a missing loved one, or those dealing with the progressive cognitive losses of a member with Alzheimer's disease (Boss, 1999).

Interpersonal boundaries define and separate family members, promoting individual identity and autonomous functioning. High-functioning families strive to maintain clear boundaries, for instance, respecting a teenager's privacy. Members take responsibility for their own thoughts, feelings, and actions. They respect the unique qualities and subjective views of others. The ability to tolerate and encourage separateness, differences, and autonomy can also foster high intimacy (Whitaker & Keith, 1981). Autonomy should not be confused with low cohesion or disengagement (Beavers & Hampson, 1993), in which family members avoid contact or distance emotionally in an insecure, pseudoindependent stance.

In enmeshed families, boundaries become blurred and confused, with members intruding into other's personal space and privacy. Parents may have difficulty in differentiating a child from themselves (Bowen, 1978). As one father explained why he hits his son, "When I look at him, I see me; he's got all my bad habits, and I try to knock 'em out of him." A parent may be inappropriately overinvolved: One anorectic college student couldn't buy clothes unless Daddy took her shopping and had her try them on for his approval.

Contrary to the myth of disconnection from families at adulthood, most families maintain strong, *inter*dependent intergenerational relationships throughout life. Although most adult children and their parents prefer to live in separate households, they value proximity and contact—a pattern that has been aptly termed "intimacy at a distance" (Walsh, 1999a). Family therapists and relational scholars (e.g., Jordan, Kaplan, Miller, Stiver, & Surrey, 1991) affirm the value of connectedness across the life course for well-rounded human functioning and the ability to form and sustain collaborative and intimate relationships.

Generational boundaries maintain hierarchical organization in families. Boundaries are established by parents or kin caregivers to reinforce leadership and authority, and to differentiate rights and obligations.

They also protect a couple's relationship from intrusion by children or extended family. Three or even four generations may be actively involved in family functioning. Intergenerational tensions can arise around authority issues. A variety of arrangements can be workable if the social organization and generational hierarchy are clear and consistent. In a two-parent family, a strong parental alliance with clear generational boundaries is important. Yet cultural preferences vary and should be explored in each case. For instance, in Latino families, the parent–child bond may take precedence over the couple relationship as the dominant dyad (Falicov, 1998).

In early family systems theory, parentification of a child was assumed to be dysfunctional. However, in underresourced single-parent or large families, especially in troubled times, it may be necessary and functional for older children to take considerable responsibility to assist with housekeeping, child care, and financial demands. When a parent is absent or has a disabling illness, a child may be thrust into premature responsibilities, such as a caregiving role or a job to help out. Such role assignment is best delegated with children assisting adults, who remain in charge. These responsibilities can foster early competence and are not necessarily harmful, as long as the burden is not excessive and other family members share tasks to the best of their ability. Boundary blurring becomes dysfunctional if adults abdicate leadership. It is most harmful if a child is exploited, emotionally embroiled in adult conflicts, or sexually abused (Scheinberg & Fraenkel, 2001).

Collaboration: Good Teamwork

In well-functioning families, members form multiple and varied alliances around shared interests, concerns, and responsibilities. They avoid triangulation (Bowen, 1978; Minuchin, 1974), when two members (often a couple) draw in a third (typically a child) to deflect tension between them. This is problematic in hostile divorces when a child is drawn in as a go-between for warring parents, or tugged back and forth in loyalty or power struggles. Distress increases when members become embedded in multiple triangles, for instance in stepfamily conflicts.

For resilience under stress, flexible alliances and teamwork are essential. Well-functioning families organize around individual strengths and interests to share and allocate tasks. Progress is tracked with members held accountable for their part. Family members flexibly fill in for one another as need arises. It is important that no one is overburdened, with others underfunctioning.

SOCIAL AND ECONOMIC RESOURCES

Mobilizing Extended Kin and Community Resources

In many traditional cultures, all villagers participate in some way in the construction of every house. By contributing a part of themselves, they all support the firm foundation of the community. Similarly, in rural areas worldwide, neighboring farm families pitch in to help each other in harvesting crops. When families are open and generous, assisting others in need, they in turn can count on neighbors and friends in times of adversity. In our era of social fragmentation and self-reliance, we need to help families build these vital networks for resilience.

Founding family therapists (e.g., Satir, 1988; Whitaker & Keith, 1981) viewed well-functioning families as open systems with clear yet permeable boundaries, much like a living cell (Beavers & Hampson, 1993), cohesive within its borders yet permeable enough for satisfying interchange with the outside world. Members are actively involved in the world, relate to it with optimism and hope, and bring varied interests and resources back into the family.

Extended kin and social networks provide practical assistance, emotional support, and vital community connection. In times of crisis or hardship, they offer information, concrete services, support, companionship, and respite. They also promote a sense of security and solidarity. Community activities and religious congregations support individual and family well-being—for instance, through regular participation in church suppers, choral singing, seniors' clubs, and parent–teacher associations. Research suggests that there is something life-protective in belonging to a group and having regular social activity of any kind, especially for singles and seniors to avoid isolation.

After my mother's death, with no family members nearby, my father was quite lonely. Increasing involvement in his men's organization brought him meaningful activities and structured social gatherings for many years. Living modestly on his Social Security check, he devoted his full time and energies to volunteer work, going daily to the staff office to assist in fundraising events on behalf of hospitals for children with disabilities. My father had suffered disability himself as a child, so this involvement held special meaning for him. As my esteem rose for my father, so too did my recognition of the value in such groups, which I had earlier derided as "men marching in parades in funny hats." When my father died, all his lodge brothers, in their hats and full regalia, turned out for his funeral and gave him a glorious send-off.

Linkages with the social world are vitally important for family resilience in times of crisis. Stinnett and colleagues (Stinnett & Defrain, 1985) found that strong families have the strength to admit they have difficulties and need help. When they can't solve problems on their own, they are more likely to turn to extended family, friends, neighbors, community services, and/or therapy or counseling. Conversely, family isolation and lack of social support contribute to dysfunction under stress. Research has documented what clinicians have long known: It is not simply the size of the network or the frequency of contacts that makes a difference; the helpfulness of contacts depends on the quality of the relationships. Some are better with practical assistance; others with emotional support; and some make matters worse. A dense network can provide varied kinds of support without overburdening anyone. Since most people come for help when they are in crisis, our assessment of social networks should also identify conflicts or cutoffs that might be repaired. It's important to search for hidden resources and foster potential new connections. We also need to offer information about community resources and facilitate linkages.

Formal and informal kin networks in African American and many ethnic and immigrant families are lifelines for resilience. These richly textured bonds have enabled struggling families to survive the ravages of poverty, racism, and inner-city violence (Boyd-Franklin, 2004). Such resources are particularly vital for single parents (Anderson, 2003). As one single mother said, "I have no family nearby. I don't know what I'd do without my friends. They are everything I could wish for in kin: when I don't know how to go on, they believe in me, and so I regain my courage."

For immigrant families in transition between two cultures, family processes that may have been functional in their country of origin may not fit adaptive challenges or norms in their new culture (Falicov, 1998; Landau, 2005) and supportive kin and community networks may have been lost. Families may become caught between two social worlds, with tugs in incompatible directions. Here especially, we must assess the fit of individuals, couples, families, and their sociocultural contexts. Our objective should not be solely to help them to "fit into" their new world; we need also to help families preserve valuable linkages with their kin, community, and cultural bonds.

Where kin and community ties have become frayed or lost, as when families relocate for job and economic opportunities, we need to help them forge new connections. Many communities link isolated elderly persons with young people by providing needed assistance in understaffed child care centers (Walsh, 1999a). Both young and old reap tremendous benefits from this involvement. The children love the special "grandparenting" attention through such pleasurable and growth-enhancing activities as storytelling, games, and skill building. Older persons become energized, productive, and valued for their knowledge, wisdom, and care.

Multifamily groups are serving as valuable networks for distressed families—for example, by linking undersupported single parents or families coping with the strains of a serious illness. The Internet has also become a vital source of information and networking for those concerned about the special needs of a family member.

It's important to pursue many kin and community options in seeking out models, mentors, and inspirational others, especially for at-risk youth. When a parent is unavailable or unable to provide a positive influence, other mentoring relationships can be cultivated in the extended kin and community network. Programs such as Big Brothers/Big Sisters are demonstrating powerful results in preventive efforts with urban children at risk: Involved youths are less likely to join gangs or to take alcohol or drugs, and show higher school performance. The key in such a relationship is spending time together, engaging in chores and productive responsibilities, as well as fun activities, with a caring, positive role model, someone to look up to, learn from, and be inspired by. We also need to expand the narrow dyadic view of the relational base of resilience, and not expect one caregiver or mentor to meet all needs. When children are raised in a thick network of caring relations in family and community, the possibilities for nurturance and mentoring are many and varied. The African adage "It takes a village to raise a child" (Clinton, 1996) holds true today more than ever.

Gaining Financial Security and Family–Work Balance

To strengthen family functioning, clinicians need to take financial resources into account and examine the structural supports and balances linking family and work systems (Fraenkel, 2003). In today's highly stressful life, two-earner and single-parent households experience tremendous role strain with the pressures of multiple, conflicting job and child care demands and inadequate supports (Hochschild, 1997). Many parents are too harried to attend to their couple and individual needs. One working mother and father described their lives as being "like two speeding commuter trains pausing briefly at the station to refuel and racing on." Surveys repeatedly find the leading issues of concern to working parents are the constant difficulty of balancing job and family obligations and the lack of affordable, high-quality child care. Many overburdened parents manage to keep their families and children functional only at a high cost to their own well-being; too many overloaded families break down as strains leave them more vulnerable to conflict and dissolution. If families are to thrive, the workplace must be restructured to help all workers achieve a better balance in their lives.

We can look to other nations' examples in developing new models to sustain family resilience. Although all industrialized countries have been experiencing recent social and economic upheaval, disruptions elsewhere are cushioned by social policies that safeguard family well-being, child and elder care, and expanding roles for men and women. Throughout Europe, family policy is part of general economic policy, and governments provide a range of supports for families across income groups and without stigma attached. In Scandinavian countries, family life and child welfare are considered crucial to the well-being of society. Public policies actively encourage a balance between family life and paid work based on two assumptions: (1) that men and women are equally responsible for the financial support, daily care, and well-being of their children; and (2) that involvement in parenthood should not disadvantage people in job security, earnings, or advancement. Parental leave and a variety of child care arrangements are guaranteed *child* entitlements.

We must counter the myth of family self-reliance that has grown out of society's individualistic strain. The major problems of families today largely reflect difficulties in adaptation to the social and economic upheavals of recent decades and the unresponsiveness of larger community and societal institutions. These structural problems make it difficult for families to sustain mutual support and control over their lives.

With mothers, fathers, and other caregivers in the workforce today, and with diversity in family structures and resources, families require a national commitment to affordable, high-quality child and elder care, universal health care, and more flexible job structures and schedules, in order to support healthy family functioning and the well-being of all members. Employers need to develop innovative options—including job sharing, a shorter work week, and home-based employment—to meet the childrearing needs of both fathers and mothers, and to fit the abilities and constraints of older people who want or need to keep working through their later years. The whole concept of the "normal family" has to be expanded so as to legitimize and optimize the varied experiences of most families. Some countries, such as Britain, are ahead of the United States in legislation that recognizes family diversity and ensures that parental responsibility for a child's well-being always outweighs parental rights over a child. We also need to grapple with economic disparity and the impact of poverty and disempowerment on families and their members—particularly on women, children, the elderly, and people of color.

In clinical work, family assessment and interventions must not be limited to the interior of the family, but must also attend to the family's interface with other systems and resources. It's important to inquire about income, financial situation, and major shifts in employment. A parent may benefit from coaching to negotiate a pay raise or a change in job schedule. Children may exhibit symptoms that reflect family concerns; for example, a son's school failure often coincides with his father's job loss.

In one family assessment interview, Bill and Alice presented a tirade of complaints about their son's failing grades and stealing of Alice's savings from under their mattress. In exploring recent stresses, we learned that Bill had recently lost his second job, severely straining the family's finances, jeopardizing their home ownership, and fueling marital tensions. Feeling deficient as a provider, Bill was at a loss as to how else he could be a "good" husband and father. We examined expectations about what a "good father" meant for family members, and how their Italian American cultural beliefs equated "good father" with "successful breadwinner." We explored qualities and achievements other than a paycheck for which family members valued the father. Bill hadn't realized before how much he meant to them and how many ways he could contribute to raising his children well. Couple sessions focused on ways to support each other's efforts, better budget their expenses, find ways they could both contribute to strengthening the family's financial security, and tap kin support until they regained solid footing.

With major shifts in the economy, companies have displaced workers at all income levels and life stages. Those with the least education and skills are hardest hit, and their families are seriously affected. Rates of alcohol and drug use increase, along with couple and family conflict. Family support is crucial for displaced workers to regain confidence and build new areas of competence. (see Chapter 7 for a model family support group project developed by our Chicago Center for Family Health.)

The crisis in many families today reflects not merely structural problems *in* the family, but structural problems in society. Scarce resources, institutional barriers, and a pileup of employment, health care, and social problems burden too many families, especially those living in conditions of poverty and urban decay. Harry Aponte (1994) has spoken out on the serious effects, especially for the poor. Societal fragmentation, with its climate of stress, isolation, and distrust, has increased vulnerability, violence, and despair. The poor "have all the personal and family problems everyone else has, along with the complications of a personal, family, and community ecosystem weakened by chronic social and economic problems" (p. 9). Teen pregnancy, single-parent families, divorce, substance abuse, and violence are not limited to the poor; however, Aponte sees the poor as our "canary in the mines," warning us of our unsafe environment. Because the same conditions are also hurting everyone else, addressing larger structural problems may also heal and strengthen our whole society.

STRENGTHENING ORGANIZATIONAL PROCESSES IN PRACTICE

No family form or style is inherently healthy or dysfunctional. Each family, influenced by its cultural values, resources, and social context, develops its structure and preferences for certain transactional patterns. Whether those organizational processes are functional depends largely on their *fit* with family challenges. We need to extend our attention beyond the household to significant relational networks: All individuals are members of kinship groups, whether formal or informal, living under the same roof, within a community, or scattered at a great distance. The myth of the isolated nuclear family, intact and self-sufficient, should not blind us to the intimate and powerful connections among kin living apart. We need to recognize the significance of intimate partnerships and friendship networks, and to do all we can to rebuild our communities.

Leading clinicians, as well as researchers, have noted the importance of key organizational patterns for healthy family functioning. Early structural–strategic family therapists considered a strong generational hierarchy and clear lines of parental authority to be essential for optimal functioning. Bowen (1978) emphasized the importance of differentiation of self in relationships. Whitaker described the healthy family primarily as maintaining an integrated whole, characterized by appropriate separation of parent and child generations and by flexibility in power distribution, rules, and role structure (Whitaker & Keith, 1981). Above all, Minuchin (1974) urged us to view the family as a social system in transformation. With this orientation, many more families in distress can be seen and treated as average families in transitional situations, suffering the pains of accommodation to new circumstances.

Family and social networks are natural "shock absorbers" in times of crisis, as an anecdote from family therapy pioneer Carl Whitaker vividly illustrates. Whitaker once presented a videotape of an interview with a "healthy family" at a meeting of the American Psychiatric Association. Many in the audience challenged him, pointing out a host of pathologies they detected. Labeling the father an "obsessive–compulsive personality," they saw him as rigid and peripheral to the family, absorbed in his work. Whitaker rose to their challenge: He met with the family once a year over the next 5 years and then returned to the conference to present his findings. All family members were still functioning well. Most remarkable, for Whitaker, were their responses to crises that had occurred, as they do in all families. When the maternal grandmother became critically ill, the mother turned her attention to providing the needed care, while the father made more time for the family. Rallying in response to the crisis, he showed unexpected role flexibility in taking over most household and child care responsibilities during those difficult months, and was able to comfort and support his wife and children through the illness and death of the beloved grandmother. As Whitaker noted, this family summoned its resources and showed its greatest strengths when challenged by crisis. We therapists need to share Whitaker's conviction that in all families, such resources can be brought forth to strengthen family resilience.

CHAPTER 5

Communication Processes

Facilitating Mutual Support and Problem Solving

The important thing is to be capable of emotions,
but to experience only one's own would be a sorry limitation.
—ANDRÉ GIDE, *Journals*

Good communication is vital to family functioning and resilience. The complex structures and demands in contemporary family life make good communication ever more important yet more difficult. In times of crisis, disruptive transitions, or prolonged stress, communication is more likely to break down—at the very times when it is most essential.

Communication involves the transmission of beliefs, information exchange, emotional expression, and problem-solving processes (Epstein et al., 2003). Every communication has a "content" aspect, conveying facts, opinions, or feelings, and a "relationship" aspect, defining, affirming, or challenging the nature of relationships. For instance, the statement "Take your medicine" is a command with the expectation of compliance. All verbal and nonverbal behavior conveys messages, including silence, withdrawal—or spitting out the medicine, which might mean "I don't like it!" (feelings); "It won't help!" (belief/opinion); or "I won't obey you!" (relationship statement).

A growing body of research on couple and family interaction has

106

focused on key elements in good communication. Olson (Olson & Gorell, 2003), for instance, assesses such specific skills as speaking and listening, self-disclosure, clarity, continuity tracking, respect, and regard. Speaking skills involve speaking for oneself and not for others. Listening skills include empathy and attentive listening. Self-disclosure involves sharing information and feelings about oneself and the relationship. However, cultural norms vary considerably and family members also differ: Parental demands for open communication may be viewed by adolescents as prying and intrusive.

Because communication facilitates all family functioning, intervention efforts with families in crisis aim to increase family members' abilities to clarify their crisis situation, to express and respond to each other's needs and concerns, and to negotiate system changes that meet new demands. As we will see, clarity, open emotional expression, and collaborative problem solving are crucial keys for family resilience (see Table 5.1).

CLARITY

Clear, Consistent Messages

Numerous studies have found that communication clarity is essential for effective family functioning (Beavers & Hampson, 2003; Epstein et al., 2003; Olson & Gorall, 2003). Satir (1988) observed that, even allowing for cultural differences, communication in healthy families is direct, clear, specific, and honest. In short, members say what they mean and mean what they say. Most communication is fairly straightforward, with messages conveyed to the person(s) they concern and not deflected onto other family members or transmitted through them. Verbal and behavioral messages are consistent and congruent, yielding shared understanding. Even with interruptions, members can pick up the thread and effectively resume discussions over a period of time. Contextual clarity enables members to distinguish reality from fantasy, facts from opinions, and serious intent from humor.

The clarity of family rules is as important as the rules themselves, since they organize interaction, set behavioral expectations, and define relationships (Minuchin, 1974). Members need to be especially clear about what they expect and think of each other, and what their transactions mean. For instance, what does it mean when a single mother calls the oldest son the "man of the house" after the father has left? When communication is vague, distorted, or left unresolved, it breeds anxiety, confusion, and misunderstanding. Members may operate on faulty as-

TABLE 5.1. Communication Processes: Facilitating Family Functioning

Clarity

- Clear, consistent messages (words and actions)
- Clarify ambiguous information, expectations
- Truth seeking/truth speaking

Open emotional sharing

- Sharing wide range of feelings (joy and pain; hopes and fears)
- Mutual empathy; tolerance for differences
- Responsibility for own feelings, behavior; avoiding blaming
- Pleasurable interactions; humor, respite

Collaborative problem solving

- Identifying problems, stressors, constraints, options
- Creative brainstorming; resourcefulness
- Shared decision making: negotiation, fairness, reciprocity
  - Managing conflicts: repairing hurts, misunderstandings
- Focusing on goals; taking concrete steps
- Building on success; learning from failure, mistakes
- Taking a proactive stance: preventing problems; averting crises; preparing for future challenges
  - Devising "Plan B"

sumptions or attempt "mind reading." Persistent ambiguity in messages about role expectations and blurred boundaries can foster depression and block mastery of challenging situations. Such ambiguity occurs commonly in caregiving for a family member with dementia (Boss, 1999). Communication unclarity can also adversely affect recovery from crisis events or the course of serious physical and mental illnesses by increasing anxiety and confusion (see Chapter 9).

Cultural differences must be taken into account. For instance, nonverbal communication is especially valued in Japanese culture (Shibusawa, 2005). Japanese children are taught to infer what others are trying to communicate from the context and the way in which something is conveyed, and to notice what is *not* said, in the belief that words cannot adequately capture meaning or emotions.

Clarity about Adverse Situation, Options

In facing adversity, it is important to clarify the situation as much as possible. Often family members glean different understandings of events and their implications, based on bits and pieces of information or hearsay. They may fill in the blanks with their best hopes or worst fears.

Shared understanding and acknowledgment of the prognosis of a life-threatening illness or the facts about a possible suicide are crucial for coping and adaptation. When family members have limited or conflicting information it's important for therapists to encourage them to gather more facts and perspectives to gain clarification. As we have seen in Chapter 3, family members do best when they can make meaning of their adversity, clarify how it came about, and appraise their options so they can determine how best to deal with it and prevent future difficulties. The experience becomes more comprehensible and manageable when information and perceptions are shared, and when the meanings of events and their implications for family members' lives are discussed openly and fully. With sudden, unanticipated crisis events, such as a school shooting, "crisis debriefings" immediately after the event can provide some initial information and support for affected families, but studies caution that group sessions that intensify raw emotions or push for premature "closure" can be harmful (see Chapter 11). Meaning making and emotional working through require support over time.

Truth Seeking/Truth Speaking

Family members may try to protect one another from painful or threatening information through silence, secrecy, or distortion, creating barriers to understanding, authentic relating, and informed decision making. When members avoid contact and block communication of knowledge, memories, or fears, the unspeakable may go underground, becoming expressed in emotional or physical symptoms (Griffith & Griffith, 1994) or surfacing in other relationships or life contexts.

Most members are usually aware of unspoken tensions in the family, like having an elephant in the room that can't be talked about. Sometimes family members postpone any discussion until they feel certain of facts or a dreaded outcome. It is usually more reassuring, especially for children, when adults relate what information they can and acknowledge the uncertainties they are dealing with. It's helpful for parents to encourage children to come to them if they have more questions or concerns. When a situation is uncertain, such as a life-threatening illness, children may become hypervigilant for further clarification, reading bad news into any hushed conversation between parents. It's important for parents to let them know that they will fill them in when more is known. We can be helpful by coaching parents on ways to share potentially upsetting information with children—facts of an adoption, a parent's absence, or a move to a new community—and by advising them not to assume that their children aren't worried if they haven't asked. Truth telling is a vital process in coping with crisis, transitions, and traumatic experiences, as we will see in Chapters 11 and 12.

OPEN EMOTIONAL SHARING

Studies of emotional intelligence (Goleman, 1995) show the importance of open emotional expression for successful coping and adaptation in life. Such abilities develop through transactions in significant relationships and can be facilitated in couple and family therapy.

Empathic Sharing of a Wide Range of Emotions

In well-functioning families, transactions are notable for a warm, cheerfully optimistic tone, with joy and comfort in relating (Beavers & Hampson, 2003). Members are able to show and tolerate a wide range of feelings—from tenderness, love, hope, gratitude, consolation, happiness, and joy to such troubled feelings as anger, fear, sadness, and disappointment. Moderately well-functioning families may show occasional constriction in expressing feelings, or a member may under- or overrespond, without disrupting family functioning. Here again, we need to be mindful of cultural differences in emotional expression.

A climate of mutual trust (see Chapter 3) encourages and is reinforced by open, empathic sharing of emotions (Beavers & Hampson, 2003). Messages are spontaneous, yet conveyed in a considerate way to respect the feelings and differences of others. With acceptance of uncertainty, ambivalence, and disagreement, members risk little in being known and open. Each shows interest in what others have to say and an expectation of being understood. Yet active listening may not be sufficient when change is also needed. When a family member is upset or expresses unmet needs, others best demonstrate empathic concern by responding in both word and deed.

The emotional health of children is affected by the emotional climate between their parents (Epstein et al., 2003). Research has consistently found that children are more likely to be healthy and happy when the couple relationship is warm and supportive, with each partner feeling loved, admired, and valued. In intact families where parental conflict is high, children fare more poorly than most do in divorced families (Hetherington & Kelly, 2004).

Couple relationships thrive when partners can discuss their needs and differences, show their own enjoyment, and take pleasure in satisfying each other. If sexual intimacy wanes under stress, or with illness or disability, couples can sustain pleasurable and soothing physical contact, such as touching and hugging, which reinforces closeness. Influenced by traditional gender socialization, women seek to build rapport by emphasizing connection and understanding, whereas men tend more to focus on factual reporting and instrumental problem solving. Women often complain that their male partners don't listen to them, share feelings, show affection, or talk about their relationship enough. Men more often complain that their female partners are too demanding and are more likely to become flooded or to withdraw from emotionally laden interactions (Gottman & Silver, 1999). In times of crisis, men who are uncomfortable revealing vulnerability, fear, or sorrow tend to stonewall or distance emotionally from their partners. They may sexualize needs for closeness, comfort, and support in affairs or submerge feelings in substance abuse or workaholism.

In some patriarchal cultures, such as many Asian and Middle Eastern cultures, women may risk emotional or physical harm when they voice concerns. Because harmony is so highly valued, assertion can be reframed as a path toward a higher level of harmony in family relationships. Therapists can affirm how much love already is present in the family and that fear blocks loving connections. To speak truthfully and respectfully, a woman must feel safe enough to share her deepest thoughts and feelings. Men can be advised that listening is a crucial leadership skill that successful men possess and can bring enhanced intimacy (Markman & Halford, 2005).

Loving Tolerance for Differences and Negative Emotions

As families go through various phases in adaptation to prolonged challenges, as with family migration, their communication will shift with emerging priorities. Different feelings may surface at different times and be expressed in varied ways by different family members. Loving tolerance and mutual support will be required, especially when feelings are out of sync. For instance, a teenager's delayed anger at the loss of a parent may erupt just when other family members are emotionally ready to move on with life.

Owning Feelings and Actions, Avoiding Blame and Scapegoating

Resilient families show strikingly little blame, personal attack, or scapegoating. Members take responsibility for their own feelings and actions and acknowledge their contribution to difficulties. In poorly functioning families, a climate of fear and mistrust is perpetuated through criticism, blame, and scapegoating. Emotional expression then becomes highly reactive, critical, and attacking (Bowen, 1978). Conflict can escalate out of control. A vicious cycle may ensue, for instance, when a parent overreacts to a son's misbehavior with threats to send him away, increasing his anxiety and provocative behavior, which then push the parent beyond tolerance and result in his expulsion.

Communication may be closed and secretive to avoid sharing painful feelings. Often this is done with good intentions of protecting children or other vulnerable family members, but consequences can be disastrous. For example, Mark, a man in his 40s, didn't tell his parents he was terminally ill until a week before he died; as a result, they had no time to anticipate and prepare emotionally for the loss of their only child. His death was so shattering that it triggered a heart attack in his father.

Commonly, when parents are concerned or upset about a serious issue, they try to spare their children from worry by covering up their own feelings and putting on a cheerful facade, as if all is "normal." However, children readily pick up underlying tension. When parents don't explain the source of their distress (e.g., a precarious job situation), children may blame themselves for being bad or unlovable or they may be on their best behavior so as not to burden a parent further. When children's own feelings and needs become submerged and unvoiced, they can erupt in physical or behavioral symptoms of distress. Yet the crisis of a child's problems can also jolt family members into the need to deal with unexpressed feelings and needs. An adolescent's drug overdose can be the impetus for important conversations and changes to take place.

In a crisis situation, the unacknowledged or ambivalent feelings within individual family members can become split between partners, siblings, or branches of a family. For example, members may differ on whether to terminate life support for a critically ill family matriarch and become increasingly polarized in intense, bitter conflict. After a tragedy, one sibling may carry all the sadness in a family while another becomes a clown to cheer up others. Enmeshed families may try to suppress mixed emotions or deny negative feelings and behaviors, while playing up the positive ones, presenting a false united front, or pseudomutuality. In more disengaged families, individuals may be strong in expressing negative or angry feelings, but wary of praise or affectionate messages. Family sessions can be valuable in all these situations, helping members to get in touch with their own mixed feelings and to hear and accept the various feelings of others.

Open communication is essential in dealing with a prolonged ordeal. One couple reflected on the importance of sharing their feelings through their son's cancer diagnosis, subsequent treatments, remission, and uncertain long-term prognosis. The husband said that his greatest lesson had been not to be afraid of fear; he had learned that bottling up his fears only increased them, but that expressing them to his wife eased his mind and brought the couple closer.

Open communication does not mean constantly talking about suffering experienced or catastrophic fear. It's essential to acknowledge the reality of an adverse situation and encourage family members to turn to one another for meaning making, support, and reorganization of their lives. Yet, over time, they also need respite from focus on their ordeal. What's crucial is that communication not be blocked so that members can feel free, as needs arise, to voice what is on their minds and in their hearts.

Fostering Positive Interactions

Open expression of positive feelings is vital to counterbalance negative interactions. Relationships can tolerate considerable conflict as long as it is offset by much more positive communication, through expressions of love, appreciation, respect, and pleasurable interaction (Gottman & Silver, 1999; Markman & Notarius, 1994). Thus, therapists need to aim beyond reduction of negative transactions, such as criticism and blaming, to active encouragement of positive interactions.

In the aftermath of a shattering experience, family members may feel numbed; chronic stress may generate "battle fatigue" and a deadened sense in relationships. It can be helpful to revive pleasures that were once shared and to envision new possibilities for satisfying connection. Couples or families can be encouraged to plan activities together that give them a pleasurable shared focus, such as a movie or a sports event; that provide an opportunity for collaboration, such as a family cookout; or that offer a spiritually renewing experience to transcend their immediate distress and draw strength for coping.

Mrs. Lamm and her four children were being seen in a therapy that was stuck in their shared depression. They came for help after 12-year-old Jeffrey attempted suicide by drinking some cleaning solvent. Family therapy focused on their depression and anger at the father, who had "disappeared" 3 months earlier without any word, leaving his family uncertain of his whereabouts or whether he would return. The father, who had a serious drinking problem, had drifted off several times in the past, each time showing up a few weeks later as if nothing had happened. This time it seemed that he might never come back. The more family members talked about their helplessness and hopelessness, the more weighted down the therapy became. The therapist, like the family, was unsure where they were headed. The therapy seemed to be in limbo, waiting for the return of the wayward father.

Invited in as a consultant, I asked the mother and children how things had changed with the father absent, and listened to their dilemma. I noted that they seemed to have lost the life of the family when the father wasn't around. Although his leaving and possible return might be beyond their control, they could, if they pulled together, regain their liveliness. I asked what they had enjoyed doing together. Hearing that they had the most fun going fishing, I asked if they might plan to go fishing one day over the coming weekend. They nodded, but they all seemed to be waiting for someone to make it happen. It was important not to put all responsibility on the shoulders of the mother, who was depleted by job and family demands. I asked each child what he or she might do to help make it possible. One child said he could clean the fishing poles in the basement; another offered to dig for worms; the two others agreed to make sandwiches and pack a picnic lunch. The mother brightened and offered to drive them to a favorite fishing spot on Saturday morning. She and the children became animated in discussing the plans and remembering past times. I asked if they could imagine anything that might keep them from going, in order to help them anticipate possible obstacles (such as bad weather or a child's misbehavior) and reduce the risk of disappointment by planning an alternative "rain date." Since the father's unpredictability in his comings and goings was so problematic in this family, it was especially important for expectations and plans to be clearly communicated; for all members to take responsibility for their own parts; and to agree that they would count on each other to follow through. The family arrived at the next session energized, with spirits revived from their outing. After this "jumpstart," the Lamms were better able to take active initiative in other steps toward coming to terms with the ambiguous loss of the father and moving forward with life.

Sharing Humor

Abundant research attests to the importance of humor in times of crisis and hardship. Humor helps families cope with difficult situations, reduce tensions, and accept limitations. Finding humor in the midst of despair can help family members to detoxify threatening situations and lessen anxiety. It can offer respite from unrelenting stresses. It can facilitate conversation and express feelings of warmth and affection. It can reduce tensions, put members at ease, help them cope with stressful conditions, and restore a positive outlook. Humor can ease a direct confrontation, melt a defensive reaction, help to accept failure or mistakes, and lighten heavy burdens. Sharing a life story with both humor and pathos can be a profound experience, drawing members closer.

When told by doctors that he would die within months from a rare disease, Cousins (1989) posited that if negative emotions can produce harmful chemical changes in the body, then positive emotions should have a therapeutic value. He checked out of his depressing hospital room and into a comfortable (and less expensive) hotel. He attributed much of his own recovery to his self-generated program, which included "laughter therapy"—watching old Marx Brothers films and *Candid Camera* vignettes. Recent medical studies are documenting that humor, indeed, can bolster our spirits and our immune systems in ways that encourage healing and recovery from serious illness.

Humor can be particularly beneficial when it points out the incongruous aspects of a harrowing situation—the inconsistent, bizarre, silly, or illogical things that happen (Wuerffel, DeFrain, & Stinnett, 1990). It can also help us to accept our failings. In high-functioning families, members realize that people can envision perfection and yet are destined to flounder, make mistakes, get scared, and need reassurance. This encourages both a sense of humor and an appreciation of paradox (Beavers & Hampson, 2003). As my mother, never at a loss for an aphorism, used to say, "Blessed are we who can laugh at ourselves, for we will never cease to be amused."

Family therapy pioneers encouraged clinicians to appreciate both the grim and the absurd, humanizing therapy in providing a context to share painful emotions as well as laughter. Whitaker stressed the importance of family humor and playfulness for creative fantasy and inventive process (Whitaker & Keith, 1981). However, humor can be destructive when used to express anger, cruelty, or contempt through biting sarcasm, or when used derisively to demean or make fun of others. In crisis-ridden families, humor may be lost altogether as family members become overwhelmed and depressed by the persistence of problems. Encouraging caring humor—members' laughing *with* one another—can revitalize families in need of respite.

COLLABORATIVE PROBLEM SOLVING

Effective problem-solving processes are essential for families to deal effectively with sudden crises or persistent challenges. Well-functioning families are *not* characterized by the absence of problems, although good fortune certainly makes life easier (Beavers & Hampson, 1990). What distinguishes family resilience is the ability to manage conflict and address problems collaboratively. This requires tolerance for open disagreement and skills for solving problems in daily living as well as crises that arise.

The practical and emotional aspects of a crisis situation are intertwined. When family functioning is disrupted by basic instrumental problems, such as the loss of a job and income, the ability to deal with emotional needs is also strained. In turn, emotional distress impairs problem solving.

A negative emotional tone between family members—anger, frustration, discouragement, or defeat—can block them from dealing successfully with serious or persistent problems. Both practical and emotional tasks of a major transition must be addressed. In divorce, for instance, a family must make decisions about household reorganization, financial support, custody, and visitation, as well as deal with the grief of losses and other complicated feelings such as anger, hurt, betrayal, or abandonment (Walsh, Jacob, & Simons, 1995). Where family members are constrained by traditional gender-based expectations for men to handle instrumental problem solving and for women to be responsible for emotional expression and caregiving, fuller participation and sharing in these processes can be encouraged.

The McMaster group (Epstein et al., 2003; Ryan et al., 2005) has outlined several steps in effective problem-solving processes. Family members first need to recognize a problem and to communicate with those involved and those who might be potential resources. Collaborative brainstorming enables them to weigh and consider possible options, resources, and constraints, and to decide on a plan. They then need to initiate and carry out action, monitor efforts, and evaluate their success. Well-functioning families manage to resolve most problems efficiently; communication, decision making, and action flow reasonably smoothly. In reviewing results, they can fine-tune or revise their efforts as needed.

Identifying Problems and Related Stressors

When help is sought for a presenting problem—a wife's depression, a husband's drinking, a child's misbehavior—family systems therapists are careful to explore other recent or ongoing stressors in family life that may be reverberating throughout the system. A child or adolescent's behavior is often a barometer of family feelings and provides ample opportunities to draw fire from parents, thereby deflecting concern from other painful family crises that require attention and assistance.

> Mrs. Wolff requested therapy for her 15-year-old son, Paul, stating that she feared that he "needed to be institutionalized" because his behavior was out of control. He had become surly and defiant in recent months, and she felt increasingly angry and helpless in dealing with him. The family assessment revealed that 8 months earlier, the maternal grandmother, with deteriorating Parkinson's disease, had moved in with the family. Mrs. Wolff became tearful in describing her mounting difficulties in caring for her mother at home. She had had difficulty sleeping since finding her mother one morning on the floor, where she had fallen during the night. Alarmed by her mother's progressive loss of motor control, she felt helpless to prevent a potentially fatal accident.
> When asked whether the family had considered placing her mother in an elder care facility, Mrs. Wolff replied that "institutionalization" was out of the question and had not even been discussed, since her father, on his deathbed a year earlier, had asked her to promise that she would always take care of her mother. Feeling alone in her dilemma, she deflected her conflicted feelings and sense of helplessness into struggles with her son. In a vicious cycle, the harder she tried to control him, the more defiantly out of control he became.

It's important to explore how the response of a spouse or other family member may be contributing to the dilemma, and to encourage the potential resource their relationship can provide in meeting the challenges.

> Mr. Wolff had increasingly withdrawn into his work over recent months, avoiding contact with his family. The therapist explored the strain of caregiving challenges on family relationships and asked Mr. Wolff what blocked his ability to offer more support. He choked up as he described how the current situation was reviving his feelings of guilt: When his own mother had become critically ill, he had left all caretaking responsibilities to his sisters. He secretly blamed his own inattention for her rapid decline. Seeing his wife care for her mother rekindled his own felt deficiency and sorrow at his mother's death—uncomfortable feelings that he pushed away by distancing from contact.

Creative Brainstorming

When problems are identified, it's important to involve family members in creative brainstorming. In well-functioning families, parents act as coordinators and coaches—bringing out others' ideas, voicing their own, and encouraging choice wherever possible. Family members speak up, and the contributions of all members, from eldest to youngest, are respected as valuable (Beavers & Hampson, 2003).

By understanding impasses to problem solving, we can find ways to overcome them. We can encourage family members to discuss both resources and constraints, and to consider a range of options, weighing the costs and benefits for all family members and for the family as a whole. Openness to trying new solutions is a hallmark of well-functioning, adaptive families. This flexible and inventive approach builds resourcefulness.

> Intervention efforts with the Wolff family addressed both practical and emotional aspects of the family's problems. Joining with Mrs. Wolff's intentions to provide the best care for her mother, the therapist opened discussion to possible ways to accomplish this aim besides doing it all on her own. She encouraged the parents' collaborative brainstorming and information gathering to consider a range of home-based services and placement options for "Nanna."
>
> Mr. Wolff's involvement, which brought needed support to his wife, was framed also as an opportunity for him to share more fully in caregiving arrangements, as he wished he had done for his own mother. The therapist provided a caring context for this emotion-laden problem solving, exploring each partner's conflicted feelings and encouraging mutual empathy. A family session explored the son's mixed feelings as well—his love for Nanna and sadness at her decline, along with his guilt for wishing that he hadn't had to give up his room to her. Normalizing and contextualizing the many feelings of family members as natural and common in their stressful situation were helpful in reducing blame, shame, and guilt. The therapist affirmed the family's honesty and caring intentions.
>
> It was noted that perhaps the most important family member was missing from their problem-solving efforts—Nanna herself. Mr. and Mrs. Wolff were encouraged to include the grandmother in the planning for her care by having conversations with her at home and asking for her input to our next session. They were surprised to learn that she was acutely aware of the caregiving complications, but that she had been constrained from talking about them because she felt like such a burden. She came to feel more valued when her feelings and preferences were considered in making plans.

Shared Decision Making: Negotiation, Compromise, and Reciprocity

In Higgins's (1994) research on resilient individuals, she was struck by their ability to "love well" in long-term relationships, with a high degree of reciprocity and concern for others as well as themselves. They consistently tried to recognize the needs of others and to differentiate them from their own. They were active participants in efforts to withstand conflict, disappointment, anger, and frustration when the needs of either partner were not met. They actively and successfully negotiated such difficulties throughout the relationship over time.

Family researchers have found negotiation processes to be crucial for optimal couple and family functioning across a broad diversity of families. In problem solving, the process of negotiation can be as important as the outcome. Family members' input is sought on major decisions. It's crucial for therapists to observe and clarify how important decisions are reached.

Anna requested individual therapy for recent depression, triggered by the decision to move to another part of the country so that her husband, Bob, could take a better job. Because the crisis involved the marital situation, I asked the couple to come in together initially, to assess the problem jointly and determine how to be most helpful. When both were asked how the decision to move was made, Bob replied, "I told her I had this great job offer that I told them I'd probably take; what do you think about it?" Confronted with a decision all but made by Bob, Anna agreed because it was good for him, without considering her own feelings and needs. After they had made all arrangements, she became acutely depressed about leaving her family, friends, and community. Bob was angry at her for burdening him with her sadness and regrets, wanting her to pull her own weight with the difficult practical demands of the transition. They both initially suggested that she should have a few individual counseling sessions "to adjust" to the move.

I recommended that couple sessions and individual sessions with both partners be combined. The partners were strongly encouraged to revisit the decision-making process and to reconsider the various options, costs, and benefits more collaboratively. They came to realize that both held mixed feelings about the move, but that Bob had expressed only the positive side, while Anna carried all the feelings of regret and loss. As their positions had polarized, their relationship became increasingly strained. The communication process was as important as the final decision. Anna needed to participate actively in the decision making and to have her feelings ac-knowledged and her preferences weighed in the balance. Had she met with a therapist individually to "adjust" to the move, she would most likely have carried resentment along with her accommodation.

Negotiation involves airing and accepting differences while working toward shared goals. Striving for an equal partnership and working out the complex demands of dual-career family life put a premium on negotiating, with comfort and skill in open communication and conflict management. To be successful negotiators, family members need to learn how to talk and listen with compassion and understanding. They need to interrupt negative cycles of criticism, blame, and withdrawal—the attacks and defensiveness that corrode relationships. Those who sustain happy relationships learn how to repair conversations that go badly and how to soothe each other when hurt or upset. One person might say, "This isn't working; let's try talking about this again," or "Let's both cool down and try to resolve our differences more calmly when we can hear each other." Such nurturing, monitoring, and support strengthen relationships as problems are resolved.

Quite often, negotiation and compromise are hindered by struggles over power and control. Battles over the relationship aspect of communication keep substantive issues from being addressed and resolved. Accommodation may be viewed in terms of winning versus losing, or having power over others versus being controlled or "one-down." Positions become rigid and nonnegotiable when compromise is felt to be "giving in" to the other. When there is a skewed deference–dominance imbalance over time, the overaccommodating individual may become increasingly resentful. A lack of trust in reciprocity breeds short-term "tit-for-tat" exchanges, or a withholding on one person's part until the other "evens the score" between them. Lack of nurturing and supportiveness contribute to resentment. Multiple stresses heighten tensions and conflict.

Differences in gender socialization and power strongly influence negotiation processes and outcome. In situations such as divorce mediation, professionals need to be alert to skews in power, influence, and financial resources when negotiations aren't conducted on a level playing field. Moreover, men and women often enter into negotiation with different basic premises and aims. Individuals reared for success in the workplace are more likely to argue their positions forcefully and convincingly, with the aim of winning—meeting their own needs as fully as possible. Women who are reared to put the needs of others before their own more often defer and accommodate. It can be helpful in therapy to contextualize this skew in terms of these differing premises.

> As Anna and Bob began to address their dilemma, Anna observed, "Somehow I always seem to defer to him. Maybe it's just my problem." I noted that this happens quite commonly between men and women because of the different ways we're raised and different rules we learn about negotiation. We explored how this might be happening for them: "Let me see if I understand your positions. It seems that for you, Bob, good negotiation means making the strongest case on your own behalf and pushing to win your case. Is that so?" Bob nodded. "That's true; sure." "And for you, Anna, good negotiation means consideration of Bob's needs and compromise of your own." Anna nodded, adding, "And since I never play by his rules and he never plays by mine, things always end up his way." I commented that it seemed to operate like "the subtle pull of gravity." Bob agreed, saying, "Right. It's like the norm is in my head. It's real comfortable." Anna added, "But this decision is too important—I want my feelings to count, too."

Such skewed communication patterns and power dynamics often come to the fore at a major life transition and trigger a relationship crisis, as in this case. Discussing the patterns in their larger social context without blame helped the couple to work toward more balanced negotiation, for Anna to assert her needs more effectively and Bob to be more considerate and mutually accommodating. Increased reciprocity can greatly strengthen a relationship and the ability to navigate transitional challenges collaboratively.

Conflict Management and Resolution

The process of making major life decisions or resolving crisis situations, often doesn't proceed smoothly and may involve intense conflict, pain, and anger. We try to help families experience these tensions as expectable, transient disruptions that don't result in long-term despair, perceptions of failure, or family dissolution. Tolerance for conflict allows for overt disagreement and acknowledgment of differences, with resolution through agreement, compromise, or new framing of the problem. Resilient couple and family relationships require effective conflict resolution without a sacrifice of empathy. Mixed feelings are accepted as a part of life and of all relationships. Families handle them by acknowledging both sides, or many aspects, of a dilemma and acting *on balance*—for instance, to serve the greater good of the family or the best interests of the children over the long run.

Catastrophic fears from past experience, such as violence or traumatic separation, can lead to unspoken family rules to avoid all conflict. Unfortunately, this protective strategy heightens risks that unresolved tensions will build up and explode in violence or family breakup. In couple relationships, destructive cycles of criticism and stonewalling, generating contempt and despair, have a corrosive effect: They lead over time to withdrawal, loss of hope of repairing the relationship, and marital dissolution (Gottman & Silver, 1999).

The best predictor of relationship success is not the absence of conflict, but its management: how differences that are bound to arise are handled and resolved or repaired. Conflict avoidance may be needed in the midst of crisis, but it becomes dysfunctional over time, heightening the risk for later relationship breakdown. Most divorces occur in the first 5–7 years, with the greatest difficulties occurring in the first 2–5 years as unresolved conflicts pile up and resentments grow (Driver, Tabards, Shapiro, Nahm, & Gottman, 2003).

To understand these corrosive interactions, the Gottman team observed couples in early marriage (Time 1) and again 4 years later (Time 2). Spouses likely to separate or divorce by Time 2 were already unhappy and separating emotionally at Time 1. Both were more defensive, making excuses and denying responsibility more than couples with a successful marital course. The researchers could predict with 90% accuracy which couples would be separated by Time 2 based on a vicious cycle in handling conflict. When conflict arose, the husband became very physiologically aroused and stonewalled his wife, then eventually withdrew. Over time he became overwhelmed by his wife's emotions and avoidant of any conflict. The stonewalling was very aversive and physiologically arousing for his wife. She initially tried to reengage him but, unsuccessful, was put off. This led to her emotional detachment and withdrawal, with expressions of criticism and contempt. Their lives became increasingly separate and parallel, as some wives described: "like two train tracks that never touched." As both withdrew and became defensive, the relationship was on its way to separation and divorce.

Gender differences were found. "Hot" marital interaction led to significantly more aversive physiological arousal and stonewalling by men than by women. Stonewalling predicted a man's loneliness and deterioration in his health over time. An interesting finding was that men who did housework were far less overwhelmed by their wives' emotions, less conflict avoidant, physiologically calmer, and healthier. The researchers considered the possibility that there is some hidden benefit in doing housework (!) but surmised that the significant variable was a more egalitarian relationship and fewer traditional masculine concerns about issues of competition, control, and vulnerability.

Even if conflicts are upsetting at the time, they can be necessary and beneficial to a relationship in the long run. Conflict is not destructive of a relationship if it is repaired and offset by positive emotional expression, particularly by affection, humor, positive problem solving, agreement, assent, empathy, and active nondefensive listening. Gottman found that the ratio of positive to negative interactions exceeded 10:1 for a marriage on a trajectory of increasing satisfaction.

Effective conflict management requires open disagreement with good communication skills for resolution. It's important to learn how to confront without being abrasive and how to accept influence. In both conflict-avoidant and high-conflict couples, therapeutic interventions need to increase skills for handling conflict to stop the corrosive process that leads to disintegration of the relationship. To help partners manage negative emotions and respond compassionately to each other, Markman and his colleagues (1994) have developed the Prevention and Relationship Enhancement Program (PREP), which teaches couples how to fight constructively. Such approaches provide ground rules for handling conflict. Difficult issues must be controlled; partners may mutually call "time out" whenever needed; escalating conflicts are slowed down; arguments should be kept constructive; withdrawal should be avoided; and involvement must be maintained. Partners can be coached to accomplish these aims. Couple therapy builds relational resilience by providing a safe context where partners can become more tolerant of differences and more skillful in managing and resolving conflict, so that the needs of both are heard and met. The building of communication skills empowers a couple to "fight for the relationship."

Focusing on Achievable Goals; Taking Concrete Steps

For resilience, the powerful belief in active mastery must be put into practice, focusing on achievable goals and taking concrete steps toward them. Basketball superstar Michael Jordan brought intense focus to the challenge of winning each game. This ability was relationally nurtured in Jordan's family. His parents, in raising their five children, emphasized the need to "focus, focus, focus" on their goals in order to achieve them (Jordan, 1996).

This total involvement in immediate actions toward the pursuit of goals is remarkably like the experience of "flow" observed by Csikszentmihalyi (1996) in highly creative and successful people who find great satisfaction in their achievements—as much in the process as in the outcome. Moreover, for a family, as for a team, success is fostered by collaboration. As basketball coach Phil Jackson emphasized: "Winning has to do with a connectedness that's going on between people, an alertness and awareness that happens because there is positive energy in the community" (quoted in Simon, 1997, p. 63).

Building on Success; Learning from Failure

With each small, shared success, family members' confidence and competence grow exponentially, enabling them to meet larger challenges. The acceptance of mistakes allows individual members to fail without being attacked or defined as inadequate. Accountable for their own part when something has gone wrong, they learn not to repeat mistakes that might have contributed to a problem situation. Indeed, failed experiences can become instructive as family members recalibrate efforts or try a new tack to solve problems. As Albert Einstein remarked, "Anyone who has not experienced failure has not known success."

Taking a Proactive Stance: Preventing Problems, Averting Crises

When a potential problem looms on the horizon, families do best if they face it fairly quickly, discuss it in a clear and open way, and address both its practical and emotional aspects. In this proactive way, a crisis can be averted and few unresolved problems will lie dormant to pile up over time or complicate attempts to deal with major disruptions that arise. In facing new problems, well-functioning families excel in their ability to give and accept directions, organize themselves, elicit input from one another, negotiate differences, and reach closure coherently and effectively (Beavers & Hampson, 2003). Not all problems can be solved; in such cases, resilient family members find aspects of the situation where they can make choices and take action, accepting what can't be resolved.

Families can falter at various steps in a problem-solving process. Members may be constrained from sharing their feelings and opinions or they may avoid bringing up a problem or a difference of opinion if they fear that conflict will escalate out of control and lead to violence or family breakup. It can be helpful to reassure family members, by normalizing, that all relationships are bound to have disagreements, and noting that research shows that couples and families do best overtime when they voice their differences and work constructively to resolve them.

Couples can be proactive in the earliest phases of their relationship, assessing their own areas of strength and vulnerability. Relationships at risk for breakdown can be identified even before marriage. PREPARE, a self-report inventory for premarital couples (Olson & Gorell, 2003), has been found to predict with 80–85% accuracy which couples will be happily married and which will be unhappy, separated, or divorced within 3 years of marriage. The inventory identifies areas of vulnerability for early intervention, and can encourage thoughtful consideration of commitment plans. Olson's group has found the strongest predictors of discord to be poor communication and conflict resolution, fueling unrealistic expectations and disappointment. Of note, the researchers could not discriminate those who would divorce from those who would stay unhappily married, underscoring the complexity of this decision, including religious convictions and family considerations.

We can foster resilience by encouraging couples and families to view a conflict, crisis, or setback as a meaningful, manageable challenge. As they approach it in a respectful, collaborative way, invested in mastering their challenge, they can emerge stronger for having done so. It's important to encourage them to look ahead, to surmount the inevitable obstacles all families face on their life journey. We can suggest they might devise a "Plan B" to keep in their relationship "vault" just in case their best efforts and plans must be altered. This proactive stance, like buying car insurance, brings a sense of security for family members who, while hoping for the best, are prepared to meet life's disappointments and unanticipated turns in the road. Fortunately, there are many, varied pathways in resilience.

In sum, as family process research has documented, clarity of communication, open emotional expression, and collaborative problem solving are vital elements in family resilience. Regardless of the specific problem that brings a family into therapy, it is crucial to strengthen communication processes to relieve family pain and enhance family resourcefulness. In accord with the key beliefs for success described in Chapter 3, it is important to help families set realistic, achievable objectives in line with their larger vision; take concrete steps and build on small successes; learn from experience and mistakes; experiment with innovations; prepare for anticipated challenges; and above all else, expect the unexpected.

PART III

Practice Application

CHAPTER 6

Practice Principles and Guidelines to Strengthen Family Resilience

The horizon leans forward
offering you space to place new steps of change.
—MAYA ANGELOU, "On the Pulse of Morning"

A family resilience–oriented approach extends strength-based practice by fostering family capacities to master adversity. This chapter first highlights key processes in family resilience to inform clinical assessment and intervention. Next, core practice principles are presented for reducing risk and vulnerability and strengthening resilience in distressed couples and families. Recommendations are then offered in Chapter 7 for more responsive family-centered service delivery and prevention efforts. That chapter will also address the resilience needed by helping professionals in our challenging work and practice environment.

KEY PROCESSES IN RESILIENCE: A FRAMEWORK FOR ASSESSMENT AND INTERVENTION

No "single thread" distinguishes well-functioning from dysfunctional families, as pioneering studies have found (Beavers & Hampson, 2000,

2004). When clinical formulations reduce the richness of family interaction to simplistic labels, such as "an enmeshed family," "an alcoholic family," or a "codependent relationship," they both stereotype and pathologize families. Instead, mental health professionals must attend to the many strands that are intertwined in family functioning, and need to assess strengths and vulnerabilities on multiple system dimensions.

The growing body of research on individual resilience and well-functioning families can inform practice approaches to draw out, enlarge, and reinforce family resources for resilience. While we must be aware of our own subjectivity in mapping a territory we all inhabit, we can distill a set of key processes in family resilience to guide family assessment and interventions. In Chapters 3–5, major research findings and clinical insights have been integrated into three domains of family functioning—belief systems, organizational patterns, and communication processes—to provide a framework for identifying family strengths and vulnerabilities. It can also serve as a useful map to orient professionals to attend to important elements in family functioning and bring coherence to intervention planning. It can help us target key processes to strengthen family resilience as presenting problems are addressed. Table 6.1 outlines these processes from the discussion in previous chapters. A brief summary is provided below.

Family Belief Systems

Family belief systems, influenced by cultural beliefs, emerge through family and social transactions. They powerfully influence our view of a crisis, our suffering, and our options. They organize family approaches to crisis situations and they can be fundamentally altered by such experiences. Adversity, in crisis events or prolonged challenges, generates a crisis of meaning and potential disruption of integration. Resilience is fostered by shared beliefs that increase options for effective functioning, problem resolution, healing, and growth. Clinicians can foster these facilitative beliefs by helping family members make meaning of crisis situations, gain a hopeful, positive outlook, and tap transcendent or spiritual wellsprings.

Making Meaning of Adversity

High-functioning families value strong affiliations and approach adversity as a *shared* challenge. Professionals can foster this *relational view* of resilience: in joining together, individuals strengthen their ability to overcome adversity.

TABLE 6.1. Key Processes in Family Resilience

Belief Systems

Making meaning of adversity
- Viewing resilience as relationally based – versus "rugged individual"
- Normalizing, contextualizing adversity and distress.
- Sense of coherence: viewing crisis as challenge: meaningful, comprehensible, manageable
- Explanatory attributions: How could this happen? What can be done?

Positive outlook
- Hope, optimistic bias; confidence in overcoming odds
- Courage and en-courage-ment; affirming strengths and building on potential
- Seizing opportunities: active initiative and perseverance (can-do spirit)
- Mastering the possible; accepting what can't be changed

Transcendence and spirituality
- Larger values, purpose
- Spirituality: faith, healing rituals, congregational support
- Inspiration: envisioning new possibilities; creative expression; social action
- Transformation: learning, change, and growth from adversity

Organizational Patterns

Flexibility
- Rebounding, reorganizing, adapting to fit new challenges
- Stability through disruption: continuity, dependability, rituals, routines
- Strong authoritative leadership: nurturance, protection, guidance
  - Varied family forms: cooperative parenting/caregiving teams
  - Couple/coparent relationship: equal partners

Connectedness
- Mutual support, collaboration, and commitment
- Respect for individual needs, differences, and boundaries
- Seeking reconnection, reconciliation of wounded relationships

Social and economic resources
- Mobilizing kin, social, and community networks; models and mentors
- Building financial security; balancing work–family strains
- Institutional supports

Communication Processes

Clarity
- Clear, consistent messages (words and actions)
- Clarity about ambiguous information; truth seeking/truth speaking

Open emotional expression
- Sharing range of feelings (joy and pain; hopes and fears)
- Mutual empathy; tolerance for differences
- Taking responsibility for own feelings, behavior; avoiding blaming
- Pleasurable interactions; respite, humor

Collaborative problem solving
- Creative brainstorming; resourcefulness
- Shared decision making; conflict resolution: negotiation, fairness, reciprocity
- Focusing on goals; concrete steps; building on success; learning from failure
- Proactive stance: preventing problems; averting crises; preparing for future challenges

Families function best when they gain an evolutionary sense of time and becoming—of a continual process of growth and change across the life course and the generations. Clinicians can offer this family life cycle orientation to help members see disruptive transitions also as milestones or turning points on their shared life passage. By *normalizing* and *contextualizing* distress, practitioners can help family members enlarge their perspective to see their difficulties as understandable in light of the adversities they face. We can reduce blame, shame, and pathologizing by viewing their problems as human dilemmas and their feelings and vulnerability as "normal," that is, common and expectable among families facing similar predicaments.

In grappling with adversity, families do best when helped to gain a *sense of coherence*, by recasting a crisis as a challenge that is meaningful to tackle and facilitating their efforts to make it comprehensible and manageable. With a sudden crisis, ambiguity and future uncertainties complicate recovery. We can support families' efforts to clarify understanding of their situation and to appraise their challenges and options ahead.

Positive Outlook

Research documents the strong psychological and physiological effects of a positive outlook in coping with stress, recovery from crisis, and overcoming barriers to success. *Hope* is essential to the spirit: It fuels energy and efforts to rise above adversity. Hope is a future-oriented belief: No matter how bleak the present, a better future can be envisioned. In problem-saturated conditions, helping professionals need to rekindle hope from despair, tap into potential resources, and encourage active striving and perseverance.

With repeated experiences of futility and failure, people stop trying and become passive and pessimistic, generalizing the belief that bad things always happen to them and that nothing they can do will matter. Despair robs them of meaning, purpose, and a sense of future possibility. It's essential for professionals to hold an optimistic bias, identifying and building on family strengths and potential to master their challenges. Unlike denial, there is awareness of a grim reality or a poor prognosis, and a choice to believe they can overcome the odds against them. This positive bias fuels efforts that can reduce risk and maximize the chances of success.

By affirming strengths and potential in the midst of difficulties, we help families to counter a sense of helplessness, failure, and blame as it reinforces pride, confidence, and a "can do" spirit. Our encouragement bolsters courage to take initiative and helps families persevere in efforts to master their challenges. We help them build confidence and competence through experiences of successful mastery, as they learn that their efforts can make a difference.

Initiative and perseverance—hallmarks of resilience—are fueled by unwavering shared confidence through an ordeal: "We'll never give up trying." This conviction bolsters efforts and makes family members active participants in a relentless search for solutions. By showing confidence that they will each do their best, families support members' efforts and build competencies.

Mastering the art of the possible is a vital key for resilience. Clinicians can help families take stock of their situation—the challenges, constraints, and resources—and then focus energies on making the best of their options. This requires acceptance of that which can't be changed. When immediate problems are overwhelming or events are beyond control, family members can be encouraged to carve out parts that they can master. Instead of being immobilized, or trapped in a helpless position, it involves playing the hand that is dealt as well as possible. Although past events can't be changed, they can be recast in a new light that fosters greater comprehension, learning, and healing.

Transcendence and Spirituality

Transcendent beliefs and practices provide meaning and purpose beyond a family's immediate plight. Most families find strength, comfort, and guidance in adversity through connections with their cultural and religious traditions. Rituals and ceremonies facilitate passage through significant transitions and linkage with a larger community and common heritage.

Suffering, and any injustice or senselessness, is ultimately a spiritual issue. Spiritual resources, through deep faith, practices, and congregational involvement have all been found to be wellsprings for resilience. It's also important to understand how religious beliefs, such as punishment for sins, may contribute to distress. Medical studies find that faith, prayer, and meditation strengthen healing and well-being by influencing the immune, cardiovascular, and neurological systems. Many find spiritual nourishment outside formal religion, through deep personal connection with nature, music and the arts, or a higher power.

The paradox of resilience is that the worst of times can also bring out our best. The experience of adversity and suffering can inspire creative expression through the arts, as in jazz. It can awaken family members to the importance of loved ones or nudge them to heal old wounds and reorder priorities for more meaningful relationships and life pursuits. They may emerge from shattering crises with a heightened sense of purpose in their lives, gaining compassion for the plight of others. The experience may spark community activism to spare other families suffering, and even lead to a life course committed to helping others or working for social justice. It's most important for professionals to help families envision a better future through their efforts and, where hopes and dreams have been shattered, to imagine new possibilities, seizing opportunities for invention, transformation, and growth.

Family Organizational Patterns

Families with diverse forms must organize their resources in varied ways to meet life challenges. Resilience is bolstered by a flexible yet stable structure, by strong connectedness, and by social and economic resources.

Flexibility: Bouncing Forward

Flexibility, a core process in resilience, involves adaptive change. The ability to rebound is thought of as "bouncing back" like a spring, to a preexisting shape or norm. However, after most major transitions and crisis events, families can't simply return to "normal" life as they knew it. Rather, their challenge involves "bouncing forward," constructing a new sense of normality and adapting to meet new challenges. Practitioners can help families to navigate new terrain, recalibrate relationships, and reorganize patterns of interaction to fit new conditions.

At the same time, families need to buffer and counterbalance disruptive changes and regain stability. Children and other vulnerable family members especially need assurance of continuity, security, and predictability through turmoil. Daily routines and meaningful rituals can assist in such times.

Firm, yet flexible authoritative leadership is generally most effective for family functioning and the well-being of children through stressful times. It's especially important to provide nurturance, protection, and guidance. We can help families with complex or dispersed structures, forge collaborative coparenting and caregiving teamwork across households. Couple relationships work best as equal partnership with mutual respect and sharing of joys and burdens.

Connectedness

Connectedness is essential for effective family functioning. A crisis can shatter family cohesion, leaving members unable to rely to each other. Resilience is strengthened by mutual support, collaboration, and commitment to weather troubled times together. At the same time, individual differences, separateness, and boundaries need to be respected. Members may differ in the meaning of events and the nature and timing of their response. When family members are separated, it is helpful to sustain vital connections with family networks through photos, keepsakes, e-mail, letters, visits, and links to their cultural and religious heritage.

Family therapists can facilitate reconnection and repair of wounded and estranged relationships. Intense pressures in times of crisis can spark misunderstandings and cutoffs. Yet, a crisis, such as a life-threatening event, can also be seized as an opportunity for reconciliation.

Social and Economic Resources

Kin and social networks are vital lifelines in times of trouble, offering practical and psychosocial support. The significance of role models and mentors for resilience of at-risk youth is well documented. Involvement in community groups and faith congregations also strengthens resilience. Families who are more isolated can be helped to access these potential resources.

Community-based coordinated efforts, involving local agencies and residents, are essential to meet such challenges as neighborhood crime or a major disaster and to lower risks of future threats. Multisystemic and multifamily group approaches facilitate both family and community resilience.

Financial security is crucial for resilience. A serious illness, job loss, or natural disaster can deplete a family's economic resources. Families also need help navigating conflicting pressures of job and family responsibilities.

We must be cautious that the concept of family resilience not be misused to blame families that are unable to rise above harsh conditions by simply labeling them as not resilient. Just as individuals need supportive relationships to thrive, families require social and institutional policies and programs that foster their ability to rebound and rebuild after major crises and to thrive in the face of prolonged challenges. It is not enough to help families overcome the odds; professionals must also work to change the odds.

Communication Processes

Communication processes facilitate resilience by bringing clarity to crisis situations, encouraging open emotional expression, and fostering collaborative problem solving. It must be kept in mind that cultural norms vary widely in terms of informational sharing and emotional expression.

Clarity

In times of crisis, communication and coordination can break down. Ambiguity and uncertainty fuel anxiety and block understanding of what is happening and what can be done. By helping families clarify and share crucial information about their situation and future expectations, we can facilitate meaning making, emotional sharing, and informed decision making. Shared acknowledgment of the reality and circumstances of a painful event fosters healing whereas denial and coverup can impede recovery.

Well-intentioned families often avoid painful or threatening subjects, wishing to protect each other from worry. However, anxieties about the unspeakable can generate catastrophic fears and are often expressed in somatic and behavioral problems. Parents can help by keeping children informed as the situation develops and by being open to discussing questions or concerns. Parents may need guidance on age-appropriate ways to share information and can expect that as children mature, they may revisit issues to gain greater comprehension or bring up emerging concerns.

Emotional Expression

Open communication, supported by a climate of mutual trust, empathy, and tolerance for differences, enables members to share a wide range of feelings that can be aroused by crisis events and chronic stress. Family members may be out of sync over time; one may continue to be quite upset as others feel ready to move on. Parents may suppress their own emotional reactions in order to keep functioning for the family; children may stifle their feelings and needs so as not to burden parents. When emotions are intense or family members are overwhelmed by a pileup of stressors, conflict is likely to erupt and spiral out of control. Clinicians can offer a safe haven to share and process difficult feelings.

Masculine stereotypes of strength often constrain men from showing fear, vulnerability, or sadness, increasing the risk of substance abuse, destructive behaviors, conflict, or withdrawal. For relational resilience, couples and families can be encouraged to share their feelings and comfort one another. Finding pleasure and moments of humor in the midst of pain can offer respite and lift spirits.

Collaborative Problem Solving

Creative brainstorming and resourcefulness open new possibilities for surmounting adversity and for healing and growth out of tragedy. Therapists can facilitate shared decision making and conflict resolution through negotiation, with fairness and reciprocity over time. We can encourage families' efforts to set clear, attainable goals and take concrete steps toward them. We can help them build on small successes and use failures as learning experiences. When dreams have been shattered, we can encourage them to survey the altered landscape and seize opportunities for growth in new directions.

To meet future challenges, we can help families shift from a crisis-reactive mode to a proactive stance, to strive toward aims and also anticipate, prepare for, and avert problems and crises. Encouraging them to have a "Plan B" aids resourcefulness when met by unforeseen challenges.

Synergistic Influences of Key Processes in Resilience

These keys to resilience are mutually interactive and synergistic. For example, a relational view of resilience (belief system) fosters connectedness (organizational patterns), as well as open emotional sharing and collaborative problem solving (communication processes). A core belief that problems can be mastered both facilitates and is reinforced by successful problem-solving strategies. A counterbalance of processes is also important, as in the fluid shifts between stability and flexibility required for both continuity and change through disruptive challenges.

Various approaches to family therapy have emphasized processes in different domains (Sluzki, 1983). For instance, the structural model attends primarily to organizational patterns; cognitive-behavioral approaches address belief systems and communication processes; and postmodern approaches focus on the social construction of meaning. In practice, most family therapists are attentive to processes across the three domains. Professionals of diverse theoretical orientations can foster these key processes for resilience.

A family resilience framework provides a flexible map for assessment and intervention, allowing us to identify and target core processes in effective family functioning (Chapters 3–5) while also keeping a contextual view and recognizing the viability of many different pathways in resilience. Resilience requires varied strengths and strategies to fit the demands of particular adverse situations over time, from a single crisis event to multiple stresses and prolonged challenges (as illustrated in Chapters 8–11). The processes in healing from shattering loss are very different from those needed to cope effectively with a chronic condition, such as illness or poverty, over time and require a practice approach attuned to each situation.

An ecological–developmental perspective is essential to assess functioning in both social and temporal contexts (see Table 6.2). It is crucial to assess family strengths and vulnerabilities in relation to each family's particular socioeconomic situation and developmental priorities. We must always be mindful that key processes may be organized and expressed in varied ways, depending on diverse cultural values and family structures. For example, open emotional expression varies with different ethnic norms. Roles and boundaries that work best for an intact family may differ from those needed for an effective single-parent household with extended family involvement, or for a stepfamily spanning two or more households. The key processes in resilience can be applied to diverse situations and through varied adaptational pathways as they fit family challenges, resources, and aims.

A family resilience approach requires an evolving view of family challenges and responses over time, rather than a cross-sectional view at one point in time. To meet the demands of different phases of adaptation, we need to help families draw upon the varied strengths needed to approach an impending crisis proactively, to manage disruption during the crisis period, to rebound in the immediate aftermath, and, where necessary, to reorganize and rebuild their lives over the long term. With an acute crisis, families need to rally their resources but may be able to resume "normal" life. Recurrent or persistent stresses pose different

TABLE 6.2. Family Resilience: Framework for Practice

- Relational view of human resilience
- Shift from deficit view of families
  - From damaged to challenged by adversity, with potential for repair and growth
- Grounded in developmental systemic perspective
  - Biopsychosocial–spiritual influences
- Crisis events impact family system; family response influences
- Recovery of all members, relationships, and family unit
- Contextual view of crisis, symptoms of distress, and adaptation
  - Family and sociocultural influences
  - Temporal influences
    - Timing of symptoms and family crisis events
    - Pileup of stressors, persistent adversity
    - Varying adaptational challenges over time
    - Individual and family developmental phases
    - Anniversary, multigenerational patterns

psychosocial challenges over time. Some situations require families to re-peatedly shift gears over a roller-coaster course, while others challenge families to adapt to progressive decline. The challenges of adversity in-teract with emerging issues in both individual and family developmental passages. They are strongly influenced by past experiences with adver-sity in the multigenerational family network. A holistic assessment of each family aims to clarify members' challenges, resources, and con-straints, and to understand their past experiences and their future hopes and dreams.

CORE PRINCIPLES FOR
STRENGTHENING FAMILY RESILIENCE

A family resilience approach has much in common with many competence-based family therapy approaches: emphasizing a collaborative process and seeking to identify and build on strengths and resources. This ap-proach builds on these developments to strengthen families challenged by adversity. It links symptoms of distress with distressful events and contexts. It focuses therapeutic efforts to enhance coping, mastery, and growth out of those challenges.

A basic premise guiding this systems-based approach is that serious crises have an impact on the whole family, and that, in turn, family coping processes influence the recovery and resilience of all members and the family as a unit. How a family confronts and manages a disruptive experience, buffers stress, effectively reorganizes, and reinvests in life pursuits will influence adaptation for all members. Interventions aim to build family resources to deal more effectively with stresses and to rebound strengthened, both individually and as a relational system. Fostering the family's ability to master its immediate crisis situation also increases its capacity to meet future challenges.

To promote resilience in vulnerable children and families, Rutter (1987) has identified four general protective mechanisms that can be strengthened through interventions. Applying his schema to family systems, we can specify the ways in which key processes in family resilience can be mobilized:

1. Decrease risk factors.
   • Anticipate and prepare for threatening circumstances.
   • Reduce exposure or overload of stress.
   • Provide information; alter catastrophic beliefs.
2. Reduce negative chain reactions that heighten risk for sustained impact and further crises.
   • Buffer stress effects; cushion impact, overcome obstacles.
   • Alter maladaptive coping strategies.
   • Withstand aftershocks, prolonged strains; rebound from setbacks.
3. Strengthen protective family processes and reduce vulnerabilities.
   • Enhance family strengths; increase opportunities and abilities for success.
   • Mobilize and shore up resources toward recovery and mastery.
   • Rebuild, reorganize, and reorient in aftermath.
   • Anticipate, prepare for both likely and unforeseen new challenges.
4. Bolster family and individual pride and efficacy through successful problem mastery.
   • Gain competence, confidence, and connectedness through collaborative efforts.
   • Manage challenges over time for sustained competence under duress.

Clinicians should inquire routinely about recent and anticipated change events, the family's response (or approach), and their impact, noting complications that pose risks for immediate or long-term dysfunction. Therapeutic efforts should be attuned to each family's challenges and resources that can be mobilized to meet them. We can help families assess their crisis situation and identify ways to reduce risks rendering challenges less threatening and more manageable. For instance, parents and other caregivers can be helped to provide leadership, guidance, nurturance, and protection in the face of disruption or loss. In anticipation of a crisis, through its midst, and in its aftermath, our aim is to strengthen key interactional processes to foster coping, recovery, and resilience, enabling the family and its members to integrate their experience and move forward in life.

Tracking Stressors and Adaptational Processes over Time

In all clinical assessment, a timeline is essential to track presenting symptoms in relation to past, ongoing, and threatened stress events, their meanings, and family coping strategies. Families don't simply react to stressful life events; their approach to potential stressors can either buffer or intensify their impact. Did members notice and discuss potential threats looming on the horizon? How effectively did they mobilize resources to head off a crisis or lessen its impact? Strains can be compounded by catastrophic fears and maladaptive coping processes, which can contribute to individual and relational distress. Often family members and professionals become so focused on presenting symptoms that they may not connect them to stressors on the system, as in the following case:

> Over the past month, Jimmy, age 12, had been frequently absent from school and dropped to failing grades. School authorities presumed that he was out in the streets and that the family, like many in their inner-city neighborhood, was either uncaring or unstable when no one responded to notes sent home. When a family counselor visited their apartment to assess the situation, she learned that Jimmy and his three siblings lived with their grandmother—their legal guardian since their mother's sudden death 4 years earlier. The grandmother had been hospitalized recently with a serious liver disease; although she was now at home, she required kidney dialysis several times a week. Jimmy, who had been very close to his mother, was now extremely anxious that he might also lose his grandmother. He was missing school to watch over her. Moreover, all were aware that the burden of

responsibility for four children added risk for the grandmother's fragile health. No one talked about the grandmother's condition, about the threat of another loss and dislocation for the children, or about what arrangements could be made for their care in the event of her further disability or death. As Jimmy said, "It was all just too scary to talk about."

In terms of Rutter's (1987) model, several steps were required in helping Jimmy and the entire family with their crisis situation. Most immediately, the counselor needed to decrease the risk factors, reduce negative chain reactions, and shore up resources for both the grandmother's care and the children's care. The grandmother's husband, who had never been involved in the children's care, was encouraged to take a more active role with them to relieve the burden on his wife. A maternal aunt was recruited to take the children out for a movie or to run errands together on weekends, while appreciating her limited availability due to her own job and child care responsibilities. The children's father, who had been out of contact since their mother's death because of a long-standing conflict with the grandmother, was contacted to assess his ability and desire to assume an active role with his children, and encouraged to put old grievances aside and to become more involved in raising his children. He surprised everyone by rallying to this challenge; he had longed for more contact with his children, but had held back until called upon in this crisis. Additional resources were found in an after-school tutoring program for Jimmy, currently the most vulnerable child. As the immediate stress was reduced, with family members managing more effectively and benefiting from new and strengthened relationships, attention could then be directed to address the family's future concerns and options for the children's residence and care. Heightened concerns about losing their grandmother due to her poor health, along with loss issues from the mother's death, were also addressed.

This case illustrates how resilience-based intervention taps into the three domains of family functioning: meaning and mastery of the crisis; reorganization of family structural patterns; and development of effective communication and problem-solving strategies. Most serious life crises aren't limited to a single moment in time, but involve a complex set of changing conditions with a past history and a future course (Rutter, 1987). Thus, efforts to strengthen resilience must attend to coping and adaptation processes over time.

We need to pay particular attention to the cumulative impact of a pileup of stressors, as in the following case:

Mike and Maggie, on the verge of divorce, were seen for a marital evaluation. The couple's conflicts had escalated over the past 3 years, with increasing volatility and recent violence. When they first sought help, Mike had moved out of the house, due to concerns for his wife's safety and attended a group for men who batter. Maggie was referred to a women's group, where she was encouraged to leave the marriage, even though no couple assessment or intervention had yet been attempted. The couple had four young children, and, with the violence under control, they requested couple consultation to see if they could salvage their marriage and keep their family intact.

As a consultant, I tracked recent patterns in the family, finding that the onset and escalation of violence had occurred in the context of a pileup of crisis events and major losses, beginning with the sudden death of Mike's brother, with whom he'd always had a stormy relationship. Overcome with grief, his father had a stroke. Maggie's mother, who had been a mainstay in helping with childcare, broke her hip, requiring Maggie's caregiving. With the local economy faltering, Mike's small business, which he had run with his father and brother, failed, and they feared losing their mortgage. To add to pressures, Maggie found she was pregnant again. Shortly thereafter, Mike lost control while driving and wrecked the family car, with the entire family barely escaping serious injury.

Mike had never mentioned this traumatic chain of events in his men's group, which focused on behavior control. He couldn't recall ever letting out his feelings to anyone, including Maggie, who had turned to her sisters for support. She noted that this was the first time they had ever talked openly about all that had happened, or had put it all together. After each event they had just tried to keep on going, although they were reeling under the series of shockwaves and the pressures of attending to the needs of four young children, as well as worries about their precarious finances. In Mike's words, he felt "assaulted"—bombarded from all sides by events beyond his control. Once they took stock of these events, they were able to make meaning of the strain on their relationship, their frayed emotions, and Mike's assaultive outbursts. It was crucial that in normalizing and contextualizing the distress, the therapist not normalize violence as an acceptable response. Work on communication skills was important to prevent a recurrence of violence; yet that focus alone was insufficient without attending to the crucible in which the violence had flared up. When Mike and Maggie were encouraged in couple therapy to share their feelings about their many losses and to comfort each other, they were able to pull together to heal emotionally and rebound to meet their family challenges.

As in the cases above, resilience-oriented assessment involves a series of questions to assess both risk and protective variables. A genogram and timeline are essential tools in noting the following:

- Recent—and threatened—stress events and their meaning.
- Pileup of stressors.
- Loading from past experiences: success or complications with similar stressors.
- Family coping processes and potential resources.

Making Meaning of Crisis Experiences

It is crucial to explore the meanings a crisis holds for a family, and to be careful not to make assumptions based on our own experience or concerns. We might ask: "What stood out for you as most challenging or upsetting in the crisis situation? What was the impact on the family? How did you try to deal with the challenges?" Such inquiry acknowledges the unique experience of each family and the subjective views of various members on what is most meaningful, troubling, or remarkable (Wright et al., 1996). It's especially important to coach families to help children and vulnerable members make sense of a crisis or threat and to provide reassurance that they will be cared for. Family members do best when they understand more fully what's happening, how it came about, the future implications, and what steps they can take to adapt best. Resilience is fostered as we help them gain a sense of coherence, rendering their crisis experience more comprehensible, manageable, and meaningful.

Compassionate Witnessing: Stories of Adversity, Suffering, and Struggle

As family members grapple to make meaning and come to terms with their challenges, we need to be fully present and listen openheartedly to their accounts of their experience and assure them that we can bear their pain and suffering and provide a safe context to contain and process intense feelings. In approaching the suffering of others, we need to be comfortable with the strong emotions that may be stirred in us. When pain and suffering are expressed, tears may come to my eyes. It can be helpful for family members to see that in human encounters there is no shame in expressing vulnerable feelings or need to keep them locked away under control. At the same time, if strong emotions are conveyed in hurtful ways to others or conflict threatens to spiral out of control, it is our responsibility as therapists to interrupt negative transactions and try to help family members find more constructive ways to express their pain and needs as we encourage empathic support of other family members.

Clarifying Ambiguity

It is important to facilitate family members' clarification of their situation: what they have been told by whom, and what they each believe. Often family members hold quite different perceptions and assumptions. In one family, heated conflict erupted over concern about the mother's medical condition. She had been diagnosed with lupus, but little information had been given to her or the family about her prognosis or what might be done to best manage her chronic illness. Some family members worried that she was working too hard and that it would kill her; others thought she was doing too little and playing on everyone's sympathies. Amid all the bickering, she finally took to her bed—fearful and unsure about what to do, and feeling unsupported by her family.

Helping family members to gain information eases anxieties and helps them to adapt. We can encourage them to actively pursue and share information, and can coach them on locating reliable sources, such as medical or public records, news articles, and reputable Internet sites. We can coach members to press medical professionals to help them sort out complicated or conflicting information about illnesses or disabilities, and convene a family consultation to clarify management guidelines. We can also encourage clients to seek out information to bring greater clarity to past traumatic experiences, as in the following case:

Dennis was having recurrent nightmares about the death of his brother Al ten years earlier in a car crash. He now worried constantly about the safety of his own son—named after Al—and imagined every sort of traffic accident. The circumstances of Al's death were ambiguous; his parents had arranged a closed-casket funeral, and afterward no one in his family had wanted to talk about it. As we worked together, I encouraged Dennis to locate a friend of his brother's who had been in the car and had survived the accident. At first he was pessimistic about finding him, saying it was "like a needle in a haystack," but I urged him to ask relatives and friends and he managed to reach the friend within a few weeks. The friend was open and informative: Their buddy driving the car had been drinking and swerved out of control, striking a tree. Al had died instantly of a skull fracture. It brought some solace for Dennis to learn that his brother had not lain helpless in pain before dying. Having a clearer comprehension of the accident helped Dennis gain greater peace of mind. It also reduced his global anxiety that "anything could happen at any time" to his son. Drawing lessons from the incident, he took more realistic precautions himself, and he taught his son never to mix drinking and driving.

Normalizing, Depathologizing, and Contextualizing Distress

A normalizing orientation heightens our appreciation of each family's unique set of experiences and beliefs, as well as commonalities with other families in similar life circumstances. We offer information and new perspectives to see individual symptoms, strained relationships, or breakdown in family processes as understandable and common under the stressful circumstances the family is undergoing.

Parents often feel deficient when they have a problem they are unable to resolve. Often they are referred for family therapy because they are told (or it is implied) that the family is the real problem. Often the symptomatic family member responds wonderfully to the therapist/ expert and only displays the problem behavior in family transactions. The therapist's immediate success reinforces parental feelings of deficiency. They may leave the session feeling worse than when they arrived. Blame and shame can lead them not to return; they may then be written off as dysfunctional and resistant.

In a culture that readily pathologizes families and touts the virtues of self-reliance, family members often approach therapy feeling abnormal for having a problem and deficient for not resolving it on their own. The confusing changes and pressures in family life today compound such beliefs. Furthermore, referrals for family therapy are often based on the faulty presumption that the family is the cause of any individual distress, or that such distress must serve a function for them.

A fundamental tenet of strength-based approaches to family therapy is that most families do not seek suffering or intend harm to their members. Most parents want desperately to do the best for their children, but they may need help finding viable solutions to their distress. It is crucial to explore any blaming and stigmatizing experiences families may have had in contacts with other mental health professionals, schools, or courts. Families then expect therapists to judge them negatively and may mistake a silent or neutral stance for confirmation of that view. We need to disengage assumptions of pathology from the rationale for involvement in therapy and make it clear that we regard family members as essential resources in problem solving.

The aim of normalizing is to depathologize and contextualize family distress. It is not intended to reduce all problems and families to a common denominator, and it should never trivialize a family's unique experience or suffering. We must be careful neither to oversimplify the complexity of family life nor to err by normalizing truly destructive family patterns. Violence and sexual abuse should never be normalized as acceptable, even though they are all too common. Likewise, respect for diversity is not the same as "anything goes" when family processes are destructive to any member. Family therapists have moved beyond the myth of therapeutic neutrality to address serious ethical concerns and therapeutic responsibility.

Using Respectful Language and Constructs

Effective intervention requires learning the language and perspective of each family, in order to see problems through its members' eyes—to understand the values and expectations that influence their approach to handling the problem or their inability to change. Narrative therapists have heightened our awareness of the power of words: they may reflect pessimism and foster blame, shame, guilt, and failure; or they can express hope, pride, and confidence about ability and potential.

Increasingly, for families' costs for therapeutic services to be even partially covered by third-party payment, an individual member is labeled with a psychiatric diagnosis fitting categories in the DSM-IV. While family resilience–oriented practice is grounded in a biopsychosocial orientation, we find it most useful to broaden our understanding of problems in relation to transactional processes, stressful events, and contextual influences. Systemic descriptions focused toward solutions open up more possibilities for change. We eschew demeaning labels for persons (e.g., "she's a borderline") and pejorative assumptions about "dysfunctional families" (see Chapters 9 and 10). Because the very language of therapy can pathologize a family, we take great care in framing problems, questions, and responses in a way that is respectful of distressed individuals and their families.

Reframing and Relabeling

Through such techniques as reframing and relabeling, a problem situation can be redefined in order to cast it in a new light and to shift a family's rigid view or response. In the early days of family therapy, strategic therapists used techniques such as paradoxical intention as clever tactics to outwit families (Nichols & Schwartz, 2005). When used genuinely and respectfully, reframing techniques, such as positive connotation, can help to alter a destructive or blaming process, overcome impasses to change, and generate hope. Problems can be depathologized when viewed as normative, expectable, transitional stresses. Symptomatic behavior can be viewed as a survival strategy—an attempt to live with an unbearable situation or to prevent a feared outcome. We note the helpful intentions, albeit misguided ways, of caring members trying to help one another.

Reframing distress contextually helps clients view themselves, their problems, and their strengths in a more positive and hopeful light. Symptoms of acute traumatic stress are normal responses to abnormal, traumatic events (see Chapter 11). A problem presented as "inside" an individual, such as a character trait, may be redefined behaviorally in context. For example, a label of "controlling personality" may be recast in terms of a mother's tenacity in her struggle to get an unresponsive school system to provide needed services for her child with serious learning disabilities. In a vicious cycle, the more she complains, the less responsive the school becomes, viewing her as the problem. By recasting the set (Watzlawick et al., 1967), the mother's efforts are validated and more effective dialogues can be facilitated.

Narrative reauthoring serves as a means through language and perspective to reframe problem situations—to present them in more empowering terms that facilitate problem resolution (Freedman & Combs, 1996). In Michael White's technique of externalization (White & Epston, 1990), the therapist recasts a problem (often a child's problem) as an external force that is responsible for wreaking havoc in family members' lives. The therapist aligns with the child and family as partners who together will defeat this negative force, leaving the child and family feeling victorious. Clinicians must be mindful that an attitude adjustment may not be enough to surmount overwhelming obstacles; knowledge, skills, and opportunities to succeed are also required.

Instilling Hope and Optimism

While being empathic with the suffering of our clients, we must also instill hope and optimism that they can triumph over their adversities. For example, I may say,

"I understand that you're experiencing a lot of pain and conflict right now. I'm also convinced that you have many strengths as a family. I believe that beneath the pain and upset, you care deeply about each other. One sign of that caring is that you all made an effort to come in and meet to solve your problems. I'm quite hopeful that if you will work together on these issues, you have strong potential to make things better. I'll be glad to work with you, to support your best efforts."

When clients have lost hope to global pessimism, we might ask: "Has there ever been a time when you felt more hopeful about your situation? What was different then? Who was most helpful? How?" "How might you harness that positive energy now?" Conversations can explore what might be learned and applied to the present dilemma, as well as what they imagine could help them regain hope. What might their partner, parents, or others say or do that might reinvigorate them? Often one spouse or partner will turn to the other and say, "I just need you to hold me and tell me you love me. That will keep me going through this crisis." A family bear hug at the end of a session can bolster an overwhelmed parent. One of my students told a beleaguered family that he understood how it was hard for members to feel hopeful at that moment, but that he firmly believed that they would weather their crisis and had enough hope for all of them. He told them, "Let me lend you some of my hope until you regain yours."

Refocusing from Complaints to Aims

Distressed couples and families can become caught up in a vicious cycle of negativity, focused on each other's deficiencies and constantly finding fault. Despite our inclinations to support the underdog and to interrupt scapegoating, therapists must be cautious not to adopt a critical stance toward a critical parent or spouse; this only reinforces cycles of blame and widens the sense of deficiency. Asking a parent, "Why are you so hard on your child?" or commenting to a wife, "It seems like you can't see anything good in your husband," only criticizes them for being critical. Instead, it's important to understand the stress, pain, and frustrations underlying such criticisms, and to help family members refocus from complaints (what's wrong) to positive aims (what would be better) and how they might achieve them. What would improve an unbearable situation? How would a couple's relationship need to change for the better for a spouse on the edge of divorce to reinvest? What would a more satisfying family life look like? What changes would they need to make to achieve it? What commonalities can help them to bridge their differences?

After hearing family members' complaints in an assessment interview, it's important to ask what they hope to *gain* through counseling. We shouldn't assume that the desired change is simply solving presenting problems or reducing distress. I'm frequently surprised, as I was in this case:

> In a family evaluation, the parents, Manny and Sylvia, presented a tirade of complaints about their son's troublesome behavior. After listening to their descriptions of frustrating, unsuccessful attempts to deal with the situation, I asked what they most hoped to gain in our work together, expecting to hear that the son should shape up. Instead, Manny replied, his voice choked up: "I'd like to learn how to show love to my kids." When I asked to hear more about that, Manny responded, "My dad had a temper—he only knew how to yell." I asked what that had been like for him as a kid, and noticed how attentive the children were, realizing that he had felt as bad as they did with him now. When asked what that experience had taught him, he said, "I don't know any other way, but I'd like to do better by my kids."

Here again, in linking past experience with present distress, a future vision can become a positive force to break destructive patterns and achieve healthier relationships.

Identifying, Affirming, and Building Strengths

All competence-based approaches are, at their core, about bringing out the best in people (Waters & Lawrence, 1993). A stance that sees and appreciates their best helps them to do their best. We can affirm strengths by finding something worthy to commend about each family member. Although no family is strong in every area, all families possess strengths and resources. Amid very real limitations, we can foster resilience by noticing members' assets and potentials, and by finding ways to nurture and praise their positive intentions, efforts, and achievements. They may believe that they are drowning in an ocean of inadequacy, but everyone has "islands of competence" that are, or could be, sources of pride and accomplishment (Brooks, 1994).

Overcoming Culture-Based Gender Barriers

Women are more likely to seek professional help, to acknowledge distress, and to assume responsibility when problems arise in the family. Professionals often need to work harder to engage men in therapy, because myths of masculinity cast vulnerability and need for help as signs of weakness and inadequacy. We can encourage men's involvement by tapping into their desire to be responsible and loving spouses and parents and strong role models for their children. We can help couples to transcend traditional gendered role constraints and to develop creative new patterns that better fit their situations, needs, and preferences.

Therapists need to be sensitive to ethnic or religious values that uphold the role of fathers as head of the family while not sanctioning the denigration of women in the family. Men in traditional cultures are often more reluctant to come for therapy if they anticipate shaming experiences, especially in front of other family members. Resilience-oriented practice, because it is so respectful of clients, is more likely to successfully engage men. When we focus on their strengths and potential, in my experience, they are also more likely to acknowledge any faults, fears, and vulnerabilities and be open to positive change efforts.

Crediting Positive Intentions

Resilience-based approaches help family members to develop in ways that bring forth their deepest desires for mastery and belonging. I prefer to err on the side of assuming that members' intentions are positive, or at least benign, even when their actions may be ineffective or hurtful. For example, we can affirm a father's desire to be a better parent, aligning with his healthier core to help him gain control over his explosive temper. The assumption of a positive intent behind or alongside problematic behavior helps family members to become less defensive and more open, and to strive for their best.

Praising Efforts and Achievements

It's important to see families as struggling as well as they can with very difficult situations. Although disagreeing with an adolescent's mishandling of a risky situation, for instance, we might credit his astute observations of the predicament he faced and ask how he might draw on those insights if he faced another danger. It's important to note small, concrete examples of caring efforts and actions, such as making it to a session despite a snowstorm. In every session, alongside problem solving, we must make sure to ask how new endeavors are going (e.g., a teen parent's job training program) and to applaud progress. Every family member has some talent or special interest to express; we can let them know we care about their lives and pursuits beyond their problems. The praise offered must be genuine and connected to their words and deeds. Empty praise will only ring hollow.

Wherever possible, we can try to shift a vicious cycle to a virtuous cycle. For example, even though a teen mother at times loses control or lashes out at a child, I may share my observation of other signs that she loves the child and has the capacity to be nurturing. I may praise the parenting skills and bonds I observe in a session, such as tenderness in cradling her infant, and point out how responsive the baby is to her loving care. She may initially respond with disbelief ("I am? She is? Really?") and then caress the child, who then breaks into a smile. So often family members comment that coming to sessions has helped them realize they're really not as bad off as they thought.

We can honor the relational base of resilience as we celebrate individual success. I once gave a long-stemmed rose to a single mother on the occasion of her daughter's graduation from college, to honor her important contribution to her child's success. Another time, I took a photo of beaming immigrant parents and their son, holding up his GED certificate. At the end of therapy, I gave the parents and son each a framed copy of the photo, so that they could always keep in mind—in good and bad times—the son's hard-won achievement and the parents' pride and love.

Drawing Out Hidden Resources and Lost Competence

When families are in distress, their view becomes problem-saturated. They most often seek help when they have reached an impasse, coping and problem-solving efforts are exhausted, and they feel overwhelmed and inadequate. Their abilities to solve their problems may be hidden, inaccessible, or forgotten. Family members benefit from therapeutic conversations that bring into awareness untapped resources or strengths to which they have become blinded. We can help them to regain lost competence and to recognize loving concern that may be overshadowed by their current distress. Solution-focused and narrative therapists search for *exceptions* to a problem situation—positive interactions or abilities shown at other times or in other parts of their lives that can be drawn upon now (Freedman & Combs, 1996). For instance, asking spouses about their ways of finding pleasure together before troubles arose can help to rekindle lost intimacy or bring to the foreground positive aspects of their lives that may have been trampled on by persistent adversity.

Highlighting Strengths in the Midst of Adversity

Even more valuable than finding positive exceptions *apart from* presenting problems, a family resilience approach highlights strengths *in the midst of* adversity. For example, we might commend family members' perseverance in struggling to overcome a financial setback or their courage in rebuilding their lives after a shattering loss.

Adversity can bring out the best in family members. Yet, in distress, they may not see or access these strengths. By highlighting them, we help families to recognize their own resources and potential; in doing so, we increase their confidence that they can draw on these strengths if future need arises. As we support their efforts to manage a crisis well, family members often discover resources they never knew they had and forge new areas of competence. A husband may develop new tenderness in caring for his wife after her serious accident. A father who may have been uninvolved with his children can learn new parenting skills and achieve closer ties when forced to manage on his own as a single parent. We search for strengths in the worst of times, striving for meaning making and mastery.

Ray and Barbara sought help for intense conflict in the seventh month of her second pregnancy. The therapist's attempts to refocus on happier times and future visions for the new baby fell flat. As a consultant, I explored the meaning of this pregnancy. I learned that Ray and Barbara had lost their first child shortly after birth and now were fearful that the worst would happen again. They tried to push that experience out of their minds and avoided talking about it. Yet they were quite anxious and found themselves arguing over plans for the baby's room. I asked them to share their memories of the first pregnancy—from their initial hopes and dreams, their preparations, and the anticipatory joy of family and friends to the unexpected, shattering loss on what should have been their happiest day. The tears came anew as they recounted the details of the birth, the hushed voices of the medical staff in the delivery room, and their utter devastation in learning that the baby was anencephalic and would not survive. In the wake of that loss, each partner had tried to process the events and their grief separately, but they had never looked back together or shared their pain. Well-meaning friends told them to put it behind them and move on—a faulty approach to resilience. Now Ray and Barbara found themselves hesitant to share feelings or invest in plans for the child soon to arrive.

Acknowledging their sorrow, I shared my admiration for their love and their courage in trying anew for a much-desired child and encouraged their mutual support for the weeks ahead to the birth. We also discussed how they might communicate their wishes and needs to friends and family members, who in their anxiety either distanced or hovered nervously around them.

Their contacts with health care professionals were also explored. Much of their anxiety came from ambiguous generalities from their doctors, who said that "there was nothing to worry about" this time. They were encouraged to meet with a genetic counselor together to gain fuller comprehension. Worried that in their high anxiety they might not ask all the questions on their minds, or clearly understand the responses, they decided to write down questions in advance and take a tape recorder. It was clarified that the new baby's fetal development was normal and that future children were at no higher risk than normal. In more fully sharing and integrating their past crisis with their current concerns, Ray and Barbara approached the impending birth joyfully.

Helping Families Live with Uncertainty

Many families need help in living with uncertainty. When recent or past events remain murky, we can help family members to clarify as much as possible about the situation and find a way to live with persisting ambiguity. In many cases, we need to help a family cope with uncertainty in the future course and outcome of a threatening situation, such as the loss of their home due to job and financial insecurity. Counselors will increasingly be called upon to help family members grapple with life decisions, such as childbearing, when they undergo genetic testing and learn that they carry risk for a genetically influenced condition that poses high risk for disability and/or early mortality but the probability and the timing of onset and progression of the illness can not be predicted (Rolland & Williams, 2005).

In many instances, family members may be helped to come to terms with a serious situation beyond their comprehension, clarity, and control by drawing on their spiritual resources to find a sense of purpose, comfort, and solace. Exploring faith beliefs and practices should become part of all efforts to help families dealing with adversity.

Seizing Opportunities in the Midst of Crisis

As therapists and families work to solve presenting problems, we can seize opportunities for personal and relational growth out of the crisis that brings them for help. We can help clients cast their crisis situation in a new light that opens possibilities. When facing a crisis, it's helpful to look back to past family experiences with adversity, for lessons that can be drawn about both helpful and unhelpful responses. In the aftermath of a crisis, we can help family members explore what can be learned from their situation. There may be important lessons about risk and vulnerability, or about the need to anticipate pitfalls and take more precautions in the future. In building resilience, we help families strive to integrate the fullness of their crisis and recovery experience.

Often something valuable is gained from a crisis that might not have been learned or achieved otherwise. Adversity may bring a startling recognition of the importance of relationships that had been taken for granted or written off. A crisis can lead family members to question, review, and redirect their lives. A disruptive family relocation can also be a milestone for taking time out to reassess life and relationship priorities, or to affirm and strengthen commitments. A woman who had oriented her life around her husband was devastated when he left her. Therapy facilitated her life transformation from an initial sense of emptiness to the development of new talents and confidence in her own identity and ability to lead a fulfilling life on her own. We can open these pathways to growth out of shattering loss.

Building Empathic Connections

We work with families most effectively when we build empathic connections with members and between them. Often therapists find it hard to be empathic with a family member who has been neglectful or is abrasive. Yet a mother's hard edge, for instance, might be seen in terms of the feistiness she developed in order to keep her family afloat through tough times and her ex-partner's bouts of drinking. We can identify with her hard struggle as a single parent and applaud the fact that, given the obstacles she faces, she's managing much better than she's given credit for.

We can also help family members gain greater compassion for one another through asking them to share their life stories, the painful experiences they have suffered, and the sparks of resilience they have shown in weathering those ordeals. A mother who is resented for overprotecting her children can be seen in a new light—as wishing to spare them the harm that she herself endured in childhood sexual abuse. The confusion of a father who is at a loss in dealing with a teenager is clarified when he describes how his own father wasn't there for him; we can be empathic with the challenge of becoming a good parent without having had a good role model in his father. We might also ask who else in his family network had been a good father or surrogate, such as an uncle or grand-father, and explore their qualities that he might aspire toward. Viewing current dilemmas in the light of life experience can make them more un-derstandable, and flawed individuals, such as his father, can be seen, with compassion, as struggling as best they could.

The following case presented intergenerational tensions common in immigrant families.

Stavros brought his 17-year-old only son, Stavros, Jr., for therapy to "straighten him out." An immigrant, Stavros was furious that his son had left their church, was hanging around with "no-good" friends, and was on the verge of school dropout. Steve (as the son preferred to be called) sat respectfully quiet in the session, yet de-fended his friends and was obstinate that he didn't care about school or religion. Steve felt constantly pressured by his father to succeed academically and go to college to get a good job. He looked down on his father's work history of low pay and long hours, and felt badgered to make up for the father's "failure" in life.

I asked Stavros whether he had ever shared his full life story and the difficulties of immigration. In a hushed voice, he revealed that he felt ashamed of his humble beginnings in the United States and his poor English. Encouraged to tell his story, he described the brutal military regime that he had fled; he was forced to leave school at 17 with his brother to escape being drafted. Although he had excelled in school, when he arrived in this country he took the only work he could find, as a janitor, and added odd jobs in order to send money back to his aging parents. Like many immigrants, he realized that he would have to start from scratch and struggle for a living, but his determination was kept strong by his hope that his ef-forts would enable his children to have a better life. Things became even harder when Steve's mother died after a long illness, when the boy was 12. Spending nothing on himself, Stavros secretly put away a few dollars whenever he could for his son's college education. He was so proud to have such a smart son. How could Steve not care about his future?

Steve, although initially claiming lack of interest in his father's story, listened intently. His voice broke as he said he hadn't realized what his father had been up against, how much courage it had taken to do all he did, and how he had struggled for the sake of his parents and his son. Steve began to see his father not as a failure, but a hero. Moreover, he hadn't been aware of his father's pride in him; he had only felt his disapproval and disappointment. For his part, Steve needed his father to be more tolerant of his friends, activities, and beliefs, so different from the father's experiences and world view in the old country. Through their conversations over several sessions, and the therapist's reframing, Stavros was able to hear how Steve's differences were less a rejection of his father and more about seeking to find himself in another culture. Stavros reflected, sadly, that in demanding that Steve do everything *his* way, he had become no different from the military dictator he had fled. Father and son were helped to find a better balance. While coming of age, Steve still needed his father's encouragement and support in making his own choices for a good life. Cast in a new light, the very possibility of choice meant that Stavros had truly succeeded in his dream of a better life for his son. He had given him the gift of freedom.

In addressing Stavros's harsh and overbearing treatment of his son, it was crucial to learn (and to help his son to appreciate) how he came to that position, and to understand its protective function. I admired his concern for his son's future so that Steve would have a better opportunity for success in life. Reaching greater mutual understanding enabled him to be less controlling and more accepting of Steve's autonomous strivings. In turn, Steve became less likely to make bad choices for himself out of angry defiance. To foster family resilience in cases such as this one, it's essential to help members reach new understanding and esteem for one another.

Encouraging a Positive, Future-Oriented Focus

The poet Audre Lorde reflected, "When I dare to be powerful—to use my strength in the service of my vision, then it becomes less and less important whether I am afraid." People coming for help are often stuck in a vision of their lives that is narrow and joyless, filled with adversity, suffering, and fear. Approaching clients about their hopes and dreams encourages them to imagine a more satisfying future and seek to achieve it (Penn, 1985).

For instance, families approaching later life can be encouraged to consider and prepare together for such challenges as retirement, transitional living arrangements, and end-of-life decisions—discussions that are commonly avoided. Future-oriented questions can also open up new possibilities for later-life fulfillment. One son was concerned about how each of his parents would manage alone on the family farm if widowed, but he dreaded talking with them about their death. Finally, on a visit home, he got up his courage. First he asked his mother, tentatively, whether she had ever thought about what she might do if Dad were the first to go. She replied, "Sure; we've never talked about it, but I've thought about it for years. I'd sell the farm and move to Texas to be near our grandkids." Her husband scratched his head and replied, "Well, if that ain't the darndest thing! I've thought a lot about it too, and if your mother wasn't here, *I'd* sell the farm and move to Texas!" This conversation led the couple to make plans to sell the farm, which had become increasingly burdensome, and move to Texas, where they enjoyed many happy years.

In work with distressed couples and families, a positive, future-oriented focus shifts the emphasis of therapy from "What went wrong?" to "What can be done for enhanced functioning and well-being?" Together, we and our clients can then envision possible options that fit each family situation, and optimistic yet realistic aims that are reachable through shared, constructive efforts. This involves imagination, a hopeful outlook, and initiative in taking actions toward desired goals. A future-oriented focus is valuable even when a current crisis reactivates past traumatic experiences, as in the following case:

Joanne and Ralph were seen in family consultation after their 22-year-old son, Joey, had a serious drug overdose on the eve of his wedding. Asked how she felt about her son's leaving home and getting married, Joanne noted that it was harder for her than it had been with the other children, but she didn't know why. Consulting on the case, I asked whether Joey had been named after her (he had), and asked about her own experience of leaving home and getting married. Joanne told of running off to marry her husband against her father's strong objections. She had been furious at his opposition, and he, in turn, had refused to speak with her again. He died 6 months later of a heart attack without reconciliation. At this point in her story, Joanne became tearful and said, "Somehow it feels the same now."

It was crucial to inquire beyond the obvious dyadic relationship between Joanne and her father to explore other system patterns that might also be fueling current difficulties. Joanne had been very close to her mother, who, once widowed, spent the rest of her life depressed and lonely. When I asked her whether she ever worried that history might repeat itself, Joanne admitted that she worried about her husband's health and his disregard of his overweight condition. In recent months he had complained of chest pains, but had refused to see a doctor. Joey's leaving aroused her fear that something terrible would happen to Ralph and she would end up like her mother.

With Joanne's catastrophic expectations and lacking a model for later-life marriage (Ralph's mother had also been widowed), she and Ralph had never discussed any dreams or plans for their future together after launching their children. Brief couple therapy focused on exploring their future possibilities. Ralph had a medical workup and started to take better care of himself. They celebrated their son's wedding and then spontaneously took a "refresher honeymoon" on their own.

In helping a family to move forward, it's important to make overt the covert connections between the past, present, and future so that family members can understand current distress and integrate their experiences. They can't change the past, but we can help them learn from it to chart a better future course.

Accepting Human Limitations

The Navaho say that the way to tell that a rug has been made by human hands is by its flaws. As helping professionals, we can cultivate acceptance of imperfections within families—as well as acceptance of our own limitations—by viewing flaws not as defects, but instead as part of being human. If a family member has been wounded by life struggles, we need to diminish blame and shame and, instead, foster compassion.

Our therapeutic approach is based on the belief that mistakes and failures are normal aspects of life and can be expected in efforts to succeed, especially under stressful conditions. We can help family members to own errors and to view them as valuable learning experiences, rather than as demoralizing defeats. It's useful, in whatever ways possible, to attribute mistakes to factors that members can change, such as insufficient effort or an unrealistic goal, rather than to innate deficits that can't be modified. This is most challenging, yet essential, when families have experienced many crises or chronic difficulties and have come to feel beaten down by repeated adversity.

Involving Families in Recovery from Individual Trauma

Even when a crisis strikes an individual and other family members are not directly touched by the event, a systemic approach considers how all are affected by it and how the family response influences recovery. Other members may not currently be showing symptoms of distress, but may hold hidden concerns and be at heightened risk for later problems. A family resilience approach draws members together for mutual support and healing. All can benefit from family interventions and become better resources for one another.

> Heather, a high school freshman, had been raped by a 17-year-old football player at an unsupervised party. Her family, wanting to help her recover, arranged for her to have individual therapy. At home, they said nothing about the incident so as to not upset her, even though it preoccupied their thoughts. They tried to lift her spirits by being cheerful and acting "normal" as if nothing bad had happened. Her therapist was very caring, yet after two months she remained withdrawn from family and friends and took a handful of Valium in a suicide attempt. Heather had misinterpreted her family's silence and forced cheer as covering over condemnation of her. She believed that her family members were being "phony" and were really talking about her behind her back, thinking she had invited the rape and was the one at fault.
>
> A family session was held, where Heather's parents revealed deep concern for her well-being and regret that they hadn't known how to show their support. None of her family members blamed her for the assault; instead, they blamed themselves and each other. Her parents fought over the decision to let her go to the party. Her older brother Brian felt especially guilty, because he knew the boy's bad reputation and felt he should have protected his sister. Other concerns surfaced as well: Heather's 11-year-old sister silently worried that it could happen to her; could boys and friends be trusted?
>
> A relational resilience approach brought a cascade of positive benefits. Heather's healing was facilitated by open, honest communication with her family. Also, the guilt, regret, and concerns of other family members could be addressed. Family members became better able to show their support; they mobilized to take action with Heather in filing sexual assault charges. Brian and Heather together organized a crisis hotline for any students feeling at risk in a social situation to call for a ride home. The parents organized a parents' association meeting at the school, where the family therapist and the school counselor were invited to discuss information about rape and the important roles family members can play in recovery and prevention. Families were encouraged to network better to ensure safety at social events. The initiatives generated by this crisis fostered a sense of empowerment and healing for Heather and her family, strengthening their bonds and sense of community.

Thus, even when an individual suffers a traumatic experience, the impact of the crisis reverberates through the network of relationships and affects others; in turn, the family can be essential in therapeutic efforts for healing. This case also illustrates two common findings in the resilience research. One key to resilience involves mastering the art of the possible: acknowledging what can't be changed (the assault that occurred) and putting efforts and actions into possible options (mobilizing to bring the assailant to justice and prevent future harm). A related key to resilience involves transcendence from personal tragedy and suffering to efforts to reduce future risk and prevent similar suffering for others. Further, the inspiration to organize a hotline is empowering as it benefits other teens in high-risk situations.

Encouraging Teamwork for Competence, Confidence, and Success

Just as negative interactions can have a destructive cascading effect, small successes build on one another in a ripple effect, increasing family members' confidence in their ability to master more difficult challenges. To foster family resilience, we need to create a therapeutic climate that maximizes the possibilities for members to be successful and to experience success as largely due to their shared efforts and abilities. These affirming beliefs and successful experiences generate realistic hope and optimism that through supporting one another, they can master their challenges.

Several guidelines are useful to strengthen family teamwork for competence, confidence, and success. First, we can encourage all members' responsibility and pride in their contribution to the process. We recognize their efforts and offer to facilitate more effective joint strategies for coping and problem solving. Second, it's important to help families initiate and follow through on concrete, achievable steps toward objectives, and to persevere when challenges loom as overwhelming and goals seem remote. As my colleague Carol Anderson tells families in her psychoeducational approach, "Yard by yard, it's just too hard; inch by inch, it's a cinch." Small successes can be sources of pride and accomplishment to build on, with increasing confidence and competence.

Second, it's crucial to attribute successes to family members, so they come to believe that their collaborative efforts can make a difference. As good coaches affirm after a winning game, the victory goes to the "team." As they become successful more of the time, they will come to believe that these shared efforts can make a difference, as in Seligman's "learned optimism" (see Chapter 3). Experiences of success in one arena of life enable enhanced coping with other life crises (Rutter, 1985). Foremost, throughout our efforts it's essential to convey our genuine caring for every family and our confidence in their abilities to master their challenges.

Pathways in Resilience

Families most often come for help in crisis. When they are overwhelmed and their presenting problems skew attention toward deficits, a resilience-based framework offers a positive and pragmatic focus for intervention. This approach normalizes distress as understandable in the context of a family's life challenges and it generates hope in the future while grounding changes in specific, reachable objectives. Table 6.3 summarizes major practice guidelines to strengthen family resilience.

In our work with families facing adversity, we must remember that resilience does not mean bouncing back instantaneously or always maintaining cheerful optimism and steady progress. Dealing with adversity may be a matter of taking three steps forward, two steps back—and then taking a breath and attempting to move forward again. Family members are bound to have times when they falter or need respite, when they take a wrong turn, or when they sink in despair. When family members experience setbacks, we need to encourage them to rebound, persist in their efforts, or seek a new pathway.

My colleague Carlos Sluzki once offered the metaphor of climbing a mountain to describe the therapeutic process. He noted that you don't

---

TABLE 6.3. Practice Guidelines to Strengthen Family Resilience

- Convey conviction in potential to overcome adversity through shared efforts.
- Use respectful language, framing to humanize and contextualize distress.
  - View as understandable, common in adverse situation (normal response to abnormal conditions).
  - Decrease shame, blame, pathologizing.
- Provide safe haven for sharing pain, fears, challenges.
  - Show compassion for suffering and struggle.
  - Build communication, empathy, support of members.
- Identify and affirm strengths, courage alongside vulnerabilities, constraints.
- Tap into kin, community, and spiritual resources to deal with challenges.
- View crisis as opportunity for learning, change, and growth.
- Shift focus from problems to possibilities.
  - Gain mastery, healing, and transformation out of adversity.
  - Rekindle, reorient future hopes and dreams.
- Integrate adverse experience into fabric of individual and relational lives.

go straight up to the top, but you make a plan that fits the contours of the mountain, the rigors of the climb, and your own skills. Much like a mountain road with hairpin turns, you choose an easy climb first to one side and then back across a little higher, forging a zigzag path ever closer to the summit. At each plateau, you gaze out over the horizon to appreciate the distance you've come. When rest and refueling are needed en route, you make a base camp where you gather strength for the next phase of the journey. Should the next stretch prove too arduous, you return to the base camp to regroup, and then try again, either on the same path or a new one. This image resonates with my experience of the therapeutic journey—and the journey we take in life. We may not reach the goal we first set out toward, and we may travel in unforeseen directions, forging new pathways. In any event, we can find meaning and joy in the journey and gain new perspective at each plateau we reach.

CHAPTER 7

A Family Resilience Framework for Community-Based Programs and Services

A hero is one who does the best of things
in the worst of times,
seizing every opportunity.
—JOSEPH CAMPBELL, *The Power of Myth*

This chapter describes the utility of a family resilience framework for community-based programs for intervention and prevention services. It also addresses the resilience needed by helping professionals to meet the demands of our challenging work and the profound changes occurring in our practice environment.

BROAD UTILITY OF A FAMILY RESILIENCE FRAMEWORK

Resilience-oriented practice facilitates the family's ability to rebound from crises and master life challenges, strengthened and more resourceful. This perspective can serve as a broad meta-framework for the training and practice of mental health, health care, social service, and pastoral care providers, and for the design and delivery of community-based programs.

164

A family resilience framework has broad utility for practice application in a wide range of adverse situations:

- Recover from crisis, trauma, loss.
- Navigate disruptive transitions (e.g., job loss, migration, separation/ divorce).
- Manage persistent stresses, master overwhelming challenges (e.g., multistressed families; serious illness, disability).
- Overcome barriers to success (e.g., at-risk youth, school dropout).
- "Bounce forward"—adapt to changing conditions, new challenges.

Family Resilience–Oriented Programs at the Chicago Center for Family Health

At the Chicago Center for Family Health (CCFH) (an affiliate of the University of Chicago that I cofounded and codirect with John Rolland, MD), over the past 15 years our faculty has developed a range of training, clinical, and community services grounded in this family resilience framework. Programs have been designed to address a wide range of crises and challenges, including:

- Serious illness, disability, end-of-life challenges.
- Family adaptation to loss.
- Major disaster and terrorist attacks; recovery and preparedness.
- Refugee and migration challenges.
- Divorce, single parenting, and stepfamily adaptation.
- Job loss, transition, and reemployment strains.
- Family–school partnerships for the success of at-risk youth.
- Challenges of stigma for gay and lesbian youth, couples, and families.

Many of these approaches are described in the following chapters, which address loss, chronic illness, multistressed families, major trauma and catastrophic events, and reconnection and reconciliation. One program illustration is offered here, focused on strengthening family resilience around major employment transitions.

Transitional Stresses of Job Loss and Employment

A family resilience–based service program was directed to the transitional adjustment of displaced workers whose jobs were lost due to factory closings or company downsizing. Our center designed and provided resilience-based support groups and counseling services in partnership with a community-based agency, Operation Able, that specializes in job retraining and placement services. Agency staff sought our approach because the ability of workers to rebound from job loss involved multiple transitional stresses in retraining and job search, and in their ability to gain, succeed at, and retain new employment. Job and income loss, as well as anxiety and uncertainty about reemployment success, often fueled depression, substance abuse, and both couple and family conflict. This pileup of stresses over many months, in turn, reduced the ability of family members to support worker efforts.

In one case, with the closing and relocation of a large clothing manufacturing plant, over 1,800 workers lost their jobs. Most were African American or Latino breadwinners for their families, many single parents, with limited education or skills for employment in the changing job market. Psychoeducational family workshops, ongoing support groups, and counseling addressed the personal and familial impact of losses and transitional stresses from a resilience perspective. This approach also addressed family strains and rallied family members as a resource to support the best efforts of the displaced worker. Group sessions focused on keys to resilience, such as identifying constraining beliefs (e.g., "No one will ever hire me") and shifting from preoccupation with deficits, such as lack of skills, limited education, and English language deficiencies of immigrants, to identify and affirm strengths, such as pride in doing a job well, and personal qualities of dependability and loyalty. The group offered support and encouragement to take initiative and persevere in job search efforts. When a group member didn't get a job or lost a position, he or she was supported to "bounce forward": to view it as a setback to be learned from and to redouble efforts to overcome obstacles and seize other opportunities. A "can do" spirit was contagious in the group process, turning a vicious cycle of hopelessness and despair to a virtuous cycle of hope and determination to succeed. Group members were both a cheering team and a sounding board. The ability to find humor in grim situations was uplifting, as was the genuine interest and respect shown to all members. Family impact and support issues were addressed and family members were welcome and encouraged to attend.

A similar resilience-based program was developed to address the adaptational challenges of single mothers in the Welfare-to-Work government program. Most of those mothers had to overcome vulnerabilities and multiple barriers to sustained employment, many involving their families and household. These mothers are too often seen through a deficit lens as unmotivated and underfunctioning, and too readily labeled as character disordered. In contrast, the resilience approach viewed these mothers as underresourced and overwhelmed by multiple crises and persistent stressors in all aspects of their lives. A family-centered approach took into account child care arrangements that must be managed around new employment demands. Counseling assisted them in mastering particular challenges associated with raising a special needs child, caring for disabled elders, stabilizing a chaotic household, or ending a troubled relationship with a boyfriend who heightened risks of substance abuse or violence. Potential kin and social supports, including religious/spiritual resources, were identified and tapped. The resilience-based orientation shifted mothers' outlooks from hopeless despair to affirm their strengths and potential. It encouraged their active initiative, perseverance, and mastery of the possible in their efforts to make a better life for themselves and their children.

International Research and Practice Initiatives

The concept of family resilience and its practice application have been drawing increasing attention in research, clinical services, and program design in many parts of the world. In 2005, I took part in an international congress on family resilience held in Zurich, Switzerland (Walsh in Welter-Enderlin, 2006). In Sweden, Cederblad, Hansson, and colleagues (Hansson, Olsson, & Cederblad, 2004) have been longtime pioneers in systems-based resilience research and "salutogenisis" (in contrast to pathogenesis); they currently design and evaluate resilience-oriented services for high-risk adolescents. In Canada, Michael Ungar, a systems-oriented researcher on resilience of at-risk adolescents, has developed an international network of researchers working on resilience-oriented practice approaches (Ungar, 2005).

In each country, the meaning and value of the concept of resilience is adapted to fit the culture. In Japan, my colleague Dr. Shin-Ichi Nakamura sees resilience in the image of a willow tree, firmly planted yet with boughs able to sway and bend in response to the wind. In Korea, Yang, and Choi (2001) studied the application of a family resilience framework, and the related Korean concept of *han*, in the development of a resource-based model of mental health and social services to foster positive growth through dealing with adversity. On a recent visit to Seoul, I expressed curiosity about the wide interest in resilience among Korean mental health professionals. My colleagues replied that although the word "resilience" is new to them, the Korean people have a long tradition of pride in their ability to rebuild their nation, time and again, after invasions and destruction. Their concept of han means suffering that is deep and yet not without hope.

Government programs in New Zealand have been applying a family resilience approach in child welfare services. In Argentina, a community psychiatrist found a relational resilience approach valuable in a community's reconstruction after their livelihood in fishing had been destroyed by the construction of a dam. In Brazil, studies of family resilience are being applied in programs to strengthen low-income families and efforts to prevent abandonment of children to the streets. Research is currently being conducted using the family resilience framework to understand the challenges and resources for Chinese and Eastern European immigrant families in Portugal. Family-centered, resilience-based health care and mental health service networks are being developed in Kosovo (see Chapters 9 and 11). These are but a few of the many inspiring systems-based resilience-oriented programs springing up internationally.

RE-VISIONING SERVICES
TO STRENGTHEN FAMILY RESILIENCE

A family resilience practice approach is both pragmatic and growth-oriented. This approach targets key family processes to strengthen family functioning and resourcefulness as presenting problems are addressed. Core principles include: collaboration and teamwork; multisystemic, community-based interventions; flexible service delivery; and prevention/early intervention. Just as there are many varied pathways in resilience, a family resilience meta-framework can be applied with a variety of systems-oriented practice models and modalities.

Collaboration and Teamwork

A family resilience approach emphasizes the value of collaborative efforts in surmounting life challenges. In crisis, mutual support is most likely to break down as members hunker down in isolated, self-reliant modes of coping or in adversarial positions. When we encourage mutual support, empathic communication, and shared problem solving among family and community members, we strengthen relationships as problems are tackled together. Couple and family conjoint sessions as well as community forums, set a collaborative context. More explicitly, we can invite members to think of themselves as partners or teammates, who become more resourceful through shared efforts.

Collaboration is also essential between the family and helping professionals. Some early practice approaches depicted therapy as an adversarial struggle, with therapeutic skills taught as powerful tactics to overcome family resistance and reduce family pathology (Nichols & Schwartz, 2005). Implicit in such power-based approaches was a skewed relationship between the competent expert/helper/healer and the deficient or pathological family. With the recognition that successful interventions depend on family resources, more recent approaches to family therapy work in partnership with families, building on existing and potential strengths.

In addition, helping professionals are encouraged to work more collaboratively on teams and across disciplines, both within and across systems, in order to overcome fragmented and unresponsive service delivery. Human services have tended to be problem-centered—narrowly focused on a symptomatic individual, or perhaps a partner, parent, or identified caregiver, while the family network (and other strains and potential resources) remains only a dim backdrop. When services are family-centered, efforts can be better coordinated and proactive in helping all family members through concerted efforts.

Multisystemic, Community-Based Interventions

If families are to sustain themselves and meet their challenges successfully, they require environmental support. Therapists are urged to expand their focus beyond the interior of the family to build linkages between individuals, families, their social networks, and larger systems (Imber-Black, 1988). For instance, our Chicago Center for Family Health developed a Family–Schools Partnership Program to reduce the high rates of school failure and dropout of at-risk youth and to promote their resilience and success (Walsh, 2002a). Such partnerships, encouraging positive, proactive involvement of families with school professionals can make all the difference. A community-based family resource perspective is especially needed in work with multistressed, vulnerable families. Interventions aimed at enhancing positive interactions, supporting coping efforts, and building extrafamilial resources work in concert to reduce stress, to enhance pride and competence, and to promote more effective functioning (see Chapter 10).

Flexible Service Delivery

Our health care and social service delivery systems must be more flexibly organized to be responsive and proactive to family challenges over time. Recovery from crisis or loss and adaptation to multiple challenges can't happen all at once in four to six sessions. Yet this doesn't mean that we must swing to the other extreme of vague, open-ended contracts with unlimited therapeutic horizons. One of my colleagues has worried that attending to adaptations over time would mean that once a couple or family is seen for help, they remain in treatment for life. Part of the problem lies in the way we have traditionally viewed mental health and psychotherapy. A resilience-based approach more closely fits the model of preventive family medicine, the ongoing role of a family doctor, and the concept of "healing." When we think of our physical health, we don't think of ourselves as patients in perpetual medical treatment. We see our physicians both in crisis and for periodic checkups, and, optimally, we develop a relationship with them (or their clinical setting) over time.

A resilience-oriented approach broadens our conception of "family therapy" to include counseling, brief consultations, and psychoeducational groups. A systemic framework guides intervention priorities: Sessions at different points might be held with a family unit, subgroups, couples, or individual members, and might even include meetings with informal kin or friends when helpful to build support networks. Community linkages are actively encouraged, such as with a family's faith congregation. We need to re-vision the traditional therapeutic contract and the rigid schedule of weekly sessions until termination, so that interventions can fit varied challenges and adaptive processes over time.

A Psychosocial Roadmap to Guide Practice

The family systems–illness model developed by Rolland (1994, 2003; see Chapter 9, this volume) has potential value as a useful psychosocial roadmap to guide intervention and foster family coping and resilience with a range of adversities. Family challenges and intervention priorities will vary, depending on the crisis patterning: onset (acute vs. gradual), course (brief vs. recurrent vs. constant vs. progressively worsening), outcome, degree of functional impairment, and uncertainty about the future trajectory. Stressors are approached as ongoing processes with landmarks, transitions, and changing demands. Each phase in the unfolding of events poses developmental tasks that may require different strengths from a family. A brief crisis requires immediate mobilization of resources; however, after the initial period of disequilibrium, a family may be able to reorganize and resume accustomed patterns in living. With longterm or permanent change or with persistent adversity, the family must grieve the loss of its precrisis identity and alter familiar patterns, as well as hopes and dreams, to accommodate a new set of circumstances. This framework can guide consultations and periodic family "psychosocial checkups" to strengthen the family's capacity to manage stress-related crises or sustained efforts over the long haul.

Therapeutic work can focus on building a family's strengths to meet immediate psychosocial demands of a disruptive transition, such as divorce, and can prepare for the anticipated course ahead. For example, in CCFH divorce mediation and post-divorce training and service, we draw on findings of longitudinal research that track families from predivorce through several years postdivorce (Hetherington & Kelly, 2002) and identify processes that promote resilience. Such research informs efforts to help parents approach separation decisions and custody, residential, and visitation options in a planful way to reduce risk and facilitate their children's positive adaptation. Following a divorce, we are proactive in helping parents to anticipate and manage transitional distress and complications that commonly occur over time, (e.g., decisions about a child's education or religious training, changes in residence, or remarriage and stepfamily formation). We link families with postdecree mediation or other appropriate services to address challenges that arise.

Just as families need more cohesion to pool resources in times of crisis, more intensive professional help is needed at such times. Likewise, just as families can shift balance to more separateness in stable periods, more intermittent therapeutic contact can sustain family functioning during plateaus of adaptation. In an initial crisis phase (which may last from a few weeks to several months), sessions can be held weekly, or more frequently if the situation is urgent. Family members can be seen separately and in different combinations—for instance, a depressed adolescent can be seen both privately and with the family. Over time, progress can be sustained by meeting at less frequent intervals (e.g., biweekly or monthly). Sessions can be scheduled for predictable stress points, such as stepfamily formation. Help can also be available as needed when unexpected problems or new disruptions occur.

Systems-Oriented Approaches: Many Pathways
in Fostering Resilience

Just as there are many pathways to healthy family functioning, our view of family therapy must be expanded from the traditional treatment paradigm to a variety of systems-based approaches and modalities to strengthen and support families. Family therapists frequently combine individual and conjoint sessions in their therapeutic work, as noted above. In the course of couple or family therapy, meeting with individual members can yield a fuller picture, particularly when communication is guarded or volatile. Careful planning, timing, and focus are important, with attention to issues of confidentiality and triangulation.

Psychoeducational models (e.g., McFarlane, 2002) and family consultation (Wynne, McDaniel, & Weber, 1986) provide valuable information, coping skills, and support to families in crisis or coping with persistent stresses and challenges. Multifamily groups, offering psychoeducation and a support network, are particularly well suited to promoting resilience for families facing a wide range of adverse situations, such as a breadwinner's job dislocation, serious illness, or bereavement (Walsh, 2002b). Pertinent research on family coping relevant to their crisis situation can inform interventions and can be shared with families, who are hungry for information and guidelines to clarify ambiguities and manage stresses. New resources are gained and distress normalized through shared experiences with other families dealing with similar challenges. Families respond positively to the energizing group aims of strengthening resilience.

Prevention: From Reaction to Proaction

In emerging priorities for mental health and health care, resources must be directed to cost-effective prevention services. Most programs for children and families in distress are reactive, focused on salvaging victims from the wreckage. It makes more sense to offer proactive, wellness-based services—to bolster those at risk or in acute distress *before* problems become entrenched and multiply. The case for preventive services, such as family life education and family support programs (Kagan & Weissbourd, 1994), is supported by mounting evidence that programs providing information, resources, and opportunities for skill and knowledge development, in an ongoing rather than a crisis-triggered manner, are both effective and cost-effective.

Resilience-building family intervention can serve as a psychosocial inoculation, to boost immunity or hardiness in facing adversity. By strengthening resilience in families before crises erupt, we decrease their vulnerability and risk, fortify their capacities to cope with stress, and increase their resources to face new challenges. Preventive actions may lower risk by modifying environmental conditions or circumstances, develop crisis prevention skills by strengthening family interaction processes, and mobilize supportive resources by building kin and community networks.

Preventive interventions may be offered before, when, or after a problem develops. Primary prevention and family life education are strategies for creating support and empowerment for individuals and families at risk (Harris, 1996). For instance, Chicago-based programs such as Family Focus and Ounce of Prevention work with new teen parents to support healthy parent–child relationships, early child development, and parents' own educational, job, and social functioning. There is need for a wide range of family-focused prevention and early intervention services in natural community settings, such as schools and neighborhood centers. Family therapists and other professionals concerned about family well-being can offer information and family coping strategies through community consultations, forums, and public speaking events.

Secondary prevention consists of early intervention, as in an early phase of crisis or initial adjustment to a stressful transition. Tertiary prevention involves actions taken later in the course of persistent problems to prevent further recurrence or exacerbation. For instance, psychoeducational approaches with chronic mental illness help patients and families manage stress to enhance coping, increase functioning, and reduce the risk of relapse and rehospitalization (Anderson, Reiss, & Hogarty, 1986; see Chapter 9, this volume).

Premarital counseling and multicouple workshops are becoming more widespread. Workshops and programs combining relationship enhancement with problem solving and communication skills training have been designed to prevent relationship distress and reduce risk of dissolution (e.g., PREP; Markman & Halford, 2005). Increasingly, premarital counseling is informed by inventories designed to assess relationship strengths and target trouble spots that predict higher risk of later marital difficulties or divorce. The PREPARE and ENRICH assessment tools have been found to have broad relevance and reliability with couples in cultures as diverse as African American, Latino, and Japanese (Olson, 2003). (David Olson has joked that, as sequels to PREPARE, an assessment for couples considering divorce could be called DESPAIR, and another for those contemplating remarriage might be named BEWARE.)

From a resilience standpoint, *all* therapeutic efforts can also be preventive if we help distressed families develop strengths to avert future crises. The treatment and healing of a knee injury offers a useful analogy. Physical therapy not only aids in recovery, but also strengthens the resilience of muscles in the vulnerable area so that future injury can be prevented. Many brief crisis intervention approaches are helpful for short-term recovery, but unless family resilience is strengthened, future crises are likely to overwhelm a vulnerable family, requiring further rounds of crisis intervention in revolving-door emergency treatment. If we organize family-centered mental health services for psychosocial care like a preventive model of family medicine or dentistry a great deal of suffering could be avoided.

In sum, resilience-based services foster family empowerment as they bring forth shared hope, develop new and renewed areas of competence, and build mutual support. We enable families not only to resolve presenting problems but also to become more proactive to meet future challenges more effectively. Every intervention is thus also a preventive measure.

STRENGTHENING THERAPIST RESILIENCE

The Human Connection

Most family therapists have shifted from emphasizing strategies and tactics for change to recognizing the essential importance of the human connection in the therapeutic relationship. For clients to be open and receptive to change, helping professionals must be genuinely interested in their life stories and concerned about their well-being. We must be understanding of their predicament, empathize with their pain, and encourage their best strivings. We need to be comfortable in bringing ourselves fully into the therapeutic relationship, modeling by example in our therapeutic transactions and sharing (as appropriate) what we've learned from our own human experiences with adversity.

The therapeutic relationship has stood out as a common denominator in research on the effectiveness of various approaches to psychotherapy over the years. This relationship is based in open communication and a trusting climate that fosters the ability to get in touch with and express a wide range of ideas, feelings, and opinions. Recent narrative approaches emphasize the healing power in therapeutic conversations.

Empathic listening, genuine interest, and respectful curiosity by the therapist encourage family members to tell their stories and consider new perspectives on their troubling situations.

As therapists have come to work more collaboratively with clients, we have also become more human in our interactions. We consider disclosing aspects of our own life experiences when we believe it will be helpful to our clients, such as a story that establishes human connections, or one to be learned from.

"Courageous engagement" of therapist and clients—a wonderfully apt phrase offered by Waters and Lawrence (1993)—is at the heart of competence-based work and collaborative efforts to build resilience. We, as therapists, as well as our clients, need courage to question and challenge constraining myths; to support attempts to move from a helpless, victimized position; and to en-courage our clients to bring out their best through the worst of times. It requires courage to expect more and take risks for better relationships and life goals. When we work from this perspective, our clients are better able to take steps toward positive change and to live with greater ease in situations that are unchangeable, or uncertain.

Our own resilience as therapists is also relationally based, bolstered through collaboration with colleagues, supportive work systems, and satisfying personal relationships. As caseloads increase in numbers and complexity while staff resources are cut back, the risk of professional burnout is heightened. I encourage students and therapists to create supportive professional networks and to seek out learning and enrichment experiences at each phase in their careers. Postgraduate family therapy training centers can offer a revitalizing professional home, nurturing contact and growth through participation in workshops, courses, and case consultation groups. Collaborative consultation teams or partners are ideal for building camaraderie, competence, and confidence. Ongoing group experiences offer mentoring relationships, collegial support, and skill enhancement. A monthly peer consultation group can sustain professional growth and connectedness.

In practice settings where teams are not feasible, a "buddy system" can readily be formed. Trusted colleagues can serve as professional lifelines: mutual resources and consultants when clients are in crisis or a professional is undersupported and discouraged. My close colleagues and I continue to turn to one another, and we always find our spirits renewed and our creative energy rekindled as a result.

A colleague once asked me to observe a session with a client after he had nearly fallen asleep in the last session. He was upset that he was becoming bored and irritated with Gloria, a middle-aged mother who was trapped in despair since her husband had left her two years earlier. Intending to show empathy for her plight, my colleague sat quietly nodding trancelike as she went on and on about her troubles, recounting everything bad that always happened to her in life. As his thoughts drifted and he looked away, Gloria increased the intensity of her drama to reengage him, which only irritated him more. This relational impasse repeated itself week after week.

As my colleague and I reflected together on the situation, it became apparent that by concentrating so intently on Gloria's sorrowful story, he was unwittingly reinforcing her passive, victimized position, her global pessimism, and her belief that others could only care about her if she evoked their sympathy. For change to occur, he needed to show genuine interest in Gloria as a lovable person who deserved a better life for herself and her children and could achieve it. As the focus of the therapeutic conversation shifted to noticing and affirming her strengths, she came alive, and he had no difficulty sustaining his investment in helping her rebuild her life after the devastation of the divorce. A resilience-promoting therapeutic relationship seeks to repair the damage from traumatic experience, to expand the client's vision of what is possible, and to support actions and relational resources in pursuit of those dreams.

Waters and Lawrence (1993) encourage therapists to see our clients' struggles and confrontations as the mythic "hero's journey"—a view consonant with the resilience approach. They note Joseph Campbell's observation that the heroes of myths are all on a quest against the odds to slay a dragon or other foe, as in the Biblical story of David versus Goliath. The hero comes to participate in life courageously and decently, in the way of nature—not in the way of personal rancor, disappointment, or revenge. When we take such a view of our clients, we can more easily appreciate the positive, competent aspects of their life journeys and our own efforts. Waters and Lawrence state:

> In our work, this goal of a courageous engagement with life guides us more than a desire to avoid the "negative" aspects of symptoms. In therapy, our clients are the heroes attempting to "slay their dragons," but if we lose sight of that and become preoccupied with their dysfunction, victimization, or handicap, we are less helpful to them. We must see that at their core is their desire for mastery and belonging. They become heroes when they—and we—have the courage to struggle against those obstacles and transform the possibilities of life. (1993, p. 58)

Balance in Our Professional and Personal Lives

Therapists are also challenged to achieve a healthy balance in our professional and personal lives. The risk of "compassion fatigue" (Figley, 2002, see Chapter 11), and the potential for spillover of painful and threatening issues, come with the territory of our chosen work. The professional and the personal each hold meanings for the success of the other, if we are able to apply them wisely and keep aware of our clients' and our own values and situations, our commonalities and differences. The safe boundaries and hierarchies of more traditional psychotherapy can become blurred in more collaborative therapeutic relationships. But the gains are worth the challenge. If we keep in mind that resilience does not mean invulnerability, we become more human and compassionate in our helping relationships and more fully engaged with our families, friends, and community.

Mending the Social Fabric: Transforming Broken Service Systems

Systems-oriented professionals, I believe, have an ethical responsibility to direct our energies beyond our office walls toward repair of the social fragmentation that heightens risks for individual and family breakdown. It would be unconscionable to help families withstand the onslaught of social and economic pressures in their lives without working to eradicate destructive social forces that heighten risks and undermine resilience. The resilience of the field of family therapy is also strengthened when we actively invest in larger system change and social movements—when we lend our expertise to help mend the frayed social fabric. Systemic changes are needed to address larger institutional and cultural influences that breed poverty and discrimination and that severely strain families. Collaborative professional and family advocacy can strengthen efforts to overcome these barriers and promote family-centered policies that enable families to thrive.

The resilience of helping professionals is essential to overcome the barriers of the for-profit managed care system in the United States, which limits access and availability of psychosocial care to at-risk and distressed families in all segments of human services. Despite these daunting challenges, systems-based, family-centered services will continue to be in demand, because of their useful application to a broad range of problems and the cost-effectiveness of helping all family members through interventions that strengthen the family as a functional unit. We need to articulate the importance of family systems–based services and marshal research evidence in support of its effectiveness. Recognizing the potential in relational resilience, helping professionals across disciplines must put aside turf rivalries and band together in collaborative efforts to transform larger systems that threaten our common mission to foster the well-being of individuals and their families. The keys to resilience for our clients are also keys to our own professional resilience.

PART IV

Facilitating Family Resilience through Crisis and Prolonged Challenges

CHAPTER 8

Loss, Recovery, and Resilience

> In coming to accept death, we can more fully embrace life.
> —VIKTOR FRANKL, *Man's Search for Meaning*

I recall my delight, as a child, in watching the celebration by the family next door when their only daughter got married. They, like other families, planned for the perfect wedding; the bride and groom looked radiant, and everyone cheered as they drove off on their honeymoon. En route to their romantic destination, they were both killed in a car crash on a rainy, winding country road. Tragedy struck at the happiest moment in the life of the young couple and their families, and it shattered all future hopes and dreams.

Coming to terms with death and loss is the most difficult challenge a family must confront. From a family systems orientation, loss is a transactional process involving those who die with their survivors in a shared life cycle, recognizing both the finality of death and the continuity of life (Walsh & McGoldrick, 2004). This perspective considers the impact of the death of a family member on the family as a functional unit, with immediate and long-term reverberations for every member and all other relationships. A family resilience approach fosters the ability of family members to face death and dying, and for survivors to live and love fully beyond loss.

This chapter first considers death and loss in sociohistorical context. It then presents a framework for systemic assessment and intervention to ease the dying process and foster resilience in the face of loss. A

181

developmental perspective is offered to view loss and recovery processes over time and across the family life cycle. Major family adaptational tasks in loss are described, identifying variables that heighten risk for dysfunction and key processes—in belief systems, organizational patterns, and communication processes—that facilitate healing and resilience. Guidelines are offered for dealing effectively with complicated situations.

DEATH AND LOSS
IN SOCIOHISTORICAL CONTEXT

Throughout history and in every culture, mourning beliefs, practices, and rituals have facilitated both the integration of death and the transformations of survivors (Walsh & McGoldrick, 2004). Some anthropologists even believe that religions were invented primarily to help people accept death, not as a final ending, but rather as a transition to continuing life in another realm (Walsh, 2004). Every culture and religion, in its own ways, offers assistance to the dying and to the community of survivors who must move forward with life. The dying and the bereaved are part of a cultural drama that asserts basic ideas about the nature of life and death (Bateson, 1994). Times of profound loss may feel unique and research has documented the wide variation in "normal" individual grief processes (Wortman & Silver, 1989). Yet, despite considerable diversity in individual, familial, and cultural modes of dealing with death and loss, mourning processes promote healing and families are crucial influences in healthy or dysfunctional adaptation to loss.

Many cultures are fortunate in having a world view that helps them to face the inescapable fact of death, including it in the rhythm of life and an abiding faith in a higher power. Some cultures rehearse loss and support the expression of grief. Others, such as the dominant Anglo-American culture, avoid facing mortality, deny the impact of loss, and encourage the bereaved to quickly regain control and closure. Many people die alone, locked into their own thoughts, which they can't communicate to others lest they upset them. Our culture has treated grief "almost like a disease, embarrassing and possibly infectious" (Bateson, 1994, p. 20). To avoid expression—viewed as "breaking down"—some impose a rigid self-control, fitting with the cultural expectation that grief should be minimized. In most cultures, loss is an occasion for family and community cohesion. In contrast, most Americans are hesitant about sharing "bad news," "burdening" others with their sorrow, or "intruding" on the grief of others. Commonly, after the initial mourning period, the phone stops ringing; visitors and invitations decline; and friends or neighbors may turn away to avoid the discomfort of contact.

Families across the ages have had to cope with the precariousness of life and the disruptions wrought by death. As is still true in impoverished communities throughout the world, death might strike young and old alike, with high rates of mortality for infants, children, and women in childbirth. Until the medical advances in the 20th century, life expectancy in North America was 47 years—an age now considered midlife. Parental death often disrupted family units, shifting members into varied and complex networks of full, half-, and steprelationships in extended kinship systems.

Before the advent of hospital and institutional care, people died at home, where all family members, including children, were involved in the preparation for and immediacy of death. Modern technological societies fostered the denial of death and avoidance of grief processes. Western medicine and nursing homes removed the dying from everyday contact in institutional settings. We lost community supports that assist families in integrating the fact of death with the ongoing life of survivors. Geographical distances and pressured work schedules increasingly have hindered contact of family members at times of death and dying. With the exception of bereavement specialists, mental health and health care professionals have been slow to deal with loss, reflecting the cultural aversion to facing and talking about death. As family therapy pioneers Murray Bowen and Norman Paul noted, death has been the most taboo subject for therapists as well as the families they see (Walsh & McGoldrick, 2004).

Currently, there is growing recognition of the importance of facing death and loss. The aging of the baby boom generation has prompted a shift in public consciousness of mortality and loss. Medical advances increasingly confront families with unprecedented decisions to prolong or end life and have raised profound questions about just what is a "natural" death. Families are actively reclaiming the dying process through involvement in palliative and hospice care to reduce suffering and enhance dignity and through advance directives, such as living wills, and meaningful memorial rites. Technology and the media have brought worldwide catastrophic events into our homes. Large-scale epidemics such as AIDS, natural disasters, war and genocidal atrocities, terrorist attacks, and ongoing threats have all jolted attention to the precariousness of life and death in our volatile and uncertain global environment (see Chapter 11).

Amid the social and economic upheaval of recent decades, families are dealing with multiple losses, disruptions, and uncertainties. This chapter focuses on loss through death; yet the family challenges and intervention priorities described here have broad applicability to other experiences involving loss, recovery, and resilience, such as migration, unemployment, family separations, divorce, foster care, and adoption. In strengthening family resilience to deal with losses, we enable all members to deepen their bonds and forge new strengths to live and love fully beyond loss.

UNDERSTANDING LOSS
IN SYSTEMIC PERSPECTIVE

Loss by death has far-reaching implications throughout kin networks because of the profound connections among members, Despite intense aversion to facing death and grief, their force will find expression, often in emotional, behavioral, relational, or somatic symptoms. Studies reveal the impact of loss on physiological functioning and altered immune system response for surviving family members, increasing their vulnerability to premature illness and death (see Walsh & McGoldrick, 2004).

Clinical attention to bereavement has focused primarily on emotionally distressed individuals who have lost a significant dyadic relationship. Nonsymptomatic family members may be presumed to be functioning normally and not in need of attention. Yet, children may cover their grief with a cheerful facade so as not to burden parents. Some members may try to escape the pain of loss through work, affairs, alcohol, or drugs. With the death of a child, a parent's suppression of grief may work well for job functioning but may block support to a grieving partner and can impair the couple's relationship and their coparenting of surviving children.

A systemic perspective is required to appreciate the reverberation of influences throughout the family network with any important loss. Family processes mediate the immediate and long-term impact of a death for partners, parents, children, siblings, and extended family. Murray Bowen and Norman Paul both observed that grief, when unrecognized and unattended, may precipitate strong and harmful reactions in other relationships—from marital distancing and dissolution to precipitous replacement, extramarital affairs, and even sexual abuse.

As I have seen in my practice, how the family handles the loss situation has far-reaching ripple effects. Therefore, it is crucial for clinicians to attend not only to the direct impact of a crisis event, but also to the family response, which can have both immediate and long-term consequences for all members and their relationships. As in the following case, children can be harmed even more by their family's inability to provide structure, stability, and protection than by the loss itself.

> Marie, a woman in her 50s, sought therapy for depression after the sudden death of her younger brother, Jim, who had been her mainstay in life. When she was 7 years old, her mother had died of cancer. She recalled that as relatives came and went on the night of her death, she dressed her brother and herself in their Sunday best, and sat holding his hand, waiting to be called in to say their good-byes. No one came for them, nor were they taken to the funeral. In the chaotic aftermath, she and her brother were separated, sent to stay with different relatives, uncertain if or when they would return home to their father, who was too bereft to care for them. When, after several weeks, they did return home, her father, isolated in his unbearable grief, drank heavily and came into her bed at night, violating her sexually. Finally, her father's remarriage brought an end to her secret trauma. She never blamed him for the abuse, feeling sorry for his sadness and loneliness. She later married a man who, like her father, was a heavy drinker and endured his abuse for many years. Her close relationship with her brother remained her lifeline until his sudden death.

As this case reveals, some families fall apart with an unbearable loss. Sibling bonds can be vital lifelines through the loss and its aftermath. For Marie, the recent death of her brother was devastating, reevoking her childhood trauma and reverberating through her relationships with her adult children. Legacies of loss find expression in continuing patterns of interaction and mutual influence among the survivors and across the generations. The pain of loss touches survivors' relationships with others, affecting even those who never knew the person who died.

Death or threatened loss disrupts a family's functional equilibrium. As Bowen (1978) observed, the intensity of the emotional reaction is influenced by the integration in the family at the time of the loss and by the significance of the lost member. The emotional shock wave may reverberate throughout an entire family system immediately or long after a traumatic loss or threatened loss. Attention to this shock wave is important in therapy. Too often, presenting symptoms are treated without understanding the relevance of loss when clients do not bring it up. Symptoms may appear in a child or other vulnerable family member, or interpersonal conflict may erupt, without the family connecting such reactions to a critical loss event. Therefore, therapists need to assess the total family network, the position of a dying or deceased member, and the family's adaptation, in order to understand the meaning and context of presenting symptoms and to facilitate a healing process. Paul cautioned that a clinician's own aversion to death and grief may block inquiry about loss issues and notice of grief-related systemic patterns. Narrow focus on observable here-and-how interactional patterns can blind clinicians to the relevance of past or threatened losses. The result is unhelpful focus on secondary problems. An active therapeutic approach is needed to confront hidden losses, foster awareness of relational connections, and encourage mutual empathy in conjoint couple and family therapy.

It is crucial for therapists to grasp the significance of loss events that are minimized or unmentioned in a client's life story. Without exploration, traumatic losses may remain disconnected, ambiguous, or distorted, as in the following case:

> Joe came to therapy to stop his drinking and extramarital affair because he feared he was on the verge of destroying everything important to him. Most of all he feared losing his son, Adam, age 8, if his wife divorced him. When doing a genogram, the therapist noted that Joe's only brother, also named Adam, had died at the age of 8. Yet Joe insisted that this was "no big deal" and had nothing to do with his current destructive behavior and catastrophic fear of loss. It was crucial for the therapist to urge him to explore possible connections, instead of simply accepting his initial denial of meaning.

Loss is a powerful nodal experience that shakes the foundation of family life and leaves no member unaffected. It is more than a discrete event; from a systemic view, it can be seen to involve many processes over time—from the threat and approach of death, through its immediate aftermath, and on into long-term implications. Individual distress stems not only from grief, but also from changes in the realignment of the family emotional field. The meaning of a particular loss event and responses to it are shaped by family belief systems, which in turn are altered by all loss experiences. Loss also modifies the family structure, often requiring major reorganization of the family system.

A death in the family involves multiple losses: the loss of the person, the loss of roles and relationships, the loss of the intact family unit, and the loss of hopes and dreams for all that might have been. A family life cycle perspective is crucial to understand the reciprocal influences of several generations as they move forward over time and as they approach and respond to loss (McGoldrick & Walsh, 2004). Each loss ties in with all other losses and yet is unique in its meaning. We need to be attuned to both the factual circumstances of a death and the meanings it holds for a particular family in its social and developmental contexts. In family assessment, we must attend to past, present, and future connections, not in deterministic causal assumptions, but rather in an evolutionary sense. Like the social context, the temporal context holds a matrix of meanings in which loss is experienced and influences future approaches to loss and to life.

FAMILY ADAPTATIONAL CHALLENGES IN LOSS

Research on loss has found wide diversity in the timing and intensity of normal grief responses (Wortman & Silver, 1989). Children's reactions to death depend on their stage of cognitive and emotional development, on the way adults deal with them around the death, and on the caretaking they have lost. Because the bereavement experience is so variable, it is more useful to think of facets of grief, rather than sequential stages. Shock and denial are often the first reactions ("No, this can't be happening"). Although denial can become maladaptive if it persists, it is a natural anesthetic and may be very useful as an initial mechanism, permitting a basic level of functioning when the full impact of grief would be devastating. Anger and rage may follow ("How could this happen to me?"), often giving way to wishful fantasy or bargaining ("If only I become a more loving child, Daddy will live"), which can yield to depression and feeling that one can't go on ("Life is not worth living"). Acceptance may be gradual. Various facets of grief may alternate and are commonly reexperienced, particularly at nodal events, such as anniversaries and family gatherings. Although painful and disruptive, grieving, in its many forms, is a healing process.

Adaptation does not mean resolution, in the sense of some complete, "once-and-for-all" getting over it. Mourning and adaptation have no fixed timetable, and significant or traumatic losses may never be fully resolved. Recovery is best understood as a gradual process spiraling over time, rather than an outcome. Thus, resilience in the face of loss does not mean quickly putting it behind you, getting "closure" on the emotional experience, or simply bouncing back and moving on. A dynamic process of oscillation occurs in adaptive coping, alternating between loss and restoration, as we face grief at times and avoid it at other times to attend to ongoing challenges (Stroebe & Schut, 2001).

Traditional psychiatric views of mourning erred in stressing the need to detach from or let go of the deceased loved one. Instead, adaptive mourning processes involve a transformation of the relationship from physical presence to continuing bonds through spiritual connection, memories, deeds, and stories that are passed on across the generations. Coming to terms with loss involves finding ways to make meaning of the loss experience, put it in perspective, and weave the experience into the fabric of one's individual and relational life passage. The multiple meanings of any death are transformed throughout the life cycle, as they are integrated into individual and family identity and with subsequent life experiences, including other losses.

While individual and cultural modes of dealing with death vary, the ability to accept loss is at the heart of all processes in healthy family systems (Beavers & Hampson, 2003). In our development of a systemic approach to loss over the past three decades, Monica McGoldrick and I have delineated four major family tasks that promote immediate and long-term adaptation for family members and strengthen the family as a functional unit (Walsh & McGoldrick, 2004). Rather than thinking of these as phases a family passes through, we prefer (as does Worden, 2002, who addresses individual mourning), to conceptualize these challenges as tasks in which families actively engage and which therapists can facilitate. They involve an interweaving of processes for family resilience in the three domains of family functioning—belief systems, organizational patterns, and communication/problem solving. If these challenges are not dealt with, they leave family members more vulnerable to dysfunction and heighten the risk of family conflict and dissolution.

Shared Acknowledgment of the Reality of Death

All family members, in their own ways, must confront the reality of a death and grapple with its meaning for them. With the shock of a sudden death, this process may start abruptly. In the case of life-threatening conditions, it may begin tentatively, with the anticipation of *possible* loss, while retaining hope, then, the *probability* and finally, the *certainty* of impending loss, as in the terminal phase of an illness (Rolland, 1994; see Chapter 9). Bowen stressed the importance of direct contact with a dying member, urging visits whenever possible and ways to include children and other vulnerable family members. Well-intentioned attempts to protect them from potential upset can isolate them and impede their grief process. They are likely to become upset more by the anxiety of survivors and their own fantasies than by exposure to death and dying.

Although individuals, families, and cultures vary in their direct expression of thoughts and feelings around death, research finds that clear, open communication facilitates family adaptation and strengthens the family as a supportive network for its members. A climate of trust, empathic responses, and tolerance for diverse reactions are especially crucial. Acknowledgment of the loss is facilitated by clear information and open communication about the facts and circumstances of the death. The inability to accept the reality of death can lead a family member to avoid contact with the rest of the family or to become angry with others who are moving forward in the grief process. Long-standing sibling conflicts and cutoffs often can be traced back to the death of a parent.

By contrast, when death and dying are faced courageously with loved ones, relationships can be deeply enriched. At the death of her partner after a debilitating illness, Bonnie was sad but also at peace:

> "The simple fact is, Jennie's body stopped. There was no unfinished business between us. I had carried a lot of fear about death. Jennie showed me how to feel more alive and more open, even in her last days. She accepted that she was dying, even though she didn't want to go. Acceptance didn't mean feeling jolly or that she liked the situation, just that this was the truth at the moment."

Facing Threatened Death and Loss

In the case of life-threatening situations such as serious illness, acknowledgment of the possibility of loss may begin tentatively, with the diagnosis of a high-risk condition. When family members don't know what to say or do, or if they wish to spare one another pain, they may say nothing and avoid contact. Uncertainty about a prognosis fuels anxiety and confusion and may make them even more cautious about sharing concerns about death and loss. The wish to deny or minimize the experience can shut down communication altogether. The unspeakable may go underground to surface in other contexts or in symptomatic behavior, as in the following case:

> An expert in child sexual abuse consulted me about a case that puzzled her. A mother had brought in her 5-year-old son, Nicky with

concern that he might have been molested at preschool, because she kept finding him fondling himself. The therapist's evaluation revealed no indication of sexual abuse. I suggested the possibility that Nicky might be expressing anxiety about other concerns, and advised her to meet with the parents and explore other stresses in the family. The mother, again coming alone, revealed that 8 months earlier the father had been found to have stomach cancer, and had undergone surgery to remove his stomach (and, reportedly, all the cancer).

It was important to understand how the family had coped with that life-threatening crisis and its aftermath. The mother reported that on the day of his discharge from the hospital, her husband had insisted that he felt fine and that he wanted to go on with life as normal, putting the incident behind them without further mention. To respect his wishes, she never brought it up. When asked how this life-threatening experience had affected her, she burst into tears, saying that it had shaken her sense of security. She had tried to push her fears of loss out of her mind until the past month, when something suspicious was noticed in her husband's checkup, raising new uncertainty about his prognosis. The parents hadn't told the children and assumed they were OK, since they never asked questions about their father's condition. After a pause she added, "Now that you mention it, last night when we said grace before dinner, Nicky added, 'And please, God, take care of Daddy's tummy.' "

In times of threatened loss, therapists can help family members to open up blocked lines of communication. It may be useful to meet with a patient or family members individually or in different combinations, working toward a larger family discussion and deciding how much to disclose to others. In the situation above, I recommended meeting first with the parents to help them share their feelings and concerns. A resilience-based approach was helpful to normalize their reactions as common in such situations and to build mutual support in dealing with the challenges and uncertainties that lay ahead. Coaching enabled the parents to plan how best to share information with their children, help them to express concerns, and provide comfort and support.

Despite a family's discomfort in opening communication about death and loss, it is imperative that veils of secrecy be lifted, particularly if any family member is showing symptoms of distress. I try to help members find ways to talk about the unspeakable—the threat of loss and the many other concerns—and age-appropriate ways to open discussion with children without overburdening or overprotecting them.

Family communication may be blocked by the superstitious belief that talking about death may bring it on. Often family members fear that if they bring up the possibility of death, the patient or others may think that they want the person to die. This concern is especially strong when a relationship has been troubled. It is common when prolonged caregiving has been burdensome and there is a guilt-laden wish for the relief that death would bring. It is helpful to explore such beliefs and feelings, normalizing and contextualizing them as understandable in the family's situation.

It is useful to discuss the dilemmas posed by uncertainty and to help members tolerate different views among them. I find it helpful to ask such questions as these: "What is it like for you to live with such uncertainty?" "While we all hope for the best, *what if* the worst were to happen?" "What if a medical crisis were to end life suddenly and unexpectedly? What would be the hardest part?" "What regrets might you have later about things left unsaid, unasked, undone?" "Without giving up hope, how might you prepare for the possibility of loss?" "What might you want to say or do with and for one another?"

Euthanasia, or assisted dying, has become a hotly debated moral, legal, and public policy issue as societies are aging and medical interventions prolong the lives of increasing numbers of persons with chronic, painful, and deteriorating illnesses. In such situations, the wish to die with dignity, by controlling or hastening the end of one's own life and suffering, poses excruciating ethical, legal, and spiritual dilemmas for patients, their families, and health care professionals. In the view of many ethicists, assisted dying should be distinguished from killing or suicide, and not labeled as such. Rather, it concerns the exercise of personal options for taking control of the dying process and the timing and manner of death. Still, these are agonizing spiritual, medical, and legal dilemmas each family must consider in reaching their own decisions. Therapists can help to open conversations to explore options and their meaning. It is also useful to broaden focus from the identified patient to consider what end-of-life decisions a spouse or other adult family members would want for themselves.

When death is highly probable, and preferably before it is imminent, families may need to be urged to confront that reality in order to make critical end-of-life decisions and to make the most of the time they may have left together. (See Chapter 12 for approaches to healing reconciliations in troubled or estranged relationships.) Drafting or reviewing advance directives and living wills in consultation with loved ones is an important way to take charge and to share important decisions. Discussions may also concern pain control and palliative care—ways to keep terminally ill persons comfortable and comforted as death approaches. Hospice care, particularly at home, benefits all involved in the dying process. It is also valuable to plan funeral or memorial rites together and to discuss wills and legacies, so that the wishes of the dying can be directly communicated. In this way, potential conflicts can be averted, and the burdens and misunderstandings of survivors can be lessened.

When family members realize that time is limited, they can reap benefits in shifting priorities and concentrating on making the most of each day and every contact, rather than postponing or putting aside important things. Indeed, couples and families often report that threatened loss sparked their most precious time together, regardless of the outcome. Acknowledging the precariousness of life and the possibility of loss can heighten appreciation of loved ones, especially when relationships have been taken for granted or blocked by petty grievances. The bitterest tears shed over graves are for words left unsaid and deeds left undone.

Western beliefs in mastery and control over our destiny make it difficult to accept death and dying, which are often experienced in terms of powerlessness, loss of control, and failure. In contrast, Eastern traditions, as in Buddhism, teach that in accepting death, we discover life (Walsh, 2004). In doing so, we can live more fully and with greater awareness of our choices to make the most of our life situation. Americans are "doers," invested in goal-oriented action, achievement, and problem solving. Many avoid contact when they believe there is nothing they can *do* to stop death. We are uncomfortable simply *being with* loved ones who are dying. When my father was terminally ill, I found visits with him difficult. A consummate "doer," I kept thinking of errands I could run for him or ways I could make him more comfortable. As I calmed my own anxieties, I became better able simply—and more importantly—to be fully present with him in his dying, sitting at his bedside, quietly keeping him company, stroking his arm, taking his hand. I still have precious memories of those long days spent together: at times chuckling over *I Love Lucy* reruns, at other times gazing peacefully out the window at the large flowering mimosa tree as the sunlight streamed through from dawn through dusk.

Shared Experience of the Loss

Rituals marking the end of a life and loss of a loved one have been central in every culture and religion over the millennia. Funeral rites serve a vital function in providing direct confrontation with the reality of death and the opportunity to pay last respects. They offer the bereaved a scripted way to share grief and to receive comfort from kin and community (Imber-Black et al., 2003). Family members should be encouraged to plan ahead for a meaningful service and burial or cremation—involving the dying person if possible, so that his or her wishes are taken into account. It is most memorable when loved ones take part in the rites—through eulogies, poems, music, artwork, and photo displays—to remember and celebrate the life passage and many-faceted personhood and relationships of the deceased. In one especially moving service, a father's son and daughter from his second marriage recounted both poignant and humorous stories from their childhood interactions with him. Then his son from a previous marriage came forward; saying he was never comfortable with words, he played a stirring song on the flute that he had composed in memory of his father.

In the Jewish tradition, as in many others, it is considered even more important to attend a funeral than a wedding, because it both honors a life and marks its loss. Key processes in resilience are movingly expressed in the following Jewish mourners' Kaddish, read aloud together by those gathered at the shiva after the burial:

> At times, the pain of separation seems more than we can bear; but love and understanding can help us pass through the darkness toward the light. And in truth, grief is a great teacher, when it sends us back to serve and bless the living. . . . Thus, even when they are gone, the departed are with us, moving us to live as, in their higher moments, they themselves wished to live. We remember them now; they live in our hearts; they are an abiding blessing. (Central Conference of American Rabbis, 1992)

Sharing the experience of loss, in whatever ways family members can, is crucial in the healing process. Families should be encouraged to press reluctant members to take part. Sometimes family members avoid a funeral and visits to the cemetery, wishing not to confront the reality of death and the pain of loss. Yet, paradoxically, the meaning of the life and the relationship can be appreciated more fully when the loss is marked.

It is becoming common to announce a death on the Internet and reach a worldwide virtual community. One 23-year-old daughter invited extended kin, friends, and acquaintances from around the globe to her website, where she had composed a moving tribute to her father at his death. She shared stories of his life journey and made an electronic photo album, with pictures from his childhood, her parents' marriage, and important relationships and milestones in their lives. Whether through conventional funerals or innovative memorial tributes, family members and loved ones are increasingly celebrating the life of a loved one, as well as honoring the death.

It is never too late to hold a memorial service, to lay a headstone at a grave, to hold a ceremony to scatter ashes, or to plant a tree in memory of a loved one. Drawing family members together on an anniversary or at a holiday gathering to remember one who has died can be a profoundly healing and connecting experience; it keeps the memory of the deceased alive as it sustains relational resilience among survivors. On the 20th anniversary of my mother's death, I wanted to find a meaningful way to celebrate her life with my husband and daughter, who had never known her. My mother's deep love of music as a pianist and organist brought to mind the carillon bells of the Rockefeller Chapel on my campus at the University of Chicago. I arranged for a simple concert in her memory, and we were invited to climb to the roof of the bell tower. As the bells pealed harmoniously, we looked out into the night sky, and I felt closely in touch with her spirit among the shining stars.

Open communication is vital for family resilience over the entire course of the loss process, but especially in the transitional turmoil of the immediate aftermath. When we take into account the many fluctuating and often conflicting responses of all members in a family system, we can appreciate the complexity of any family mourning process. Families are likely to experience a range of feelings, depending on the unique meaning of the relationship and its loss for each member and the implications of the death for the family unit. Tolerance is needed for different responses within families and for the likelihood that members may have different individual coping styles and may be out of sync with one other. They may also have unique experiences of the meaning of a lost relationship. For instance, siblings may have had quite different relationships with a parent, in part associated with gender, birth order, and their age at loss.

The mourning process also involves shared narrative attempts to put the loss into some meaningful perspective that fits coherently into the rest of a family's life experience and belief system. This requires dealing with the ongoing negative implications of the loss, including the loss of dreams for the future.

As a family experiences a loss, members are going to be touched in different ways and to show a wide range of reactions, depending on such variables as their age and individual coping styles, the state of their relationships, and different positions in the family. Empathy is needed for one another and an ability to respond caringly. Tolerance for different responses and timing is important. Strong emotions may surface at different moments, including complicated and mixed feelings of anger, disappointment, helplessness, relief, guilt, or abandonment, which are present to some extent in most family relationships. In the dominant U.S. culture, the expression of intense emotions tends to generate discomfort and distancing in others. Moreover, the loss of control experienced in sharing such overwhelming feelings can frighten family members, leading them to block all communication about the loss experience to protect one another and themselves. When grieving is blocked, emotions may explode in conflict. Some children may internalize their grief in symptoms of anxiety or depression, while others may externalize their distress in behavioral problems. Adolescents may withdraw from the family and/or engage in risky behavior and drug or alcohol abuse.

If a family is unable to tolerate certain feelings, a member who directly expresses the unacceptable may be scapegoated or extruded. Unbearable or unacceptable feelings may be delegated and expressed in a fragmented fashion by various family members. One may carry all the anger for the family, while another is in touch only with sadness; one may show only relief, while another is numb. The shock and pain of a traumatic loss can shatter family cohesion, leaving members isolated and unsupported in their grief, as in the following case:

Mrs. Ramirez sought help for her 11-year-old daughter Teresa's school problems, which had worsened in recent weeks. In order to understand "Why now?", the therapist explored recent events in the family. The oldest son, Ray, age 18, had been caught in the midst of gang crossfire. The shot that killed him had also shattered the family unit. The father, Raymundo, withdrew, drinking heavily to ease his pain. Miguel, the next eldest son, carried the family rage into the streets, seeking revenge for the senseless killing. Two other middle sons showed no reaction, keeping quietly out of the way. Mrs. Ramirez, alone in her grief, deflected her attention to Teresa's school problems.

Family sessions over the following 10 weeks provided a context for shared griefwork. Family members were encouraged to share their feelings openly and to comfort one another. It was especially important to involve the "well" siblings, who had been holding in their own pain so as not to upset or burden their parents further. The therapist helped the parents to obtain legal counsel, to gain the necessary information to navigate the court system, and to plan and carry out concerted actions, with Miguel's assistance, to seek justice for the murder. They were also helped to sort through

Ray's possessions, each family member choosing something as a keepsake—his jacket, a favorite shirt, his prized guitar. They dreaded Ray's impending birthday. The therapist encouraged them to think of something they might do together to remember him. The family decided to go to church—for the first time, in a long time, all together—and to light candles in his memory. The therapist also suggested that they invite grandparents, aunts, uncles, and cousins to join them there. This led them afterward to spend the whole evening together, telling old family stories, as Miguel strummed Ray's guitar.

Such processes repaired the family's fragmentation, promoting a more cohesive network for mutual support and healing. On follow-up, Teresa's school problems and the father's drinking had subsided. The experience of pulling together to deal with their loss had strengthened their resilience, helping them to cope better with other problems in their lives.

Reorganization of the Family System

The death of a family member leaves a hole in the fabric of family life. It disrupts established patterns of interaction. The process of recovery involves a realignment of relationships and redistribution of role functions to compensate for the loss, buffer transitional stresses, and carry on with family life. At times, structural planning requires attention before parents may be ready to deal with their own emotional grief.

One father, a recent immigrant, brought his 8-year-old daughter for therapy after the death of the mother from AIDS. The father refused to participate in therapy, not wanting to "fall apart" by facing his own grief at the loss of his beloved wife. Moreover, he, too, had AIDS and wanted to keep working and functional for as long as possible. The therapist wished to respect his decision not to come to therapy for his own griefwork. Yet, given his life-threatening condition, it was crucial to discuss plans for his daughter's custody and care if he should die. He told the therapist he had thought about it and assumed that a friendly neighbor woman, with children of her own, would take his daughter in, a common arrangement in his home village in Mexico. But he had not actually asked his neighbor and he was unaware that, legally, in the event of his death, without relatives in the United States his daughter would become a ward of the state and go into the foster care system. It was important to work with him to make appropriate arrangements.

Family roles and responsibilities may interfere with mourning. A father's role as main financial provider may reinforce his tendency to block emotional expression to keep in control and function at work. In single-parent families, children may sacrifice their own needs or collude to keep a bereaved parent strong because everyone depends on him or her. It is important to help overburdened family members structure the time and space they need for their own grieving, and to rally the contributions of others to provide the respite needed for healing.

It is important to help families pace their reorganization. Some families may take flight from losses by quickly get rid of all clothes and possessions or by moving precipitously out of their homes or communities. Further dislocations generate more disruptions and loss of social supports, as when children must adjust to a new school and the loss of friends. Some seek immediate replacement for their losses, through affairs, sudden marriages, or pregnancies. These replacement relationships are then complicated by the unmourned losses.

It's not uncommon for many families to keep the deceased member's room and possessions intact for many months. However, some hold on rigidly to old patterns that are no longer functional, in order to minimize the sense of loss and disruption in family life. Later, the formation of other attachments and commitments may be blocked by fear of another loss. Overidealization of the deceased or a sense of disloyalty may also contribute to reluctance to accept a new member who is seen as replacing the deceased, particularly when the loss has not been integrated.

After her husband's death in a car crash, Mrs. Miller vowed to carry on family life as if her husband were still "at the head of the table," and to raise their children as she imagined he would have wished. She took a stressful full-time job, yet continued to keep the house spotless and prepare meals the father had loved. His favorite family outings and holidays were celebrated in the same way, year after year. Five years after the death, the family came for therapy when the middle of three daughters was rebelling against her mother's authority. The girls, now in adolescence, voiced their wish to spend more time with friends and to give up activities they had outgrown and only pretended to enjoy, yet they didn't want to be disloyal. The mother acknowledged her constant strain in trying to be "two parents" and live up to her husband's standards, as she idealized them. We worked on finding ways to honor the father's memory and yet modify their living patterns to better fit changing developmental needs and their structure as a single-parent family.

As we saw in the case of Marie, children can suffer not only from their exclusion from the dying process and funeral rites, but even more by further separations, confusion, and lack of protection in the aftermath of loss. Families sometimes fall apart structurally as well as emotionally with an unbearable loss: Leadership and communication may falter, and parents may be unable to nurture and protect children. Preoccupied by their own loss, they may be unavailable to children or breach generational boundaries, using them inappropriately to meet their own needs. Every effort should be made to keep siblings together, as the sibling bond can be a vital lifeline (McGoldrick & Watson, 1999). As it is natural for children to worry about losing the surviving parent, reliable contact is valuable, even if they must live apart for a while. It is important to provide clear information about what will happen, when, and who will take care of them. Because family structure can break down with the loss of a parent, extended family members need to help the surviving parent reorganize daily patterns of living and provide appropriate care and protection for children through the disruption. Social supports often dwindle after the first few weeks of a loss, so it's vitally important to link those who are bereaved and isolated with kin and community support over many months to prevent inappropriate burdening, neglect, or abuse of children.

Reinvestment in Other Relationships and Life Pursuits

The process of mourning is quite variable, often lasting much longer than people expect. Many cultures ritualize a mourning period of around a year. Survivors may not be ready to reengage for much longer after sudden, traumatic, and untimely losses, whereas those who have experienced lengthy anticipatory grief in protracted illnesses may be ready to move on emotionally much sooner. And yet, each new season, holiday, and anniversary is likely to reevoke the loss and a surge of painful feelings. Joyful events such as graduations, marriages, and births may elicit sorrow at shattered dreams and milestones never to be celebrated. Overidealization of the deceased, a sense of disloyalty, or the catastrophic fear of another loss may block the formation of other attachments and commitments.

Often, family reorganizational tasks must be addressed before members are emotionally ready to reinvest in new relationships. If family members take flight from painful losses by seeking immediate replacement, they risk complications due to blocked mourning processes.

Well-intentioned friends and relatives may see the need for someone to fill the role functions of a deceased mother or father and push the surviving parent unwisely into premature remarriage "for the sake of the children." In other cases, a widow's decision to remarry may spark upset reactions by children or former in-laws if they view it as disloyal. Often, children balk at acceptance of a new stepparent who is seen as a replacement when the loss has not yet been integrated. Therapists can help families navigate these challenges.

After a period of grieving the loss of a significant family member, a new and unforeseen life direction may open up. One woman, Denise, initially was devastated at the death of her husband and the loss of all their shared plans for the future. She knew nothing about managing money, which had been his domain, and had no sense of her own identity apart from the marriage. For 22 years she had oriented herself around her husband's needs, career, and social network and felt her life was now empty. Our therapy helped her begin to see glimpses of possibility: to build her own social network and to pursue a career, which she had years earlier set aside, and to take it in a new direction in home-based consultation, fitting her priorities at midlife as well as constraints in the workplace. She found great satisfaction—especially in managing the financial aspects of her business.

A resilience-oriented systemic approach to loss requires the same ingenuity and flexibility that families themselves need to respond to various members and subsystems as their issues come to the fore. As changes occur in one part of a system, changes in other parts will be generated. Decisions to meet with an individual, couple, or family unit at various points are guided by a systemic view of the loss process.

This practice approach encourages active steps that facilitate the mourning process over time. In my work with the Miller family (above), whose grief at the father's death had been blocked for several years, I encouraged them to sort through old sealed boxes in the basement. They discussed which keepsakes each wanted to hold on to, sent some to relatives and friends of their father, and gave the rest to charity. For the approaching anniversary of the death, the mother decided to write a tribute, which she had been asked, but unable, to do at the time of the death. This prompted one daughter to write a poem and another to make a drawing in memory of their father. With great enthusiasm, they gathered these into a booklet, which they sent to relatives and friends, reviving many valuable contacts that had been lost.

VARIABLES IN FAMILY RISK AND RESILIENCE

The impact of a death is influenced by a number of variables in the loss situation and the surrounding family processes and social context (Walsh & McGoldrick, 2004). It is important for clinicians to be aware of patterns that can complicate family adaptation and heighten risk of dysfunction (Rando, 1993; see Chapter 11, this volume). In order to work preventively at the time of a loss, or to understand and repair long-term complications, these risk factors should always be carefully evaluated and attended to in interventions that promote healing and resilience.

Nature and Circumstances of the Loss

The timing and manner of death pose varied challenges for surviving family members and need to be explored in any clinical assessment. In family assessment, a genogram and timeline are particularly useful in tracking sequences and concurrence of significant events and symptoms over time in the multigenerational family field (McGoldrick et al., 1999).

Timing of Loss in the Family Life Cycle

The meaning and impact of a death vary depending on the developmental challenges the family is negotiating. The particular timing of a loss may place a family at higher risk for dysfunction (Walsh, 1983; Walsh & McGoldrick, 2004): (1) *Untimely loss* is hardest to bear and seems unjust especially in the death of a child, which reverses generational expectations (Oliver, 1999); (2) The *concurrence of a death with other loss, major transition, or stresses* produces a pileup of stress and incompatible demands; (3) A *history of traumatic loss and complicated mourning* intensifies the meaning and response in a recent or threatened death. In each situation, the nature of the death, the function of the person in the family, and the state of relationships will interact. A developmental perspective can facilitate adaptation in ways that strengthen the whole family in future life passages.

Sudden or Lingering Death

Sudden deaths or deaths following protracted illness are especially stressful for families and require different coping processes. When a person dies unexpectedly, as in a car crash or a heart attack, family members lack time to anticipate and prepare for the loss, to deal with unfinished business, or even to say their good-byes (see Chapter 11). When the dying process has been prolonged, family caregiving and financial resources are often depleted, with the needs of other members put on hold. Relief at ending patient suffering and family strain is likely to be guilt-laden. Moreover, families increasingly face anguished dilemmas over whether and how long to maintain life support efforts (see Chapter 9).

Ambiguous Loss

Ambiguity surrounding loss interferes with adaptation, often producing depression and conflict (Boss, 1999). In one type of ambiguous loss, a family member may be physically present but gradually lose their cognitive functioning and even become unable to recognize loved ones, as occurs in Alzheimer's disease (see Chapter 9). In other types of ambiguous loss, a loved one may be physically absent but their fate unknown, such as an abducted child, the victim of a politically motivated disappearance, or those missing in combat or in a major disaster (see Chapter 11). Family members may be tormented, hoping for the best while fearing the worst. We can help them to live with uncertainty, while actively encouraging their best efforts to gain information to confirm whether their loved one is dead or alive.

Unacknowledged and Stigmatized Losses

Mourning can be complicated when losses are unacknowledged, hidden, or minimized, such as losses in pregnancy, the death of a close friend, lover, or former spouse, or the loss of a cherished pet. The bereaved can be isolated when they feel they don't have a right to their grief or that it is inappropriate, or if it doesn't fit into socially approved categories. Losses may be hidden when a relationship itself is secret and/or disapproved of by family or community, as commonly occurs in gay and lesbian relationships. When couples lack the legal standing of marriage, survivors are also denied death benefits and if they have coparented the biological child of their partner, they may lose legal rights to continue that relationship.

The stigma surrounding HIV/AIDS has contributed to secrecy, misinformation, and estrangement, impairing family and social support, as well as critical health care. The epidemic of AIDS in the gay community—

and increasingly, for men, women, and children in poor communities worldwide—is all the more devastating because of the multiple losses and anticipated losses of partners, parents, children, and other loved ones in relationship networks.

Violent Death

The impact of a violent death can be devastating, especially for loved ones who have witnessed it, may have contributed to it, or narrowly survived themselves (see Chapter 11). Body mutilation or the inability to retrieve a body complicates family mourning processes. After the loss of a family member in a major disaster, such as a plane crash, survivors commonly report their inability to begin mourning until the body, or personal effects belonging to their loved one, is recovered and the death becomes physically real. The senseless tragedy in the loss of innocent lives is especially hard to bear, particularly if it is the result of negligence, as in drunk driving, or deliberate acts of violence, as in neighborhood or school shootings.

Murders are committed more often by relatives or acquaintances than by strangers. Clinicians should be vigilant in cases of partner violence and child abuse and take threats of harm seriously. Risk of murder is heightened when an abused spouse attempts to leave the violent partner or, after separation, begins a new relationship.

Suicides are tormenting deaths for families to come to terms with, particularly when they appear impulsive, senseless, or intended to hurt or punish loved ones. In adolescence, peer drug or drinking cultures can encourage and romanticize self-destructive behavior. Clinicians also need to be alert to family influences, such as abandonment or sexual abuse, as well as job or social influences that fuel depression, guilt, or shame over misdeeds or failure, and that may pose a heightened risk of suicide.

In the aftermath, clinicians need to help family members with their anger or guilt, particularly when they are blamed or blame themselves for the death. The social and religious stigma of suicide also contributes to family shame and cover-up, which distort family communication and can isolate families from social support. Clinicians should routinely note family histories of suicide or other traumatic losses that may predict future suicide risk, particularly at an anniversary or birthday.

Daniel, age 13, and his family were at a loss to explain his recent suicide attempt and made no mention of an older deceased brother. Family assessment revealed that Daniel had been born shortly before the death of an elder son at the age of 13. Daniel grew up attempting to take the place of the brother he had never known, in order to relieve his parents' sadness. The father, who could not recall the date or events surrounding the death, wished to remember his first son "as if he were still alive." Daniel cultivated his appearance to resemble photos of his brother. When he had reached the age of his brother's death, and his growth spurt at puberty was changing him from the way he was "supposed" to look, he attempted suicide to join his brother in heaven. Family therapy focused on enabling Daniel and his parents to relinquish his surrogate position so that he could move forward in his own development.

When self-harm is a risk, psychotropic medication can assist therapeutic efforts to restore hope to a bleak outlook, to assess life constraints and options from a clearer perspective, and to find meaning and energy to reengage in relationships and life pursuits. In many cases, finding ways to reduce physical suffering or social isolation is also important in regaining the desire to live. Although a therapist or loved ones cannot always prevent a suicide, the risk can be lowered by opening communication, mobilizing the support of family and friends, and fostering a sense of coherence in the meaning of past or ongoing trauma. Helping family members support one another to integrate painful experiences and to envision a meaningful future beyond disappointments and losses is vital in strengthening both individual and family resilience.

Family and Social Network

The general level of family functioning and the state of relationships prior to and following the loss should be carefully evaluated with attention to the extended family and social network. Family belief systems, organizational patterns, and communication processes are crucial in mediating adaptation to loss. Particular note should be taken of the following variables.

Meaning Making

Beliefs about death and the meanings surrounding a particular loss are rooted in multigenerational family legacies, in ethnic and religious beliefs, and in the dominant societal values and practices (see McGoldrick et al., 2004; Walsh, 2004). Each family's belief system significantly influences adaptation to loss. In families showing the most maladaptive patterns, members may avoid painful realities through denial or distortion.

In all families, members struggle to make sense of their loss and put it in perspective to make it more bearable (Nadeau, 2001; Neimeyer, 2001). Commonly they grapple with painful questions: Why us? Why my child (or sibling or spouse) and not me? How could this have happened? Is someone to blame? Could it have been prevented? Such concerns remain salient when the cause of a death is unclear. Deaths that are sudden and unexpected or seem senseless can shatter core assumptions of normality, security, and predictability.

Clinicians need to explore beliefs that foster blame, shame, and guilt surrounding a death (Rolland, 1994). Such causal attributions are especially strong in situations of traumatic death where the cause is unclear and questions of responsibility or negligence arise. Family members often hold a secret belief that they themselves or others could have, or should have, done something to prevent a death. It is important to help members share such concerns and come to terms with the extent of their responsibility and limits of control in the situation. Western values of personal responsibility, mastery, and control can fuel blame and guilt and can hinder acceptance of death.

Hope: A Positive Outlook

It is in times of deepest despair that hope is most essential. Resilience involves mastery of the possible with acceptance of that which is beyond control. Family members may despair that, despite their best efforts, optimism, or medical care, they couldn't conquer death. Although they may not be able to stop death, they can be encouraged to engage fully in the dying process to make the most of precious time, alleviate suffering, and heal relational grievances. Although they cannot bring back a loved one, when death shatters hopes and dreams, clinicians need to help family members find new and renewed meaning to go on with life and positive legacies to pass on to future generations.

Transcendence and Spirituality

Death ends a life but a relationship transcends death and is sustained through spiritual connection, memories, stories, and deeds. Our own death and that of our loved ones can be faced more openly and courageously through symbolic ways to define ourselves as part of a larger, meaningful whole. Those who believe in a spiritual afterlife or reincarnation find comfort in accepting death as a passage to another realm and, in Eastern and Native American beliefs, part of a larger evolution-ary cycle in the universe (Deloria, 1994; Walsh, 2004).

Spiritual beliefs and practices foster resilience in the face of death and loss (Becvar, 2001; Walsh, 1999b, 2004). Research has documented the positive physiological effects of deep faith, prayer, meditative prac-tices, and congregational support at these times (Koenig et al., 2001). Many find solace in the belief that a tragic death may be beyond human comprehension but part of God's larger plan, or a test of our faith. Some turn away from their faith. One bereaved father, after the death of his newborn son, who was to be named for him and his father, cried out, "I'm angry at God—how could he take the life of an innocent baby!" In some cases, religious beliefs can be a major source of distress. One mother in an interfaith marriage believed that the stillbirth of her second child was God's punishment for not having baptized her first child. It is important for clinicians to include the spiritual dimension in the experi-ence of death, dying, and loss in both assessment and therapeutic work, and to consult with or refer to pastoral counselors as appropriate.

Suffering can be transcended through creative expression, as in writing, music, or the arts. Many honor the deceased through memorial dedications to benefit others. After the suicide of their young adult daughter, who suffered from bipolar disorder, one family organized pub-lic education programs on serious mental illness in her name. Families can transcend their personal loss through social activism or advocacy to prevent the suffering of other families. Healing is fostered by efforts to honor the best aspects of the deceased person and the relationship. As one mother stated after a reckless driver took the life of her daughter, "My daughter wouldn't want me to become consumed by grief or rage; she would want me to honor her life by taking up some meaningful pur-suit in her memory." Such impetus led several bereaved mothers to found Mothers Against Drunk Drivers (MADD).

Family Flexibility and Structure

Family organization—the system of rules, roles, and boundaries—needs to be flexible, yet clearly structured, for reorganization after loss. It is helpful to inquire about what changed and what did not change with a death and how the family can restore or adapt familiar patterns in the wake of loss. A family that becomes chaotic and disorganized with loss will need help building authoritative leadership, stability, and continuity necessary to manage the disruptive aftermath. An overly rigid family may need help to modify set patterns and make necessary accommodations to loss.

Prior Roles and Functioning in the Family

A loss is greater the more important a person and his or her role function were in family life, such as a parent, grandparent, or sibling who played a major role in childrearing, or a spouse or adult child who was the primary caregiver. The death of an only child, an only son or daughter, or the last of a generation, leaves a particular void. Families risk dysfunction if they avoid the pain of loss by seeking an instant replacement. At the other extreme, a family can become frozen in time if surviving members are unable to reallocate role functions or form new attachments.

Family Connectedness

Adaptation to loss is facilitated by strengthening cohesion and mutual support, with tolerance and respect for individual differences in response to loss. Extreme family patterns of enmeshment or disengagement pose complications. In an intensely fused family, any differences may be viewed as disloyal and threatening, leading members to submerge or distort feelings. To avoid the pain of loss, some families may use a child, a new partner, or a new baby as an emotional replacement, which can complicate that relationship and pose difficulties for attachment and later separation. Other families may avoid the pain with distancing and emotional cutoffs. When families are fragmented, members are left to fend for themselves, isolated in their grief.

State of Relationships at Time of Death

All family relationships have occasional conflict, mixed feelings, or shifting alliances. The mourning process is likely to be more complicated if there has been intense and persistent conflict, strong ambivalence, or estrangement. The death of a troubled or absent parent is difficult; an adult child may have long grieved for a parent he or she never had. The greatest sadness can come from knowing that what might have been can never be. One woman was hospitalized at age 70 with depression, following the death of her 94-year-old father. She had vied unsuccessfully with her younger sister throughout her life for her father's favor. On his deathbed, he called for her sister. Even in later life, what pained her most in his death was the loss of future possibility that she might one day win his approval.

When death is anticipated, as in life-threatening illnesses, clinicians should make every effort to help family members to reconnect and to repair strained relationships before the opportunity is lost. Often this requires overcoming members' reluctance to stir up painful emotions or to dredge up old conflicts. They may fear that confrontations could increase vulnerability and the risk of death. Family therapists need to deal sensitively with these concerns, interrupt destructive interactional spirals, and help family members to share feelings constructively with the aim of healing pained relationships, forging new connections, and building mutual support. A conjoint family life review (Walsh, 1999a) can help members to share different perspectives, to clarify misunderstandings, to place hurts and disappointments in the context of life challenges, to recover caring aspects of relationships, and to update and renew relationships that have been frozen in past conflict.

Extended Family, Social, and Economic Resources

The loss experience is buffered by supportive kin, friendship, and community networks. When long-standing conflicts, estrangement, or social stigma have left families isolated, clinicians can be helpful in mobilizing a potentially supportive network. Internet resources are increasingly tapped for information and support, offering a virtual community, but can overload, misinform, or heighten distress of family members hungry for assistance and connection. Family recovery is impaired when finances are drained by costly, protracted medical care, inadequate health insurance coverage, or the death of the major breadwinner. It is important to help families discuss such financial issues.

Clear, Open Communication versus Secrecy

When a family confronts a loss, open communication facilitates the processes of emotional recovery and reorganization. Clinicians can help members to clarify facts and circumstances of an ambiguous or unacknowledged loss. When certain feelings, thoughts, or memories are prohibited by family loyalties, social taboos, or myths, communication around the loss experience can be distorted and contribute to symptoms (Imber-Black, 1995). The cover-up of an alcohol-related accident, a drug overdose, or a suicide is common and carries its own painful legacy for survivors in further blocked communication, cutoffs, and self-destructive behavior, often fueled by a vague, pervasive depression, guilt, or shame. It is important to foster a family climate of mutual trust, empathic response, and tolerance for a wide and fluctuating range of responses to loss over time.

Gender-Related Issues

Although gender roles and relationships have been changing in recent decades, expectations for men and women in families are still influenced strongly by traditional gender-based norms. Women are vulnerable to blame and guilt when a death occurs because they are expected to bear primary responsibility for the well-being of their spouses, children, and elders. Yet, in traumatic events (see Chapter 11), men may suffer from guilt if they weren't able to protect or rescue a loved one, a coworker, or others who died, especially women and children. In bereavement, women have been socialized to assume the major role in handling the social and emotional tasks, from expression of grief to caregiving for the terminally ill and surviving family members, including their spouse's extended family. Men who have been socialized to manage instrumental tasks tend to take charge of funeral, burial, financial, and property arrangements. In the dominant U.S. culture, they are more likely to become emotionally constrained and withdrawn around times of loss. Cultural sanctions against revealing vulnerability or dependency can block emotional expressiveness and ability to seek and give comfort. These constraints contribute to high rates of serious illness and death for men in the first year of widowhood (Lopata, 1996).

The different responses of partners to loss, especially in the death of a child, can strain couple relationships. Men are more likely to express anger than sorrow and to withdraw, seek refuge in their work, or turn to alcohol, drugs, or an affair. They may be uncomfortable with their wives' expressions of grief, not knowing how to respond and fearful of losing control of their own feelings (culturally framed as "breaking down" and "falling apart"). Grieving individuals may perceive their partners' emotional unavailability as abandonment when they need comfort most, thereby experiencing a double loss (Johnson, 2002).

Individual approaches focused on the "symptomatic" partner appear to have limited impact on recovery when couple relationship dynamics are not addressed as well. Most commonly, it is women who seek treatment for depression or other symptoms of distress concerning loss, while their husbands appear to be functioning well and may see no need for help for themselves.

Marlene was being seen in individual therapy for inconsolable grief, after her only child, 18-year-old Jimmy, had collapsed and died in her arms. Marlene and Matt, a working-class African American couple, had worked very hard to raise Jimmy well and were extremely proud that he had just earned a scholarship to college. Although Matt too had lost his only child, he refused therapy for himself, saying he was fine and didn't need any help. Yet he drove Marlene to each session and waited for her in the car. When presented with clinic forms to sign, however, he balked; he did not want to fill out a symptom checklist or to be labeled as needing help. His stoic manner of maintaining control was a source of pride to him. However, he responded to the therapist's encouragement that he could be a helpful resource to his wife by sitting by her side and supporting her in sessions. It wasn't long until he gained trust in the therapist and shared his own deep pain of loss and both spouses found comfort in sharing their grief.

When one spouse has difficulty acknowledging vulnerability and sorrow at a time of tragedy, the other may then carry the emotions for both of them. Resentment may build toward the unavailable partner, who is felt to be insensitive and unsupportive. A couple approach is essential to build mutual empathy, since the relationship is at risk. Interventions can decrease relational polarization so that partners can support each other and share in the full range of human experiences in bereavement.

Loss in the Family Life Cycle

Untimely Losses

Deaths that are premature or untimely in terms of chronological or social expectations, such as early widowhood, early parent loss, or death of a child, can be immensely more difficult to come to terms with (Neugarten, 1976). Untimely losses are complicated by the lack of social norms, models, or guidelines to assist in preparation and coping. Such a loss is often experienced as unjust, ending a life and a relationship before their prime, robbing hopes and dreams for a future that can never be. Prolonged mourning, often lasting many years, is a common occurrence. Long-term survival guilt for spouses, siblings, and parents can block life satisfaction and achievements for years to come.

Early Parent Loss. Children who lose a parent may suffer profound short- and long-term consequences, including illness, depression, and other emotional disturbances. They are at risk for later difficulty in forming other intimate attachments, with catastrophic fears of separation and abandonment. A child's adaptation to parent loss depends largely on the emotional state of the surviving parent, as shown in Marie's case above. Griefwork with the surviving parent and efforts to organize and strengthen the supportive role of the extended family can make all the difference in children's ability to cope and adapt. Children need help in making meaning of the loss experience appropriate to their developmental stage. Stabilizing their home situation and providing clear reassurance that they will be well cared for and not abandoned are essential. Children also show better adjustment when not separated from their siblings and significant kin.

An inspiring portrayal of family resilience is found in the film *Crooklyn*, by Spike Lee (1994). The film looks at life through the eyes of a 10-year-old daughter in an African American family struggling to get by financially and raise five children well in a blighted urban neighborhood. The parents' relationship is not without conflict and skew; the mother is the solid bedrock of the family, and the father, although warm and loving, is often inconsistent, underresponsible, and self-absorbed. Yet, when the mother is found to have terminal cancer, the father rises to meet the challenges, drawing on previously untapped resources within himself to provide strength, security, and comfort to their children. When the daughter, devastated by the death, angrily refuses to get dressed up and attend the funeral ("What for? It's not going to bring her back!"), her father's tender empathy for her feelings along with authoritative firmness enables her to join family and friends to pay their last respects together. Her older brother, long her tormentor, moves over to sit beside her and hold hands, opening up a new bond. Heeding her mother's last request, she takes on new responsibility, keeping an eye out for her youngest brother. When weeks later she finally breaks down, frightened and sobbing, her father's arms encircle her as he helps her express her bottled-up emotions. She asks, "Will I get cancer too, like Momma?" and she then shares her greatest fear: "You won't leave us too, will you? Or send me away?" The father's responses are thoughtful, honest, and reassuring. As their conversation helps her begin to find meaning and solace in her mother's death, she asks, "Momma was in a lot of pain, wasn't she?" "Yes, she was." "Then it's good that she's gone to a place where she's not suffering any more." "That's a real nice way to put it," he tenderly replies. As the film ends, it is clear that many challenges are yet ahead, but a secure family foundation has been laid.

Child Loss. The death of a child, reversing the natural generational order, is also a devastating loss for a family (Rando, 1984). It is often said that when your parent dies, you have lost your past, when your child dies, you have lost your future. The untimeliness and injustice in the death of a child can lead family members to profound questioning of the meaning of life. In addition, of all losses, it is hardest not to idealize a deceased child; this may complicate relationships with surviving siblings.

With the loss of a child, a parental marriage is at heightened risk for discord, distancing, and divorce. However, spouses who support and sustain each other through the tragedy can forge even stronger relationships than before, underscoring the critical role of couple and family therapy in child loss. It is also crucial not to neglect the impact on siblings, who may experience prolonged grieving or anniversary reactions for years afterward. A sibling's death may also be accompanied by a sense of loss of parents who are preoccupied with caretaking or grieving. Normal sibling rivalry may contribute to intense survival guilt that can block developmental strivings well into adulthood. Some parents turn to a sibling as a replacement, as in the case of Daniel, above.

The impetus to have another child is very common and can bring solace. However, parents should be advised to allow themselves time to experience the loss so that the new relationship is not burdened by replacement needs or attachment difficulties, as in the following case:

Bill and Jean were seen in couple therapy for conflict over their inability to name their baby, now almost a year old. The solution-focused therapy succeeded in two sessions in naming the child; however, Jean then became suicidal. It was learned that they had conceived this child only 3 months after the loss of a much-desired pregnancy, for which Jean blamed herself. Upon learning that her grandfather, who had abused her as a child, had died suddenly, she was overcome by a "crazy mix of emotions." She went out all night drinking and partying "to get away from it all," and suffered a miscarriage the next day. Urged by well-intentioned relatives to have another child "to get over it," she found herself unable to attach to the new baby. It only made matters worse when, pressed to name their daughter, Bill and Jean gave her the name that they had chosen for the other baby.

Careful evaluation is needed before intervening in a problem situation. Losses during pregnancy and perinatal deaths tend to be hidden and minimized. The impact of such loss experiences will depend greatly on spousal support and on religious or cultural beliefs about the meaning of stillbirth, infertility, miscarriage, or abortion.

Loss of a Partner. Early widowhood can be a shocking and isolating experience without emotional preparation or essential social supports. Other couples and peers at the same life stage commonly distance to avoid facing their own vulnerability. Here too, immediate replacement may lead to further complications.

> Doreen and Nick were seen in couple therapy because she felt their "semi-committed" relationship was "deadlocked" and wanted either to get married or to end it. Most nights Nick came for dinner; after her girls went to bed, he and Doreen would set up a cot next to her bed, where he spent the night, returning to his own apartment each morning. The therapist learned that 6 years earlier, within a few months of the sudden death of her husband, Doreen had accepted an offer by Nick, an old friend, to move with her children to his community to start a new life. Nick found her a job and an apartment next to his own. Because they had moved too quickly into this relationship, its status remained ambivalent. Doreen, devastated by the loss of her husband, had initially found support and consolation from Nick and had found the move a welcome escape; yet she became depressed, overweight, and unhappy in her job. Couple sessions revealed Nick's ongoing casual affairs with other women and his refusal ever to commit himself fully again since a bitter divorce and cutoff from his children. Doreen decided to end the relationship and move on with her life. With this loss, she found herself dreaming nightly of her deceased husband and was flooded with intense longings for him, opening up her delayed griefwork in therapy.

It is common for unresolved mourning from a past loss to surface at the breakup of a replacement relationship. Individual sessions are valuable at that time to attend to the delayed grief process; to review the earlier courtship, marriage, and family life; and to explore the many meanings of the loss and subsequent life passages. Issues of loyalty and guilt are crucial to address. With the encouragement of the therapist, Doreen returned to her hometown to visit her husband's grave for the first time since the funeral, and spent some time at the gravesite "telling him" all she would have liked him to know about their children's development and budding talents, the memories she would carry on of their life together, and their continuing love for him as they went forward in their lives. This visit and conversation brought her a sense of peace.

Concurrence with Other Losses, Stresses, or Life Changes

The temporal coincidence of a loss with other losses, other major stress events, or developmental milestones may overload a family and pose incompatible tasks and demands. A genogram and timeline are particularly useful in tracking sequences and concurrence of nodal events over time in the multigenerational family field (McGoldrick et al., 1999). Sketching a timeline can alert clinicians to concurrence of losses and stressful transitions and their relation to the timing of symptoms. Particular attention should be paid to the concurrence of death with the birth of a child, since the processes of mourning and of parenting an infant are inherently conflictual. Moreover, as in the case of Daniel's family, a child born at the time of a significant loss may assume a special replacement function that can be the impetus for high achievement or dysfunction. Similarly, a precipitous marriage in the wake of loss is likely to confound the two relationships, interfering with bereavement and with investment in the new relationship in its own right. When stressful events pile up, mobilizing the support of family members is especially important.

Past Traumatic Loss and Unresolved Mourning

Some individuals and families emerge hardier from past traumatic loss experiences, whereas others are left more vulnerable to subsequent losses. When problems with separation, attachment/commitment, or self-destructive behavior are presented in therapy, it is crucial to explore possible connections to earlier traumatic losses in the family system, especially around nodal events, such as the birth of the symptom bearer.

It is important to note transgenerational anniversary patterns, that is, when symptoms occur at the same point in the life cycle as a significant death or loss in a past generation. Individuals may become preoccupied with their own or their spouses' mortality when they reach the same age or life transition point (e.g., retirement) at which a parent died. Many make abrupt career or relationship changes, or start new fitness regimens and feel they must "get through the year," while others may behave self-destructively. Unresolved family patterns, or scenarios, may also be replicated when a child reaches the same age or stage as a parent at the time of a prior death or traumatic loss (Walsh, 1983). It is crucial to assess a risk of destructive behavior at such times. In dysfunctional families, such linkages may be covert and disconnected from current symptoms.

An appreciation of the power of covert family scripts (Byng-Hall, 1995a) and family legacies is important to understand the transmission of such patterns in loss. Anniversary reactions are most likely to occur when there has been a physical and emotional cutoff from the past and when family rules, often covert, prohibit open communication about past traumatic events. This occurred in the case of Martin's family (page 18, in Chapter 1). Interventions are aimed at making covert patterns overt and helping family members to come to terms with the past and differentiate present relationships, so that history need not repeat itself.

In order to help families with loss, therefore, family therapists need to help them reappraise family history, replacing deterministic assumptions and catastrophic fears with an evolutionary perspective that integrates life experiences and yields meaning and hope for the future.

HELPING FAMILIES WITH LOSS: THERAPEUTIC CHALLENGES

As we've seen, healing and resilience in the face of loss are not simply matters of individual bereavement, but also involve family mourning processes. Of all human experiences, death poses the most painful and far-reaching adaptational challenges for families. A systemic framework for clinical assessment and intervention with loss is crucial to address the reverberations of a death for all family members, their relationships, and the family as a functional unit.

A family resilience–oriented approach to loss is guided by an understanding of major family adaptational challenges, variables that heighten risk, and key family processes that foster recovery. Given the diversity of family forms, values, and life courses, we must be careful not to confuse common patterns in response to loss with normative standards, or to assume that differences in bereavement are necessarily pathological. Helping family members deal with a loss requires respect for their particular religious beliefs and cultural heritage and encouragement to forge their own pathways through the mourning process. Because all family members and their relationships are affected by a loss, individual, couple, and family sessions may need to be combined flexibly to fit varied adaptive challenges over time. By strengthening key relationships and the functioning of the family unit, a healing process can reverberate throughout the system, to benefit every member.

Although open communication and mutual support are emphasized, active processes in dealing with death and loss are also encouraged. The drawing up and discussion of wills, living wills, and directives by all adult family members (not only the most vulnerable ones) are advised. Planning and participating in meaningful memorial rites are also encouraged, as are visits to the grave—not only at the time of loss, but also on anniversaries, even years later. In cases where mourning has been blocked, it's helpful for clients to sort through and bring in old photos and memorabilia, which open up memories and trigger the flow of old and new stories. They can be encouraged to share stories and mementos with children, other family members, and friends, setting off a chain of positive mutual influences for recovery and new resilience.

Dying and healing are not incompatible. To find healing in the face of death involves integrating the fullness of the life and significant relationships. Bereaved families can find strength to surmount heartbreaking untimely loss and go on in a meaningful life by bringing benefit to others from their own tragedy. Clinicians can help clients to find pride, dignity, and purpose in their darkest hours through altruistic actions such as organ donation, memorial contributions to medical research, or taking the initiative in forming support groups for families who have suffered similar losses or community action coalitions.

As clinicians, our own resilience is tested in work with loss. In turn, the profound nature of this work can strengthen our capacity to meet the most difficult human and therapeutic challenges. We need to create a safe haven where family members can open up and share deep pain and intense emotions, with assurance that we will not abandon them in their pain nor worsen it. We offer compassionate witnessing, as well as strong support, encouragement, and perseverance to overcome the many fears and protective barriers that block family members from facing death and healing from loss. Helping professionals may suffer at times from compassion fatigue (Figley, 2002), particularly in oncology and hospice settings, caring for so many individuals and families facing painful losses. It's also important to guard personal time for activities and relationships that revive the spirit. One hospice worker found it restorative to volunteer monthly to help parents with newborn infants.

Consultation teams are valuable for sharing and processing the emotional toll. One child oncology department holds an annual day of mourning and renewal for all staff at a beautiful nearby campground. In an open ceremony, staff members are invited to share experiences they've had with patients and their families that had especially touched their hearts. Music and singing are an important part of the gathering.

In dealing with life-and-death matters, we need to be accepting of the limits of our control: Despite our rescue fantasies, we cannot stop death or bring back a loved one. Moreover, we must become comfortable with the stirring of our own emotions by a tragic death and loss. One man, who had worked hard in therapy to begin to forge a relationship with his distant and critical father, came back to see me in crisis. His father had suffered a serious stroke and lay in a coma in intensive care, with the prognosis uncertain. Tears came down my own cheeks as he cried openly, saying, "I can't bear to lose him when I only just found him."

Work with death and loss brings us in touch with our own vulnerabilities. Like the families we work with, we all must experience and come to terms with our own losses and mortality. This work also brings blessings and keeps us in touch with the meaning of life. Forming caring therapeutic bonds in the face of loss deepens our humanity and offers a model to clients of living and loving beyond loss. As Robert Lifton (1979) has said, "There is no love without loss." In accepting loss, we open ourselves most fully to life and love.

It can be profoundly moving for us as clinicians, as well as for family members, to experience the creative transformations and deepening of relationships that occur in the healing process. And, in opening ourselves to loving connections, we are better able to face the challenges of loss.

CHAPTER 9

Chronic Illness
and Family Caregiving
Challenges and Gifts

All the world is full of suffering; it is also full of overcoming it.
—HELEN KELLER, *Midstream: My Later Life*

Serious physical or mental illnesses pose a myriad of challenges
for families, requiring considerable resilience in coping and adaptation.
A health crisis can also be experienced as a wake-up call about life. It
can heighten and alter our sense of priorities, which are too often lost in
the helter-skelter demands of daily living. Persistent conditions can force
us to make changes in our patterns of living and reorient our hopes and
dreams. This chapter highlights salient issues for a family resilience approach to chronic illness and disability.

LEARNING THE ART OF THE POSSIBLE:
LESSONS FROM LIFE

Over the course of the life cycle, serious illness strikes us all; therapists
are not immune. Our own experiences with illness and caregiving challenges can teach us many things about resilience. It can deepen our work

with individuals and families who are striving to live as well as possible with persistent conditions (McDaniel, Hepworth, & Doherty, 1997).

In 1985 I was hospitalized with meningitis on return home from a consultation in Morocco. I was informed of the diagnosis, but was given no information about what I might expect. The first few nights, the nurses woke me several times but never told me why, so I presumed that it was to make sure I was still alive. At the end of the week, I was informed that the crisis period was over, my EEG appeared normal, and I could go home and resume "normal activity." When I asked for guidelines, I was told only to avoid stress for a while. The next night, I hosted a dinner party for close friends; I thought that this was "normal activity"— celebratory and fun—not what I considered stressful. I collapsed before the end of the evening. At my follow-up appointment with the neurologist a few days later, I was angry. I asked for clearer guidelines: "How should I know what's too stressful?" I'll never forget his reply: "If you walk to the corner and need an ambulance to get home, then that was too much." This was not helpful. If I only found out *after* I required the ambulance, I had no guidelines to protect myself and avert a health crisis.

The year that followed was a long nightmare. I struggled to meet the demands of a flourishing career and of parenting an active 3-year-old child. I could pull myself out of bed to get my daughter off to nursery school and then teach a 3-hour seminar, only to collapse with piercing headaches, dizziness, and exhaustion for the rest of the day. I had no memory of what I had said in class. I tried to work on a book draft, only to have excruciating difficulty finding words and forming coherent sentences. My doctor was amiable but patronizing, each time telling me simply to "take it easy" and I'd soon feel better, as if I were exaggerating my difficulties for sympathy. I felt helpless and despairing. My resilient self was not bouncing back.

After a year of "taking it easy," I was still not much better. I consulted another neurologist, who performed further tests and found that I had suffered neurological damage, particularly to the vestibular system; this accounted for my persistent symptoms. Although the news was more grim, this physician was more helpful and hopeful. His approach was closer to a healing and resilience philosophy than to the traditional treatment paradigm. Its central assumption (based on growing scientific evidence) was that the human brain has considerable plasticity; it is able to repair itself and modify its wiring to compensate for injury and loss, if we actively mobilize our resources for recovery. Working collaboratively, he took time to listen to my concerns and answer my questions, gave me informational brochures, drew diagrams of the brain injury, and helped me to comprehend my illness experience. Medication controlled the pain and dizziness. Convinced that the brain, like other body parts, needs exercise to function well ("use it or lose it"), this physician started me on a program of strengthening exercises to reduce my vulnerabilities and restore my mental energy and functioning. He encouraged me to persist in my teaching and writing efforts, but in a more planful, incremental way, which would allow me to regain my proficiency gradually. He helped me not to become discouraged when symptoms worsened at times of high stress, to anticipate such times in the future, and to restructure my life to buffer stress more effectively. Months later, much improved, I asked him how he and my first neurologist could have approached the same patient so differently. He laughed and said, "I've known Dr. X for years; we play tennis together. When he has an injury, he stops playing for a few months and takes it easy. When I have an injury, I get physical therapy and get back on the court as soon as possible. It's all in our world view."

Indeed it was. Looking back, I can see that the successful approach to my persistent condition embodied many of the key processes in resilience and was based in a collaborative therapeutic partnership. Unfortunately, one link was missing: inclusion of the family. Although I came through the worst of the ordeal personally strengthened, my marriage, already strained, didn't survive. Yet the many months of quiet contemplation enabled me to gain a new perspective on my life and to deepen the precious bond with my child. I learned to reduce my work overload, focus on the things that really mattered, set aside petty things, and find more joy in my life. Over time, I had to come to grips with the long-term sequelae of the brain injury, accepting the challenges I would have to live with the best that I could. I learned to practice the art of the possible.

THE ILLNESS EXPERIENCE:
A SYSTEMIC PERSPECTIVE

A family resilience approach to serious illness is grounded in a systemic orientation; it involves language and concepts that humanize the challenges of illness and that encourage optimal functioning, as well as personal and relational well-being.

Bridging the Mind–Body Split

The development of an integrated biopsychosocial approach to both psychiatric and medical disorders requires a paradigmatic shift from the traditional Western view of mind and body as distinct and separate (Bateson, 1979). Although such theories first posited a mind–body connection in psychosomatic disorders, the label "psychosomatic" was shameful, laden with pejorative attributions of character weakness or family pathology. It has become increasingly evident that all illnesses involve a recursive interplay of biological and psychosocial influences. Emotional and interpersonal distress contributes to a wide range of physical symptoms, lowers physiological immunity, and can hasten death. Likewise, serious illness and disability are often accompanied and exacerbated by anxiety, confusion, and depression, particularly when social support is lacking.

However, mental illnesses in particular continue to be stigmatized in cultural beliefs and treated differently in health care policy and practice, despite conclusive research findings that serious mental disorders have a biological base. Managed care developments "carved out" mental illnesses, with suspicion of greater malingering and abuse of benefits. Strong efforts by the mental health professions and consumer lobbying groups are gaining some success in overcoming old prejudices and changing policies toward parity of benefits for mental conditions.

A Biopsychosocial–Spiritual Orientation

The phrase "biopsychosocial" is in wide currency, but it is often not translated into practice. Although medical training is becoming increasingly oriented toward treating the whole person, the family and social context receive insufficient attention. In most psychiatric settings, psychopharmacological treatment approaches coexist with individually focused psychodynamic and cognitive-behavioral models. A family-centered approach attends to the psychosocial bridge connecting individuals with their families and community resources.

It is now well documented that physical illness has a significant impact on family functioning and that family beliefs and practices can influence the physical and mental health of their members (see, e.g., Campbell, 2003). Early studies focused on family contributions to a negative course. Only recently have investigators been examining the impact of individual and family strengths on the illness course and on the quality of life for all family members (Weihs, Fisher, & Baird, 2001). Key family processes have important ramifications for physical hardiness and recovery from illness. For instance, since stress events have been linked to a range of health problems, efforts to strengthen family resilience can buffer stress, contribute to enhanced biological functioning, and bolster physiological immune processes. Family support also increases compliance with treatment and medication regimens.

A family resilience approach, grounded in a biopsychosocial orientation toward illness and treatment, attends to family challenges and strengthens family processes to reduce risks, promote healing, and support optimal functioning. When living with a serious physical illness (e.g., diabetes or multiple sclerosis), disability (e.g., spinal cord injury), or mental illness (e.g., schizophrenia or bipolar disorder), individuals and their families need to forge strengths to weather crises and navigate complications over the long-term course of a chronic condition.

Moreover, illness and suffering involve spiritual matters, opening questions about the human condition, our physical vulnerability, and our mortality (Wright et al., 1996). Varying cultural traditions and spiritual beliefs must be understood and integrated in a holistic approach. For instance, many traditional cultures have understood mental disturbances as forms of possession by spirits. When one Hmong family from Southeast Asia brought a young daughter to a California hospital emergency room for treatment of seizures, a cross-cultural crisis ensued (Fadiman, 1997). The family members wanted the daughter's distress alleviated, but they refused medication to avert future seizures, which they regarded as sacred connections with the spirit world. As they put it, "The spirit catches you and you fall down." The well-intentioned medical staff gained a court-ordered removal of the girl from her parents in order to treat her seizures; however, this only heightened her distress and alienated the family, who refused further treatment after her return home, leading to a tragic outcome. If the medical staff had developed a collaborative relationship with this family and sought to understand their cultural and spiritual beliefs, instead of taking an adversarial approach, their tragedy might well have been averted.

The Illness Experience in Families

As helping professionals, our approach to illness can either constrain or facilitate coping and adaptation. Our images and language matter in conveying respect and humanizing an illness experience, such as speaking of "a person with a disabling condition" rather than "a disabled person" or "identified patient." The term "chronic disorder" too often conjures up pessimistic views of hopeless cases and institutionalization. However, at the other extreme, images of superstar patients and loving families who defeat all odds can be inspiring and yet they can leave ordinary individuals and their families feeling they've failed if they can't reverse a disabling condition or prevent death. With medical advances, increasing numbers of people are living longer with chronic conditions that vary widely in their course, severity, and degree of functional impairment. Although, at present, they may not be curable or reversible, most can be managed well through individual and family efforts, with the support of health care systems and community resources (Rolland, 1994).

The needs of "well" spouses, caregivers, siblings, or other family members must also be understood, validated, and attended to. Family members who put their own needs on hold or are consumed by caregiving demands are themselves at risk for depression, illness, and premature death. Yet, when not overloaded or lacking in support, many find their relationships deepened and more intimate through caregiving.

The term "illness experience" best captures the human experience of living with symptoms and suffering (Kleinman, 1988). The illness experience refers to how impaired persons and members of their family and social network perceive, live with, and master the physical and psychosocial challenges of painful symptoms, disability, and treatments. Life-threatening conditions also present the challenge of carrying on with life in the face of an uncertain prognosis and anticipation of death and loss (Rolland, 2004). In practice, the therapeutic discussion of a woman's experience of breast cancer, mastectomy, and subsequent treatments of radiation and chemotherapy would broaden to explore how it affects her body image, her relationship with her spouse, any children they might have, and their life priorities in the face of possible recurrence and death. We explore such questions as:

How are family, work, and social functioning affected?
What is the illness experience for the spouse? Children?
How can a couple shelter their relationship to weather the strains over time?
How can parents approach their children's concerns about loss?
How can they respond to a daughter's worries about the threat of cancer for herself?
How can kin and social resources be mobilized?

When illness strikes a family member, the entire family requires attention for the optimal coping and adaptation of all. In addition, the advances in genomic science and technology pose a myriad of challenges for families with genetically influenced conditions. Clinicians increasingly will need to help individuals and their families as they grapple with decisions about genetic testing, sharing results with others, and informing children, siblings, or other family members who may be at risk for heritable disorders (Miller, McDaniel, Rolland, & Feetham, 2006; Rolland & Williams, 2005).

Resilience-Oriented Family Systems Approaches to Health Care

Family systems–based health care is a growing field of practice, regarding the family as the central unit of care (Kazak, Simms, & Rourke, 2002; McDaniel, Campbell, Hepworth, & Lorenz, 2005; Rolland & Walsh, 2005). The Collaborative Family Health Care Coalition, founded by Donald Bloch, seeks to encourage patient–family–provider collaboration in the treatment of health problems and accompanying psychosocial challenges.

Family intervention models with serious illness are grounded in a stress–diathesis model, addressing the mutual interactions of biological vulnerability and environmental stresses. Interventions aim to manage the illness, to reduce stress, and to strengthen individual and family functioning and well-being. With an approach that engages the family as an indispensable ally in treatment and taps their potential for resilience, families can more readily seize opportunities to make a difference, increasing their sense of control and quality of life (Rolland, 2003).

Meeting Varied Psychosocial Challenges over Time

The particular challenges of specific illnesses vary; yet there are many commonalities, depending on the psychosocial demands and the timing of an illness. The family systems–illness model developed by Rolland (1994) provides a useful framework for evaluation and resilience-oriented intervention with families dealing with chronic illness and disability. The model casts the illness in systemic terms according to its pattern of practical, emotional, and interpersonal demands over time. The unfolding of a chronic condition involves the intertwining of the illness phases with individual and family life cycles. How we help families think about success or mastery will vary with their challenges, their resources, and their values. The model addresses three dimensions: (1) psychosocial types of illnesses; (2) phases in their course; and (3) key family system variables.

On the first dimension, illnesses are grouped by key biological similarities and differences that pose distinct psychosocial demands for the individual and family. Illness patterning can vary in terms of onset (acute vs. gradual), course (progressive vs. constant vs. relapsing or episodic), outcome (fatal vs. shortened life span or possible sudden death vs. no effect on longevity), incapacitation (none vs. mild vs. moderate vs. severe), and the level of uncertainty about the trajectory. Each psychosocial type of condition poses a pattern of practical and emotional demands that can be addressed in relation to the style, strengths, and vulnerabilities of a family.

On a second dimension, the concept of time phases provides a way for clinicians to think longitudinally about chronic illness as an ongoing process that families navigate with landmarks, transitions, and changing demands. The crisis, chronic, and terminal phases have salient psychosocial challenges, each requiring particular family strengths or changes. For instance, the crisis phase involves the initial period of socialization to chronic illness. Family developmental tasks include creating a meaning for the disorder that preserves a sense of mastery, grieving the loss of the pre-illness family identity, undergoing short-term crisis reorganization, and developing family flexibility in the face of uncertainty and possible threatened loss. Gradually, families must come to accept the persistence or permanence of a chronic condition, learn to live with illness-related symptoms and treatments, and forge an ongoing relationship with professionals and health care systems. In the chronic phase, families must also pace themselves to avoid burnout, rebalance relationship skews (as in caregiving), and juggle the competing needs and priorities of all family members. They must find ways to preserve or revise individual and family goals within the constraints of the illness and to sustain intimacy in the face of threatened loss. With a fatal condition, they need to shift their views of mastery and control over the illness to letting go and making the most of precious time.

The psychosocial demands of any condition are addressed in relation to each phase of the disorder. The model informs the assessment of the interface of the illness with individual and family dynamics and development; the family's multigenerational history of coping with illness, loss, and other adversity; and the meaning of the illness experience for family members. Key processes in family resilience, involving belief systems, organizational patterns, and communication processes, can be targeted as they fit the evolving situation. This framework can guide periodic family consultations, or "psychosocial checkups," as salient issues surface or change over time.

As therapists, we must be flexible in helping families to meet emerging challenges over the uncertain course of a serious, life-threatening illness, as the following case illustrates:

I worked with Kate, a vivacious woman, at various phases and transitions over her 8-year journey with breast cancer. She and her husband, Wayne, showed remarkable courage and resilience through two recurrences, maintaining active initiative in searching out the best treatment options and keeping informed of medical advances. I coached them to listen and respond sensitively to their children's concerns as they emerged, and to keep channels of communication open. Wayne was supportive of Kate and flexible in shifting his work schedule to be more available in parenting their three children during difficult periods. A few couple sessions were held at a time when Wayne became remote, exploring his unexpressed fears of loss and concerns about his ability to manage parenting responsibilities on his own. Kate decided to maintain her part-time clerical job, which she experienced as "an island of normality," taking her mind off her own condition as she tackled mountains of paperwork and enjoyed socializing and light banter with coworkers. She was open in informing colleagues of major changes in her condition or treatments, and took time off when needed; otherwise, she preferred not to discuss her illness at work, keeping a boundary to preserve non-illness-focused aspects of her life. She took "long vacations" from therapy during periods of remission, wanting to "just smell the roses" during stable plateaus, but called proactively when new complications loomed on the horizon. Sometimes she came in, when, as she put it, she lost her compass and needed to reorient herself on her journey.

A year ago, when the cancer spread to her lower spine, Kate underwent an experimental bone marrow transplant, once again beating the odds and doing well over the past year. However, in the midst of her recovery, her 70-year-old mother was diagnosed with untreatable colon cancer, which progressed rapidly to death. A month later Kate called, concerned about Mollie, her 12-year-old daughter. She had found a letter that Mollie had written to a friend, saying that she was desperately unhappy and wanted to run away. We held a family session, where at first Mollie railed against her teachers, wanting to go away to boarding school because "life sucks!" When I asked how the grandmother's recent death had affected family members, Mollie's eyes filled with tears. Her parents' receptiveness helped her to share her fear: "Grandma's death scared me so much. She had cancer, and Mom has had cancer three times. If she could die, so could Mom. Sometimes I have nightmares that

the cancer hasn't all gone away. Then I just want to run away."
Both parents held her, soothing her as she sobbed. Mollie's siblings
were encouraged to share their feelings and concerns, as well. I supported the parents' efforts to talk about the dilemmas in living with
uncertainty and the wish they each had—that they could just make
the cancer go away once and for all. Both parents reassured the children that Mom indeed was continuing to do well, and vowed to be
honest with them if the situation changed. The discussion turned to
ways they could make the most of family time together.

This case illustrates how systemic therapists may combine individual, couple, and family sessions, holding a resilience-oriented systemic
conceptual map to guide intervention priorities over time. Even when
parents handle an illness experience as well as possible at one crisis
point, others will arise later that require renewed—and new—conversations. Here, the death of the grandmother shattered the shared optimism
(positive illusions) that the mother would always continue to beat the
odds. Also, developmental transitions are nodal points when new concerns often surface. As Mollie approached adolescence, she had greater
comprehension of her mother's condition and all it would mean to lose
her. She also began to worry about her own risk of breast cancer. The
time had come to talk more openly about those issues.

Coming to terms with an illness and its ramifications is never a
once-and-for-all matter, but a process that must be worked on periodically over time. The mother's long-term goal was to be there for her
daughters until they were launched and off to college. When that transition occurred, she met with me, saying, "Well, I guess I'd better come up
with a new reason to keep thriving!" We talked about meaningful pursuits for her and travel she and her husband would enjoy together. Such
life-cycle transitions can be valuable touch points for consultation.

Putting the Illness in Its Place

With the diagnosis of a chronic condition, families can't simply "bounce
back" to the old normal life, but must "bounce forward" to navigate a
new terrain, which some describe as "leaving the normal world and entering the illness world." It is crucial that families find ways to gain a
perspective on the illness so it doesn't define an individual's identity or
rule family life. The challenge is to recognize the influence of the condition, master what is possible, accept what is beyond control, and come

to terms with living with it. To do this successfully, families need to find ways to "put the illness in its place" (Gonzalez & Steinglass, 2002). Setting boundaries as to when, where, and with whom illness concerns are discussed can be helpful, just as Kate (above) kept boundaries in her work life to preserve what she called "an island of normality."

For couples, over time a chronic condition can skew the relationship between the impaired partner and the caregiving or "well" spouse (Rolland, 1994). The persistent intrusion of an illness into all aspects of family life can fuel despair, as in the following case:

Mike and Delores, in their mid-40s, came for couple therapy as growing conflict threatened the survival of their marriage. In the first session, they argued over money, sex, and Mike's whereabouts on weekend nights. Neither partner mentioned that Delores had been suffering for many years from multiple sclerosis, even though her difficulty in walking with a cane was evident. When asked about her condition, both minimized it as "nothing new" and resumed fighting over petty grievances.

Separate individual sessions were held to hear more about the illness experience for each partner and to afford each one the opportunity to express concerns more freely. Mike revealed that he was alternately depressed and furious at Delores because of her increasing disability and dependence. They had traditional breadwinner–homemaker roles in their marriage. As her illness progressed, she was less and less able to keep the house clean or to manage shopping and errands, and had lost all interest in sex. It bothered Mike to come home and find her "lying around" while he worked an exhausting construction job plus overtime to keep up with her medical bills. He harbored fantasies of leaving her, became irritated with her over small things, felt ashamed, and then drowned his frustration in bouts of heavy drinking at a neighborhood bar on weekends. As for Delores, the less she felt in control of her own body, the more controlling of Mike she became. She alternated between feeling guilty for being such a burden on him and then irritated and resentful that he wasn't more attentive to her needs.

It was important to reframe the couple's distress as not attributable to his failings or hers, but rather as a shared dilemma arising from the burdens imposed on their relationship by a progressively deteriorating illness. They were then better able to hear and comfort each other as they shared the ways in which each had been devastated by the illness and how it had ravaged their relationship, their financial security, and their hopes and dreams for the future. Strains also came from living with uncertainty about the long-term worsening of Delores' condition, as well as the possibility of her early death. Their marriage was strengthened as they banded together to find ways to reduce the intrusion of the illness in their lives and find pleasure together. Delores, realizing that Mike's night out with the boys was not an affair, encouraged him to go out when she couldn't; in turn, he agreed not to drink to excess. Feeling less trapped, he was kinder toward Delores and supported her need for outlets and visits with friends. They decided to set aside a little money each week toward a weekend trip for their upcoming anniversary.

When a chronic illness looms increasingly large—imposing heavy physical, emotional, and financial burdens, and diminishing hopes and dreams for the future—it is crucial to help clients regain a view of each person and their relationship as defined by more than the illness. Similar to White's (White & Epston, 1990) technique of externalizing the problem, the illness is framed as an unwelcome intruder; by joining forces they can regain control of their lives. Couple therapy can help each partner gain empathy for the other's position, address such issues as guilt and blame, and rebalance their relationship to enable them to live and love as fully as possible.

Terminal illness poses daunting challenges. When the dying process has been prolonged, family caregiving and financial resources are often depleted, with the needs of other members put on hold. Relief at ending patient suffering and family strain is likely to be guilt-laden. Moreover, families increasingly face anguished dilemmas over whether and how long to maintain life support efforts, at great expense, to sustain a family member who may be in a vegetative state with virtually no hope of recovery. The fundamental questions of when life ends and who should determine that end have generated controversies concerning medical ethics, religious beliefs, patient/family rights, and the possibility of criminal prosecution. In some cultures it is taboo even to plan for death or discuss it openly, so clinicians must be sensitive to family beliefs. Families can be torn apart by opposing views of different members or coalitions. Clinicians can help family members to prepare and discuss living wills, to share feelings openly about such complicated situations, to weigh the various options, and to come to terms with any decisions taken. Moreover, such decisions should be reviewed, and revisions flexibly considered over time, or as health conditions change, since people commonly change their minds over the course of an illness or disabling condition.

Key Family Resilience Processes: Navigating the Challenges of Chronic Illness

Belief Systems

The belief systems of the ill person, family, their culture, and health care providers interact to color the illness experience and all healing transactions. We need to work with causal explanations of how and why health problems have occurred and persist, as well as beliefs about the role of helping professionals and the family in the treatment process and outcome.

Epidemiological research points to the importance of maintaining hope in the face of uncertainty with a life-threatening condition, such as cancer (Taylor, 1989; see Chapter 3, this volume). Patients and their families are better able to rally when they hold "positive illusions," or selective bias toward an optimistic view that they can "beat" a poor prognosis. Unlike denial, or acting as if "everything is normal" and there is no risk, this optimistic stance is a conscious choice based on full recognition of the actual situation. It fuels active initiative and perseverance in steps to maximize the likelihood of a positive outcome; in so doing, it can make a difference in the course. For instance, hearing that there are only 20% odds of recovery, a patient and family may decide to put all their energies on the positive side, hoping and striving to be in that 20%. In beginning to help families face the *possibility* of death and loss, it is important not to undermine their hope and to encourage their best efforts for optimal chances and quality of life. If an illness progresses, sensitivity is needed in helping families to redefine realistic hope and to confront a greater *probability* of a poor outcome, such as a limited recovery or death. In the event of a terminal condition, and the *certainty* of death, they can be helped to redirect hope, prayers, and efforts for control of pain and suffering, enhanced comfort, emotional and relational well-being, and spiritual peace of mind.

It is useful to ask families what illness information they have received and what each member believes about the future course, exploring their best hopes and worst fears. Often, these beliefs are polarized among family members, which can generate strong conflict, particularly if decisions must be made about whether to pursue or forgo further treatment options. We can help families obtain clearer information about the medical prognosis, treatment options, and management issues to guide shared decision making. As the course of a condition worsens, we can help families reevaluate their options and chances, and help enable them to master the possible and accept what may be beyond their control. Although their best efforts may not result in the hoped-for outcome, they can impact the quality of life and enhance their relationships on their illness journey. One husband, afflicted with multiple sclerosis, maintained a positive outlook despite a poor prognosis: "I'm not happy I have it, but I'm a happy man living with it." Taking part in research gave his life greater meaning. "If I can help anyone it gives me pleasure. My glass is half full—I have no hope for myself, but I'm more concerned with future generations and I have great hope for them."

Organizational Patterns

Family organizational patterns may need to shift with various adaptational demands over the course of an illness. For instance, a father's heart attack generates a crisis in a family with teenagers that might have been moderately flexible and separate—patterns appropriate to that life cycle phase. With a heart attack, the family may shift rapidly to very high levels of cohesion as the illness crisis draws members together. Chaos is generated with the emotional upheaval and the disruption of many daily routines. Over the following weeks, the family attempts to bring the chaos under control and resume some routines. Several months later, family functioning may remain closer and more structured. Members may be hypervigilant and cautious not to upset the father, out of fears of recurrence. An adolescent may become constrained from launching and leaving home under pressure to support parents. Although all families change in response to a crisis, many need help in readjusting their roles, rules, and leadership to achieve a new balance that maximizes their resources and coping skills, especially if an illness enters a more chronic, long-haul phase.

Communication

Open communication is vital. Clinicians need to help families clarify an illness diagnosis, prognosis, treatment options, and management guidelines. Framing events, such as receiving a diagnosis, cast meaning on a serious illness and help in dealing with it (Rolland, 1994). Health care professionals may unwittingly contribute to blocked communication and isolation among family members by telling a spouse or another family member separately about a life-threatening prognosis, leading them to presume that it is unwise to talk openly about it together or with the patient. Such meta-communication may heighten a family's catastrophic fear that talking about the illness or life-threatening possibilities could be harmful. By contrast, when clinicians sensitively help family members to share information and clarify an illness situation and options, they are better able to support one another in mastering the challenges they face.

Clinicians also need to explore cultural differences and family preferences. In traditional Japanese culture, the family is told that their loved one is dying but the patient is not told, for fear that it will hasten death. Yet we should not assume that all Japanese would want to follow that norm. And often, patients are aware of their condition but don't talk with loved ones about it out of a wish to spare them upset.

One set of studies examined the role of communication in the adaptation and competence of families with a child with serious mental disabilities (Beavers & Hampson, 2003). Contrary to clinical lore that such families are permeated by a sense of chronic sorrow and inevitable family dysfunction, researchers found that families that dealt openly with their feelings adapted well. Members were able to express a wide range of feelings, including joy, sorrow, and frustration. Some noted that the shared experience of caring for a child with disabilities increased their mutual support. In contrast, the most dysfunctional families revealed despair, which was reinforced by a strong taboo on expressing these feelings. Such studies underscore the importance of facilitating open communication for optimal adaptation to illness and disability.

ILLNESS AND CAREGIVING IN LATER LIFE

Societies and families are rapidly aging, due to a declining birth rate and increasing life expectancy. With medical advances, more elders are living longer with chronic health conditions (Institute for Health & Aging, 1996; Walsh, 1999d). In the United States, health problems and their severity vary greatly with disparities associated with income, race, and adequate, affordable health care. Although more people are healthy through their 60s than in the past, declines in physical and mental functioning, chronic pain, and progressive, degenerating conditions are common. Physical and mental deterioration may be exacerbated by depression and a sense of loss of control. The growing numbers of frail elderly over age 85 pose increasing demands for long-term care and financial coverage.

Family caregiving for elders can be demanding and can strain intergenerational relations. As the average family size decreases, fewer children are available for caregiving and sibling support. With more people having children later, or remaining childless, those at midlife—the so-called "sandwich generation"—face multiple pressures: meeting job demands, raising children, and caring for aging parents, grandparents, and other relatives. Caregiving responsibilities have burdened women disproportionately in their roles as daughters and daughters-in-law, but men are increasingly involved in caregiving. Finances can be drained by college expenses for children just as medical expenses for elders increase. Adult children who are past retirement age, and facing their own declining health and resources, must assume responsibilities for infirm parents in their 80s and 90s.

Family and friends are the front lines of support. Growing numbers of elders with chronic conditions are receiving home-based care for daily functioning, and are requiring costly medications and periodic hospitalizations. Prolonged caregiving takes a heavy toll in depression, anxiety, and health decline. Eighty percent of caregivers provide help 7 days a week, averaging 4 hours daily. In addition to housekeeping, shopping, and meal preparation, two-thirds also assist with feeding, bathing, toileting, and dressing. Some aspects of chronic illness among elders are especially disruptive for families, such as sleep disturbance, incontinence, delusional ideas, and aggressive behavior. One symptom and consequence of such family distress is elder abuse, which, while infrequent, is most likely to occur in overwhelmed families that are stretched beyond their means and tolerance. Useful management guidelines by medical specialists, home health aides, and day care programs can greatly diminish the frustration and exhaustion family members commonly experience.

Progressive dementia is especially challenging for families. It affects 10% of persons over 65 and over 40% of those over 85. Dementia gradually strips away mental and physical capacities, with gradual memory loss, disorientation, impaired judgment, and finally loss of control over bodily functions. Alzheimer's disease, accounting for 60% of dementias, is one of the most devastating illnesses of our times. The irreversible disease course, which can persist for up to 20 years, or more, has aptly been called "the long good-bye." Families need help in dealing with ambiguous loss (Boss, 1999): the gradual loss of a loved one's former self, family roles, and relationships. It is most painful for loved ones when they are not even recognized or are confused with others, even those long deceased. It is crucial to help family members to deal with the progressive losses without extruding the person as if he or she were already dead. Finding humor can lighten spirits.

Danny, who was devoted to his parents, found his father's worsening dementia heartbreaking, and lamented the frustration and sadness it caused his mother, who tended to him despite her own medical ailments. Danny had dinner with them frequently to help out. One night, as his mother cleared the table, his father leaned over to him and said, "See that woman over there—she's a darn good cook and good-looking, too. If I wasn't a married man, I could really go for her!" Danny hugged his father and replied, "Pop, you're a lucky man—because you ARE married to her! She's your wife!" They all had a good laugh and retold the story many times to lighten their mood.

Pets can be valued companions for elders with declining health. One father, with dementia, could not follow family conversations but found contentment petting and giving treats to the family dog, who curled up close to him on the sofa. Dogs trained to assist individuals who are visually or hearing impaired or are wheelchair-bound provide companionship and enable them to live independently.

Family psychoeducational groups and support networks can provide relatives with help in meeting care-giving challenges, coping with stress, and dealing with confusion and memory lapses. Useful illness-related information and management guidelines reduce the risk of caregiver depression, commonly experienced. With prolonged strain over many years, it is important to validate the needs of a spouse or adult children to go on with their own lives while providing care. Activism and advocacy for better treatments can be a source of resilience for families with this experience.

Common Issues in Caregiving

A family resilience approach expands our society's narrow, individualistic focus on a primary caregiver to involve all family members as a caregiving team. Family intervention priorities include (1) stress reduction; (2) information about the impaired member's medical condition, functional abilities, limitations, and prognosis; (3) concrete guidelines for sustaining care, problem solving, and optimal functioning; and (4) linkages to supplementary services to support family efforts. To meet caregiving challenges, communities must support families through a range of services from day programs to assisted living and commitment to full participation of individuals with disabilities in community life.

Issues of intergenerational dependence come to the fore as aging parents lose functioning and control over their bodies and their lives. Meeting their increasing needs should not be seen as a parent–child "role reversal." Even when adult children give financial, practical, and emotional support to aging parents, they do not become parents to their parents. Despite frailties or childlike functioning, an aged parent has had over 50 years of adult life and deserves respect as an elder. Family therapists can open conversations about dependence-related issues with sensitivity and a realistic appraisal of strengths and limitations. An elderly father driving with seriously impaired vision may be unwilling to admit the danger or give up his autonomy to be driven by others. Older parents may fail to tell their adult children that they are financially strapped because of the shame and stigma of economic dependence. Adult children can be coached on ways to develop a filial role—taking responsibility for what they can appropriately do to assist their elders in living as fully as possible.

If an aging parent becomes overly dependent on adult children, who become overly responsible through anxiety or guilt, a vicious cycle may ensue: The more they do for the parent, the more helpless the parent may become, with escalating neediness, burden, and resentment. Siblings may go to opposite extremes in meeting filial responsibilities. One may assume the role of the designated caregiver and come to resent others who distance or do little to help.

Caregiving challenges can be burdensome; yet they can also become opportunities for family members to heal strained relationships and begin to collaborate as a caregiving team. When family relationships have been ruptured by past grievances, long-standing conflict, or estrangement, caregiving is more likely to be complicated. Life-and-death decisions become more difficult, as in the following crisis situation:

Joellen, a 38-year-old single parent, was deeply conflicted when her father, hospitalized for complications of chronic alcohol abuse, asked her to donate a kidney to save his life. She felt enraged to be asked to give up something so important when he had not been there for her as a father over the years. He had been a mean drunk, often absent and many times violent. She was also angry that he had brought on his deteriorated condition by drinking and had refused to heed his family's repeated pleas to stop. Yet, as a dutiful daughter and a compassionate woman, she also felt a sense of obligation and guilt: She did not want her father to die because she had denied him her kidney.

I broadened the dilemma to include Joellen's siblings, suggesting that she discuss it with them, but she dismissed that idea, saying that they had been estranged for many years and rarely were in contact. I then encouraged Joellen to talk with her mother, who informed her that her father had also asked her siblings for the kidney donation. She was furious that old rivalries would be stirred up as to who would be seen as the good, giving child or the bad, selfish ones. She now took initiative to get her siblings together. When the meeting proved hard to schedule, I encouraged her to persevere. When they met, old rivalries melted as they began to grapple with the dilemma.

I encouraged them to broaden their focus and begin to envision how they might collaborate as a team to share the many challenges likely to come up in caring for *both* aging parents and potential widowhood. With this conversation, the eldest brother then volunteered to donate his kidney for their father. He felt less conflicted because he had memories of good times with their father in earlier years before the problem drinking. The others offered to support him and agreed to keep in contact and contribute to their parents' future well-being in ways that fit their abilities and resources. The beginning of a new solidarity was forged. The oldest brother also helped the younger siblings gain a new appreciation of their father, and compassion for the life struggles that had fueled his increased drinking and explosive outbursts.

Even when family contact has been severed, my experience has taught me never to give up on relationship possibilities before trying to reengage members. Without support, a family may have become overwhelmed and burned out by persistent stresses in coping with an illness, especially if the condition has been uncontrolled by medication or exacerbated by self-medicating alcohol or drug abuse. Recurrent crises can fuel helplessness and hopelessness; escalating conflict may become destructive. Yet the immediate relief of a cutoff is commonly overshadowed by family members' continual worry about the elderly person's well-being and their abiding sorrow or guilt that they could not (or did not) help their loved one.

Family members commonly distance out of sheer exhaustion and depleted resources. Siblings may distance from painful past experiences, failed rescue attempts, anger over destructive behavior, or the fear that they will be pulled into a bottomless pit of selfless caregiving. There may also be fears of contagion or concerns of heightened genetic risk. Loss issues and survival guilt are common as well: "How can I be successful and enjoy life when my sister's life has been devastated by her illness?" "How can I continue to care for my partner with dementia, when he no longer recognizes me?" There may well be inner conflict over responsibility for being a loved one's keeper, with the sacrifices extracted by an illness. It's useful to question all-or-none assumptions of involvement: "I avoid all contact, because if I open the door an inch, I'll give over my life to endless caregiving." My work with many in this position—parents, siblings, and adult children of frail elderly—has heightened my appreciation of their many struggles. Our successful work in bridging new connections has strengthened my conviction that it is rarely too late to repair and redefine frayed bonds (see Chapter 12).

Placement Decisions

The point at which failing health requires consideration of extended-care placement is a crisis for the whole family. Placement is usually turned to only as a last resort—when family resources are stretched to the limit and in later stages of mental or physical deterioration. Nevertheless, feelings of guilt and abandonment and notions about institutionalization can make a placement decision highly stressful for families. The Wolff family case (described in Chapter 5) revealed the value of a genogram and the importance of inquiry about elderly family members. Problems presented between a mother and teenage son were found to relate to a caregiving crisis and placement decision concerning a grandmother with a deteriorating condition in the home. It is also crucial to increase support of a spouse who has distanced. In the Wolffs' case, this was due to the husband's lingering guilt over having left the care of his dying mother to his sisters.

Family sessions can enable members to assess needs and resources, weigh the benefits and costs of options, and share their feelings and concerns before reaching a decision together. Often through discussion new solutions emerge that can support the elder's remaining in the community without undue burden on any member. Organizations such as the Visiting Nurses Association can provide homebound services and inform families of community backup resources. Respite for caregivers is crucial to their well-being. When placement is needed, we can help families see it as the most viable way to provide good care, and help them navigate the maze of options.

Dealing with terminal illness is perhaps the family's most painful challenge. Clinicians need to attend to unmet needs for pain control and palliative care, and to worries about financial and emotional burden on loved ones. Family collaboration is essential to reduce suffering and make the best arrangements to keep the seriously ill person comfortable and comforted, while balancing the needs of other family members. Increasingly, families are facing agonizing end-of-life decisions. Efforts to legalize assisted dying involve medically hastening death for someone who is terminally ill to enhance dignity, peace of mind, and control over the dying process. Families will need wise counsel as they grapple with these personal, ethical, and spiritual dilemmas.

We would be mistaken to view later life only as a time of decline and loss. This period also holds potential for personal and relational change and growth (Walsh, 1999d) and the achievement of "family integrity" (King & Wynne, 2004). One father's cognitive decline was accompanied by a softening of his prickly defensives and mellowing of his affect from his former gruff demeanor, enabling his adult children to engage more warmly with him. The challenges of caregiving also present opportunities for greater intimacy and for healing relationship wounds. A terminal illness may hold unexpected gifts, particularly at life's end, when family members fully engage with loved ones and make the most of precious time.

James came to talk with me about his unbearable sorrow at his mother's terminal illness. A devout Catholic, she had done all she could to keep her family intact while enduring an abusive marriage and many uprooting relocations due to his father's alcoholism and repeated job loss. After the father's recent death, James had bought a new home for his mother in high hopes that, at last, she could enjoy her later years in comfort and peace. He was devastated that her illness so quickly shattered these dreams. "It's just not fair!"

At adulthood, he and his sisters had scattered around the country and maintained little contact. In recent months, they made several trips to care for their mother. Now she called them together, he feared, for their last good-byes. He was tormented as he left for the visit. When I saw him after his return, he seemed transformed: his inner turmoil had subsided, although his mother, indeed, had died during the visit. He told me, "I knew my mother was a strong woman, but she was most amazing as she faced her own death—she deliberately brought me and my sisters to care for her, time and again, to knit us back together. Her final request assured that we'll continue our bonds. She told us she didn't want to be buried in her town so far from her children and her roots. Instead, she asked that her remains be cremated and that we take the urn with her ashes and travel together to each town where our family had lived and scatter some of her ashes in a beautiful place we had enjoyed together. Her courage inspired us to honor her wishes even better. We told her we would save a portion and make a trip to Ireland together to scatter the last remains in the town of her grandparents, where she had always wanted to visit. She was so pleased and died

peacefully a few hours later as we sat around her singing Irish bal-
lads she had loved."

This potential for transcendence, forged in the midst of suffering
and loss, distinguishes the concept of resilience from coping and adaptation. As we've seen, resilience entails more than shouldering a caregiving
burden, bearing the sadness of loss, or adjusting dreams downward.
This moving story reveals the core of relational resilience: Family members rallied together to practice the art of the possible. They made the
most of limited time together and transcended the immediate death and
loss, inspired by their mother to carry out her wishes, thereby honoring
and sustaining her memory and spirit. In the process, they and their relationships were transformed. In resilience-oriented practice, we can facilitate such processes.

FAMILY COPING WITH MENTAL ILLNESS

Clinical approaches toward mental illness have been undergoing major
transformations over recent decades. As the mental health field has
shifted from a nature-versus-nurture controversy to a biopsychosocial
orientation, there has been a shift from shunning families as pathogenic
influences to involving them as valued resources and collaborators in the
treatment process.

Historically, the field of mental health oscillated between polarized
positions assuming *either* biological *or* social causality in schizophrenia
and other chronic mental disorders (Walsh & Anderson, 1988). Some
opposed any labeling of illness, diagnosis, hospitalization, or medication, arguing that they foster a stigmatizing "patient" identity and a
chronic course. We now have ample evidence of the complicated, mutual
influences between biogenetic vulnerability and family environmental
stress factors in the course of major mental disorders (Reiss et al., 2000;
Tienari et al., 2004). Yet, a biopsychosocial orientation remains not well
integrated into most treatment approaches.

I was fortunate to benefit from clinical training in 1968 on an experimental psychiatric inpatient unit at Yale (Tompkins 1) based on the
philosophy of milieu therapy—a patient–staff community with combined interventions of psychotropic medication, individual, group, family, and multifamily group modalities. In the early 1970s, I was family
studies coordinator in an NIMH-funded schizophrenia research program directed by Roy Grinker, Sr. Grinker, was a visionary psychiatrist

who regarded a biopsychosocial–systems orientation as fundamental to the study and treatment of serious mental conditions. Those programs put into practice a true interactionist perspective, addressing individual and family influences, as I learned in my very first family therapy experience:

> Walt brought his wife, Emmy Lou, for admission to the psychiatric inpatient unit during a psychotic episode. Emmy Lou had been suffering from manic–depressive (bipolar) disorder for over 20 years. Every spring, almost like clockwork, Emmy Lou had a manic episode: she painted her face, dressed in multihued, mismatched outfits, and went off on a wild spree. Walt, a devoted husband, took the primary role in raising their two children, by then teenagers. He took Emmy Lou to all the best treatment centers; stood by her through her recurrent breakdowns, hospitalizations, and brief recoveries; and never stopped hoping for a cure.
>
> Emmy Lou began taking lithium, a newly experimental drug treatment at the time. She and her family were also referred for family therapy as part of the multidimensional approach. A first-year psychiatry resident and I eagerly began seeing our first family case, and as Emmy Lou made an astounding recovery, we credited our skillful family therapy interventions for the great success (only joking, of course, as we admitted that lithium might have had some effect).

This family taught me an invaluable lesson. Even when a disorder is clearly biologically based and can be managed with psychotropic medication, the involvement of the family in treatment is crucial for patient and family adaptation. The family didn't *cause* her disorder, but they too suffered its impact. The family members didn't *need* Emmy Lou to be ill; nor did her symptoms serve a function for them. Nevertheless, they had structured family life around her disturbance over the years. Any recovery, while it is everyone's greatest wish, involves a disruptive transition. Although medication can reduce florid symptoms, all loved ones must reorient their relationships and patterns of living as they move forward with their lives.

> It was important to help the family to relate to Emmy Lou not as a chronic patient, but a beloved person recovering from a devastating condition. To enhance her functioning and worth as wife and mother, the family needed help to alter patterns of family functioning, set in place over the years to compensate for Emmy Lou's illness. Walt had increasingly taken over the household duties, with

Emmy Lou assigned to feed and walk the dog. To restore her competence and confidence, the parental partnership needed to be rebalanced. Walt and the kids would have to shift their expectations. They were nervous and uncertain how to relate without the illness to define their roles. Discharge planning and posthospitalization reentry sessions enabled family members to share their feelings about this major change in their lives, and to reorganize long-standing illness-centered patterns. We scheduled a follow-up family session for early spring, the time family members anticipated a recurrence, since every spring they had hovered over Emmy Lou, vigilant for signs of another episode. This session offered an opportunity to discuss fears of a setback, to ensure that medication levels were appropriate, to reaffirm confidence in Emmy Lou, and to sustain the family's gains.

To optimize functioning, reduce the risk of serious relapse, and prevent the need for rehospitalization, family members should be partners in treatment from the time of hospital admission through discharge, with planned follow-up and referral for outpatient sustaining care. The first few weeks and months following psychiatric hospitalization can be the most challenging. Families desperately need guidelines on what to expect and how to proceed. Members may share unrealistic beliefs that "normal" life can be resumed with medication and discharge. Following a "honeymoon" period of relative calm, tensions are likely to mount as difficulties arise. When family members are helped to reorganize interactional patterns and develop new communication skills, they are better able to reduce stress and support the optimal functioning of the recovering individual.

From Deficit-Based to Resource-Based Therapeutic Approaches

A focus on deficits, reinforced by psychiatric nomenclature, exerts a powerful influence in clinical practice. Policies in managed care can worsen the situation by demanding diagnosis and documentation of more severe pathology for therapy to be reimbursed beyond a few sessions. When those with recurrent emotional distress seek help, they often carry pathology-loaded baggage from previous treatment experience. A resource-based approach aims to transform this experience.

Jessie and Ted, a recently married couple in their late 20s, sought help for Jessie's phobic anxiety, which prevented her from leaving their apartment without a panic attack. She was evaluated for psychotropic medication, which lowered the intensity of her anxiety; yet she remained alone in the apartment all day, becoming increasingly depressed and ruminating about the emptiness of her life and the hopelessness of her emotional problems. The couple had recently moved from the city where Jessie had grown up, so that Ted could take a new job. In the first few sessions, Jessie talked at great length about her "dysfunctional family," her mother's chronic alcoholism and depression, and her own recurrent episodes of panic, which had led to three brief psychiatric hospitalizations. She had spent the last 6 years in psychoanalysis, with sessions several times a week until their move. Now fearing she was coming "unglued" again, she was making crisis calls to her former therapist. Ted was attentive and caring toward Jessie, yet frightened by her agitated state and catastrophic fears.

A deficit-oriented therapy might have continued to focus on past family damage and Jessie's resulting limitations and emotional fragility. Some therapists might have felt sympathy for the "normal" spouse stuck with a "damaged" partner. Or, they might have assumed both partners in a marriage to be equally dysfunctional, and searched for underlying pathology in Ted, as well. A resource-oriented family resilience approach identified and encouraged their strengths. Ted was solid, stable, and caring. His attraction to Jessie was understandable: She was a lovely woman, warm, affectionate, attractive, and smart. Ted's fears from a past failed marriage also played a part. Recently divorced by a woman who had left him to pursue her career, he was reassured by Jessie's dependency and devoted loyalty to him. However, he neither anticipated her intense suffering nor "needed" her helplessness.

As our sessions became dominated by Jessie's accounts of how her long history of emotional problems "explained" her current plight, I shifted focus to the recent transitional crisis in the life of the couple—the disruption wrought by their relocation. I asked how the decision had come about. The partners had shared their feelings, concluded that on balance it would be a good move, and arrived at the decision jointly. Still, there was a skew in the experience of the transition, generating more stress for the more vulnerable partner. The move furthered Ted's career advancement; his new job focused his attention and gave him a sense of pride. Also, the move brought welcome contact with his family, who lived nearby. Jessie, who wanted to assume a homemaker role and hoped to start a family soon, had lost her community network, a satisfying job, and her therapist. She felt isolated in long, empty days in their apartment in an unfamiliar city. The loss of structure and support fueled her anxiety, rumination, and self-doubts.

Helping the couple to make meaning of the recent symptoms in the context of this major transition was pivotal to Jessie's adaptation and the couple's resilience. I expressed my conviction that a major relocation is very stressful for a relationship as well as for individuals, and that by strengthening their resilience as a couple, they would both more likely make the best adjustment. To help them begin to form a new support network and to anchor them in their new community, I explored their interest in joining a church that fit their beliefs and lifestyle, encouraging them to make several visits. Within weeks they found a new "spiritual home" and a congregation of "kindred souls." Jessie met several women through the church who took her under their wing, helped her get oriented, recommended good neighborhood resources, and accompanied her on errands. These small concrete supports eased her insecurities and helped her gain a sense of mastery over the "foreign" environment. As her comfort increased, we talked about the library job she had left behind and her love and knowledge of books. Ted encouraged her to volunteer in the church's fund-raising sale of used books. Her success in that endeavor led to a volunteer position in the neighborhood library. That experience in turn led within a few months to a part-time job in a bookstore, a short bus ride away. With Ted's confidence in her, she overcame her "fear of becoming panicky" and excelled on the job, which she found to be a rewarding challenge.

It was vital to our work that Jessie stop defining herself as damaged, but rather broaden her identity as a likable and interesting person, with many positive attributes as well as vulnerabilities. It was also crucial that she experience therapy not as a place to nurse old wounds endlessly (as in her past therapy), but as a place to develop latent talents and abilities. Jessie came to look back on her prior therapy as an addiction: Over the years, her vulnerability and overdependence on her therapist had increased to the point that she doubted her ability to survive on her own when that contact ended.

Our therapy ended successfully after 5 months. Jessie's medication was tapered off gradually. A year later, I received a birth announcement with a very cute baby picture and a note of appreciation for helping Jessie and Ted launch their new life together. Yet life doesn't follow an orderly course. Six months later Jessie called in a panic: Ted's company had been bought out, and he might be downsized out of a job. Over several sessions, the couple considered possible options if a "worst-case scenario" required them to move again. The ax fell a few months later, but the couple was prepared and Jessie didn't panic. Ted had already begun a job search, which landed him a good position in a desirable community where Jessie planned to return to complete college. We met for a few sessions before the move, and I linked them to a trusted colleague in the new community if the need arose. Jessie's physician recommended that she resume her antianxiety medication if needed during the expectable turmoil of the move. We scheduled a follow-up phone contact, and they sent a card at holiday time expressing their pride at how smoothly the new transition had gone: With all they had learned from their previous move, they now considered themselves experts on relocation. Jessie even thought about writing an article for a magazine on the subject.

From "Schizophrenogenic Mother" to Respectful Collaboration

Clinicians and investigators have long sought to understand and effectively treat the most debilitating mental disorders, but have too readily pathologized families and excluded them from involvement. For decades, the concept of the "schizophrenogenic mother" blamed disturbances in the mother's character and parenting style for causing schizophrenia. In the late 1950s, schizophrenia research based on a family systems perspective shifted from a linear, deterministic view of maternal causality to attend to multiple, recursive transactions in the family network. Still, in the early development of the field of family therapy, the focus was primarily on dysfunctional family transactions in so-called "schizophrenic families" implicated in the ongoing *maintenance* of symptoms, if not their origins. In the 1970s and 1980s, solid research evidence of a biological base in schizophrenia and a wide range of functioning in patients' families made it clear that there is no one-to-one correlation between individual disorder and family pathology (Walsh & Anderson, 1988). Clinicians must be careful, therefore, not to label families by the diagnosis of a family member or presume them to be severely dysfunctional. There is no "schizophrenic family" any more than there is a "diabetic family."

With recognition of multiple influences in serious mental disorders, studies have looked at the role of the family in the future *course* of the illness. For instance, high "expressed emotion" (i.e., critical comments and emotional overinvolvement) predicts later symptomatic relapse for vulnerable individuals with schizophrenia, major depression, and anorexia nervosa. In studies of adopted away identical twins with high genetic risk for schizophrenia, those growing up in families with communication deviance were significantly more likely to develop the disorder (Tienari et al., 2004). Showing the importance of family protective factors, families with healthy communication patterns protected children at high risk from developing the disorder. By identifying such process elements, we can target family interventions to lower stressful interaction patterns as we strengthen both individual and family functioning.

In recent years, there has been growing respect toward individuals and families coping with major mental illnesses. However, the heavy burden on families has increased, as policies of utilization review and managed care have drastically reduced hospital stays for medication and rapid stabilization. (Can "drive-through" meds be far off?) Adequate funding has been lacking for outpatient services and community supports to sustain independent living and prevent family burnout. We see the failure of these policies in the tragic numbers of seriously troubled persons living precariously from day to day in the streets and shelters. The expectation for families to assume the primary caregiving burden over the chronic course of a mental illness, and the unresponsiveness to their stresses and concerns, have led families to mobilize (Lefley,1996). Consumer advocacy groups such as the National Alliance for the Mentally Ill (NAMI) and the Child and Adolescent Bipolar Foundation are providing valuable networks and information for families (Torrey, 2001, 2002) and lobbying for more supportive programs and community resources.

Family Psychoeducational Approaches

Research and practice developments with schizophrenia have informed family intervention with a range of serious and persistent mental illnesses. Success depends on mobilizing family and community resources through collaborative therapeutic relationships. Assessment and intervention are not aimed at searching for past causal factors, nor do they presume that an individual's disturbed behavior serves a function for the family. Family members are viewed as caring and vital resources for long-term adaptation in the community. Interventions aim to reduce stress and strengthen the supportive functioning of the family.

It is crucial for clinicians to counter the stigmatizing experiences of families who have felt blamed for recurrent symptoms or failed treatment efforts. Current family distress is not necessarily indicative of long-standing pathology or the cause of an individual's symptoms. Much of the family distress evidenced at a family member's emotional crisis or hospitalization is fueled by concerns about their loved one. The family may be coping as well as can be reasonably expected in the face of recurrent psychotic or destructive episodes and depleted resources. Referral for family therapy should be disengaged from causal assumptions; rather, it should be based on the value of family involvement in strengthening the ability to cope effectively with the stressful challenges of living with persistent mental illness.

Combined treatment strategies have been found to be most effective with serious mental illnesses. Family psychoeducation, along with psychotropic medication, has proven the most effective approach in preventing relapse in schizophrenia and in treating bipolar disorder, major depression, and other serious disorders (Anderson et al., 1986; Miklowitz & Goldstein, 1997; McFarlane, 2002). Numerous studies have demonstrated the effectiveness of this approach in preventing relapse, improving recovery, and increasing family well-being. Long-term drug maintenance may be necessary to control the severity of symptoms and to prevent repeated hospitalizations. Additionally, patient involvement in a social skills group boosts social functioning and decreases social isolation.

Psychoeducational approaches provide useful information, management guidelines, and social support. By regarding the family as an indispensable ally in treatment, these approaches correct the blaming causal attributions experienced by so many families. A connecting phase establishes an empathic alliance with families by attending in a noncritical manner to the family's needs and experiences, and to specific areas of stress in their lives. In the Anderson et al. (1986) model, a daylong survival skills workshop provides a group of families with information and management guidelines, followed by brief (2- to 3-month) family therapy focused on helping patients take concrete steps toward stable functioning in the community, and then by long-term multifamily groups to sustain gains.

The basic principles of psychoeducation have been adapted to fit varied treatment settings and practice with a range of conditions (McFarlane, 2002). Brief, focused family consultation (Wynne et al., 1986) also can be helpful in responding to family members' stress, and in setting concrete, realistic objectives collaboratively with the family. Family consumer groups, critical of more traditional treatment, have responded positively to these developments.

Brief Therapy

Brief family therapy, providing structured, focused interventions, is useful to many families challenged by a serious illness. Improved functioning along with reduced stress and conflict can be achieved through pragmatic focus on concrete, realistic objectives that can be achieved within 2–3 months. Once a higher level of functioning and stabilization has been reached, gains can be sustained and setbacks averted with monthly or periodic family consultations or multifamily group sessions.

Psychoeducational Multifamily Groups

Family psychoeducational groups have proven to be valuable with both mental and physical illnesses (Anderson et al., 1986; Gonzalez & Steinglass, 2002; McFarlane, 2002). These groups prevent or delay relapse, increase medication and treatment compliance, reduce stress, and improve both patient and family functioning. Professionally led multifamily groups, typically including four or more families or couples, focus on ways to manage situational stress, loss, and transition, while strengthening relationships and problem-solving abilities. The group context provides a social support network and opportunities for family members to learn from one another's experiences, to gain perspective on their own crisis situation, and to reduce guilt and blame. The shared experience helps to reduce family isolation and stigma, especially with such illnesses as HIV/AIDS and schizophrenia.

Psychoeducational multifamily group interventions may have a short-term or modular structure, such as a daylong workshop, or 4–6 weekly prevention-oriented modules. Monthly meetings can sustain gains, avert crises and setbacks, and address ongoing challenges and new or recurrent strains. They encourage isolated families to establish support networks that often extend beyond the group sessions. Multifamily self-help groups are also useful for sustaining care and support over the long haul of a chronic condition.

HELPING FAMILIES LIVE WELL WITH CHRONIC CONDITIONS

General Clinical Priorities

In the treatment of serious physical and mental conditions, it is vital to build family strengths, resources, and successful coping strategies. Families are better able to handle stresses and to be more proactive to prevent and ameliorate future crises when we (1) identify and address common illness and treatment challenges; and (2) offer problem-solving assistance through predictably stressful periods. Flexibility is needed to tailor interventions and respond to family members as needs arise over the course of the illness and with changing life cycle challenges. Priorities include the following:

1. Reduce the stressful impact of the illness/disability experience on the family
2. Provide information about:
   - The illness/disability, treatment strategies, and likely course
   - Patient abilities, vulnerabilities, and potential
   - Importance of compliance with medication, treatment, or diet regimens, and physical therapy/rehabilitation to reduce vulnerability and increase functioning
   - Expectable psychosocial challenges for the family over time
   - Interaction with individual and family life cycle priorities
3. Offer practical guidelines through different phases of the condition for:
   - Ongoing stress reduction
   - Managing symptoms, treatments, and complications
   - Problem solving and crisis prevention
   - Building strengths for optimal functioning and well-being
   - Respite and attention to other needs, family members, and life priorities
4. Provide links to services that support functioning in the community and the family's caregiving efforts, for example:
   - Home health care support
   - Day care, structured work programs, and social contact
   - Assisted living and group homes
   - National and local consumer groups; useful Internet resources

Family members confronting the demands of a serious and chronic illness are often unsure whether they are doing too much or too little and how to navigate unfamiliar and challenging situations. They greatly value information, management guidelines, and help in setting realistic expectations. A neglected family issue is the need for respite—time out from illness and caregiving concerns for family members to meet their own and each other's needs, replenish their energies, and revitalize their spirits.

We need also to attend to the many actual and perceived losses that can accompany a chronic condition—loss of functioning, loss of limbs or disfigurement, loss of a sense of intactness and "normality," loss of valued roles and functions in the family, loss of employment and status, and loss of personal and shared hopes and dreams for the future.

Mick, a construction worker left permanently disabled and wheelchair bound by the collapse of a building, began to drink heavily; one night Peg, his wife, found him passed out on the floor, with his hunting gun ready to be fired. In individual and conjoint sessions, we explored the multiple losses he had suddenly experienced: his family role as breadwinner, his "tough guy" image, and the active life he had always wanted to live. Realizing that he was loved, valued, and needed by his wife and children not for his paycheck, but for himself, was most crucial to his inner healing and resilience, recharging his will to go on living. With his family's encouragement, Mick found new ways to be productive and active. He eventually set up a home-based small business and began to coach his son's soccer team.

A resilience orientation embraces the whole person, helping families to see beyond disabilities to appreciate and encourage positive abilities, talents, and potential in their loved one. This is especially important in countering the stigma of serious mental disorders. Many individuals who suffer from schizophrenia, affective disturbances, and autistic-spectrum disorders have remarkable gifts and can find expression in music, the arts, and other arenas that can bring great joy and meaning. One remarkable woman with autism, Temple Grandin, achieved an advanced academic degree and channeled her hyperfocus and sensory differences into an extraordinary ability to relate to animals and take in the world as they do. She has written about the cognitive and emotional abilities of animals (Grandin & Johnson, 2004). Her sensitivity to animal suffering and well-being led to the design of more humane treatment of livestock. She has also been an inspiration to so many who have been labeled with severe deficits by describing many autistic symptoms, such as hyperspecificity, as strengths rather than weaknesses. She notes that whooping cranes can memorize long migratory routes they've flown only once using a brain capacity similar to that which some individuals with autism show in making drawings with perfect perspective. By appreciating such special abilities, families can bring out the best in their children and share joy in their interests and talents.

Crisis Intervention/Crisis Prevention

Crisis intervention should be available to families in times of acute distress, since most chronic disorders involve periodic exacerbation of symptoms. Without such guidance, many individuals and their families veer from one crisis to the next; achieve few gains over time; and risk emotional exhaustion, serious conflict, and relationship cutoff. Therapists must be active and provide enough structure to help temporarily overwhelmed families to reorganize and gain control of threatening situations. Because individuals with mental impairment (e.g., major depression, schizophrenia, developmental disorders, or dementia) may lack motivation, use poor judgment, or not take needed medication, family collaboration is crucial to sustain involvement in treatment and to reduce stress to manageable proportions. Periodic "psychosocial checkups" and prevention-oriented consultations can be timed around major changes in a condition or disruptive life transitions to help families "bounce forward" with resilience.

Community-Oriented Family-Centered Health Care

Families are essential resources in treating serious and persistent illness. We can encourage collaboration, understand their challenges, and support their best efforts. Yet families cannot carry the burden alone. Families living in impoverished conditions, especially ethnic and racial minority families, are most vulnerable to the risks of serious illness and disabilities, inadequate health care and mental health services, and caregiving strain. Continuity of care and community-based services are critically important over the long-term course of disabling chronic conditions. A report commissioned by the Robert Wood Johnson Foundation (Institute for Health and Aging, 1996) took a broad view to address these challenges for the 21st century. The report envisioned a system of care—a spectrum of integrated services, medical, personal, social, and rehabilitative—to assist people with chronic conditions in living fuller lives. A continuum of care is essential for individuals and their families to receive the care appropriate to their condition and their changing needs over time, and to sustain independent living, optimal functioning, and well-being.

Both family and community resilience can be nurtured if we, as helping professionals, reach out to persons with disabling conditions and their families, respect their dignity, and work to forge viable extended kin and social supports. In many cases, basic needs for human connection and productive functioning can be met through such programs as structured group living arrangements and sheltered workshops, tailored to the vulnerabilities and potential strengths of residents. Our efforts to sustain resilience must be relationally based, shifting from faulty expectations of self-reliance to programs that sustain functioning and spirit through interdependence.

Sadly, the current managed care system in the United States fails to meet the health care needs of most families. A for-profit, bottom-line orientation takes precedence over adequate service provision. Family-centered prevention and early intervention services have no place in the reimbursement system. Individual psychiatric diagnoses are required for reimbursement of psychosocial care and, for more than a few sessions, therapists often must document severe disorder, which pathologizes families and their members. Families and helping professionals must complete burdensome paperwork and navigate confusing and frustrating compliance and reimbursement bureaucracies. Because health care plans are tied to employment, families lose coverage with job loss; 45 million Americans have no coverage at all. The restricted access to services and the jeopardizing of client confidentiality through computerized records undermine our core professional principles. Advocates for a single-payer not-for-profit national health care system have been gaining support to ensure high-quality care for all families.

An ongoing project in Kosovo offers an inspiring model in developing a resilience-oriented family and community based health care system in a war-torn region. In 1999, a team of American family systems–oriented mental health colleagues joined efforts with Kosovar professionals to train local professionals in resilience-oriented approaches to assist families in recovery from the war-related atrocities of ethnic cleansing (see Chapter 11). With the effectiveness of that project, the team has continued to consult for the newly emerging government to establish regionwide sustainable systems for prevention and intervention in a range of health and mental health conditions, drawing upon the strengths of family, community, and culture. Attuned to the cultural value of the extended family and the community, the overall resilience-based design views families as the most important unit of change and communities as the primary units of both prevention and care. As in Landau's (2005) LINKS model, the family and community members participate in designing the systems of delivery and prevention. Family members serve as links, bringing their ill members to "health houses" in their own communities, and, if necessary, then taking them to one of seven regional mental health centers or specialty hospitals for complex cases. Through active involvement, the inherent competence and resilience of the individuals, families, and communities, as well as their cultural heritage, are mobilized. A truly resilience-based health and mental health care system has been emerging across the region, with high compliance rates in the treatment of chronic mental illness. Further efforts are being directed to develop effective mechanisms for dealing with trauma, grief and loss, violence, addiction, HIV/AIDS, and other serious and chronic illnesses, including mental illness. Such bold and ambitious programs, arising out of resilience-oriented response to tragedy, are an inspiration.

CHAPTER 10

Strengthening Resilience in Vulnerable Multistressed Families

Hope has never trickled down; it has always sprung up
—STUDS TERKEL, *Hope Dies Last*

Many families, especially those in poor communities, are buffeted by frequent crises and persistent stresses that overwhelm their functioning. A family resilience approach is most needed and beneficial with families that have come to feel beaten down and defeated by repeated frustration and failure. This chapter offers a conceptual base and practice guidelines for strengthening highly vulnerable families—for supporting their best efforts to manage their stress-laden lives and overcome the odds of high-risk situations. In focusing on their potential, such families gain a sense of hope and confidence that they can rise above persistent adversity.

UNDERSTANDING MULTISTRESSED FAMILIES

Increasingly, in a range of practice settings, helping professionals are seeing families that are chronically stressed by serious problems cutting across many dimensions of their lives. Battered by internal and external pressures, families can become overloaded and destabilized. Couples are at high risk for conflict and breakup; single parents become depleted; and more than one family member may suffer from ill health, serious emotional problems, substance abuse, violence, or sexual abuse. Recurrent crises and chronic distress carry over from year to year and can cascade from one generation to the next.

Historically, highly vulnerable families have been defined in terms of their deficits. The label of "severely dysfunctional family" reinforced the view that multiple problems are endemic to a pathological family type, prejudged as hopeless and untreatable. Focus on the interior of the family contributed to blaming mothers for faulty parenting and chastising peripheral or nonresidential fathers as "deadbeat dads." The label "multiproblem families," carries unfortunate connotations that blame families for their problems. These families are struggling to overcome many problems, which are often beyond their control and not of their making. Seeing them as "multistressed families" (Madsen, 2003) better contextualizes family distress, appreciating their precarious life conditions and overwhelming challenges.

It is important to understand how multistressed families become overloaded and undersupported, rendered vulnerable by many past and ongoing challenges and unmet needs. Crisis situations are often embedded in problems in the workplace, health care system, community, and the larger society, which must be addressed. Crises may also be fueled by reactivation of past traumas, which need to be understood and integrated for greater resilience. While many children and families are at high risk for future serious problems and breakdown, Swadener and Lubeck (1995) prefer to think of them as children and families "at promise," with conviction about their potential and investment in helping them surmount barriers to achievement.

Family Challenges of Poverty and Discrimination

In a cruel paradox, crisis and disruption may be a constant in the lives of poor families. When they live so close to the edge, each crisis—whether job loss, illness, or violence—threatens to plunge them into a financial abyss. In the United States the disparity between the rich and the poor continues to widen. Poor families, disproportionately people of color, confront relentless stresses of unemployment, substandard housing, discrimination, and inadequate medical care. Parents struggle to provide their children with the basic essentials of food, clothing, shelter, and education. When surrounded by neighborhood blight, crime, violence, and drugs, they worry constantly about their safety (Garbarino, 1997). Life prospects are bleak in communities with limited job opportunities and access to community resources. Temporary or part-time work without benefits makes it hard to break the cycle of poverty and despair. Such problems present mammoth challenges to even the healthiest families and the most seasoned therapists. In work with highly vulnerable families, the barriers may seem insurmountable.

The combined psychological, social, and economic burdens of poverty and discrimination place poor minority children and families at greater risk for multiple problems. Poor people are stereotyped and marginalized; people of color who are poor suffer doubly. Immigrant families face the additional challenges of cultural differences and language barriers. Intertwined family and environmental stresses contribute to children's school difficulties and dropout, gang and criminal activity, and teen pregnancy—all of which worsen family strains. Interventions to reduce family vulnerability must address the environmental forces that pose such immediate threats to family survival.

Pileup of Stresses and Family Developmental Challenges

Family vulnerability is heightened by a pileup of stressors over time (Boss, 2001). With a single, isolated crisis, a family must mobilize quickly but can most often return to "normal" life. Multiple traumas, losses, and dislocations can overwhelm coping efforts. Recurrent crises repeatedly disrupt family life. The demands of many persistent challenges overload the system and drain resources. A family developmental perspective helps us to contextualize family distress across the life course and the generations. Psychosocial demands change over time with the process of adaptation to each crisis and change, interacting with individual and family life cycle passages. For example, a job loss may precipitate a change in residence, which triggers multiple dislocations for family members, such as challenges for children in a new school with new peers in an unfamiliar neighborhood, as parents are preoccupied with redirecting their lives. Therapeutic response to child emotional or behavioral problems must be attuned to these multiple transitions and stresses.

We can help families to gain perspective and to pace further disruptive changes. When overstressed, family members are more likely to compound their difficulties through fatigue, diminished competence, or errors in judgment. For instance, within days of the fatal drug overdose of his oldest son, a father pressed his family to move far away. The therapist helped the parents to consider that a precipitous move might create more dislocation and later regrets, without taking time to grieve and plan their future course.

A systemic assessment of multigenerational influences, unlike a deterministic search for "the cause" of problems, yields understanding of the clustering of stressful events and family members' distress over time and explores the meaning and impact of those events for the family. In a multistressed family, a genogram often reveals multiple incidents of trauma, disruption, and loss. Although they can't all be addressed, it is important to identify the major crises and attend to recurrent patterns and their legacies. Although most counseling is brief and focused on current distress, it is crucial to understand how symptoms and catastrophic fears are fueled by such experiences. In work with one couple in crisis, a partner's fears of commitment, withdrawal, and drinking are better comprehended when he recounts the many separations and losses he experienced throughout childhood in his family of origin and foster care system. His drinking stirs his wife's catastrophic fears stemming from painful memories of her previous marriage shattered by alcohol abuse. An understanding of where families are coming from increases their ability to make meaning of their current dilemma, informing and empowering them in the future directions they take.

STRENGTH-BASED, FAMILY-CENTERED SERVICES

Core Principles

Families that present multiple, complex, and severe problems, more than one symptom bearer, and recurrent crises make up a disproportionately large segment of human services caseloads. Unfortunately, they are more likely to be ill served and to fall between the cracks (Kaplan & Girard, 1994). Traditionally, services have tended to be deficit-based, individually focused, fragmented, crisis-reactive, inaccessible, and defined by professionals for clients. In contrast, strengths-oriented services stress the following core principles:

- Identify and build on family strengths and resources that empower families.
- Take a family-centered approach to individual problems.
- Provide flexible, holistic services.
- Emphasize prevention and early intervention.
- Build community-based and collaborative partnerships.

From a Deficit-Based to a Resource-Based Model

Uri Bronfenbrenner (1979), a champion of families, decried deficit-based public policies and services that required potential recipients to document their families' inadequacies to qualify for help. Negative stereotypes of parents as destructive, hostile, and uncaring; preconceptions of them as unreachable, unmotivated, and untreatable; and thick files of past problems and failed treatments—all create adverse expectations for any therapeutic contact. Too often professionals underestimate family ability to understand and tackle their problems.

Yet these families often show remarkable strengths in the midst of adversity. Many are resilient in simply making it through each day in the face of unrelenting stress and hardship. Resourcefulness can be seen in the inventive ways they manage on meager earnings. Most parents do care about their children and want a better life for them, although a myriad of difficulties may block their ability to act on these intentions. They often know what they need to change in their lives, if we are able to value their input, listen well, and support their best efforts.

A resource-based perspective in work with multistressed families empowers them to manage their stress-laden environments (Berg, 1997; Madsen, 1999; Minuchin et al., 1998). When therapy is overly problem-focused, it grimly replicates the problem-saturated experience of family life. Interventions that enhance positive interactions, support coping efforts, and build extrafamilial resources are more effective in reducing stress, enhancing pride and competence, and promoting more effective functioning.

From an Individually Based to a Family-Centered Approach

Human service systems have tended to treat problems as individually based—for example, a teen's pregnancy or a youth's delinquency. With services compartmentalized and individuals categorized narrowly according to presenting symptoms, there is insufficient attention to the whole person or to the family and social context. Often agencies that in principle avow the importance of the family actually, in practice, only see the individual—or may hold occasional sessions with a primary caregiver. With very heavy caseloads and complicated family situations, workers may doubt whether there is any way to be helpful at all. Without training in effective family systems work, a failed experience may reinforce beliefs that multistressed families are beyond repair.

One of my students, wanting to work with families in the juvenile justice system, found that despite her agency's stated mission to work with incarcerated youths and their families, in practice no families were currently seen. She was told that over the years, agency staff had found it too difficult to get "such dysfunctional families motivated for treatment" and no longer "wasted their resources." Instead, they met individually with the youth offenders, even though most youths returned to live with or near their families. Family involvement is crucial to gain their support for the transition back into the community, to encourage educational and job training pursuits, and to reduce family stresses that could undermine success. Without such efforts, these youths are more vulnerable to being lured into street gangs. When the family foundation is strengthened, home can become a more solid anchor for at-risk youths. When parents are not able to provide this structure, we need to search in the kin network for positive models and mentoring relationships to encourage resilience in these youths (Ungar, 2004a, 2004b).

Regardless of which family member seeks help, we need to broaden the focus of our interventions to the kin network to identify and build potential resources. Maintaining a family focus doesn't require seeing the whole family together, which may not be feasible in overstressed or fragmented families. It does involve holding a systemic view that addresses the important connections between family members, their problems, and possibilities for change and growth.

From Fragmented to Holistic Services

Social service systems often re-create and intensify family confusion when problems are handled in a disorganized way. Family members must navigate a bureaucratic maze, often sent from one agency to another in search of services. Different workers and agencies lack coordination in their efforts, offering crisis-focused, individually oriented services in a piecemeal fashion. In a family, one child may be seen by a school-based professional and a sibling by a juvenile justice counselor; another family member may be in a substance abuse treatment program; a grandparent in the home may need extensive medical care; while an overloaded single parent suffers with untreated depression. With fragmented services, no one is assessing or addressing interrelated concerns.

A family-centered resilience-oriented approach aims to improve communication and coordination of service delivery across systems. For effective services, a broad, comprehensive approach is essential, with coordinated and integrated services and a pooling of resources. Services must be viewed holistically, tailored to each family's challenges, and provided in the context of community, ethnic, and religious affiliations.

From Crisis-Reactive to Prevention-Oriented Services

Mental health and health care services, as well as school contacts with families, tend to be crisis-reactive. At such times, brief interventions cannot sufficiently address more complex or entrenched problems, or prepare families to meet future challenges. A limited focus may not allow for the relationship building and restructuring of family life that are needed to consolidate and sustain gains. Flexibility and responsiveness over time are necessary to attend to persistent problems and prevent future crises.

Regrettably, prevention has received little funding in the United States, although it is far more costly to treat a crisis after it occurs. As Kaplan and Girard (1994) note

> Our shame is that we pay scant attention to children and their families and spend little money on them until it is absolutely necessary. To qualify for help, an individual or family is categorized (and) assigned a pathological label. . . . This experience is dehumanizing and stigmatizing; worse, the help often comes too late. As a society, we must undergo a philosophical shift. (p. 15)

By investing in families "up front," we increase their coping ability and prevent escalation and chronicity of problems (Harris, 1996).

Family-Centered and Community-Based Partnership

Programs based on a multisystemic strengths-oriented philosophy create family and community partnerships to alleviate distress and build capacities to thrive in the face of adversity. Services are designed to be accessible, affordable, and offered through home-based and neighborhood programs. Combined approaches address individual symptoms (e.g., a child's school problems and a mother's depression) through family and larger systems interventions, such as family–school partnerships. Efforts are made to build a strong sense of community, and to overcome fear and mistrust through informal contact, program newsletters, and family/staff activities. Active family participation is encouraged in setting priorities and seeking solutions. Head Start's highly successful program is designed to empower families and improve children's life chances. Family involvement is encouraged in all aspects of the program. Parents are active collaborators in program decision making and participate in activities as volunteers, observers, and paid support staff. By working closely with professional staff they learn how to help their own children and many parents dramatically improve their own lives.

Over the past decade, there has been a growing movement of family support and preservation programs for at-risk children and families. Founded on the belief that families are our best resource, such programs maintain that the best place for children is with their families as long as their safety is not compromised. Instead of replacing troubled families, programs aim to support and strengthen them.

Family support programs have concentrated on prevention and early intervention (e.g., Children's Defense Fund, 1992; Dunst, 1995; Family Resource Coalition, 1996; Kagan & Weissbourd, 1994). They operate at the grassroots level and are consumer-oriented. Local, accessible *family resource centers* provide a range of information and services to support and strengthen families. Professionals and neighborhood paraprofessionals assist families with stressful life cycle transitions. Most provide parenting education and support in raising young children, particularly for single teen mothers. They link families with formal and informal services and support networks and they pool efforts of communities, school systems, hospitals, and corporations.

Family preservation programs have a dual commitment to protect vulnerable children and to strengthen their families. They aim to prevent out-of-home placement through immediate, home-based intervention to defuse a crisis, stabilize the family, and teach new problem-solving skills to avoid future crises. In contrast to traditional child welfare services, in which a worker is expected to assure the safety of all children in an overflowing caseload, highly trained staff work intensively with a small number of families in their homes, identifying mutual areas of concern. There is a balance of accountability for any future neglect or abuse and many family members are actively involved in assessing risks, reducing stress, and strengthening leadership, nurturance, and protection. Additional support is available as needed. Placement is necessary when children are at high risk of serious neglect or of physical or sexual abuse, and when family interventions prove to be unworkable. Efforts are made so that residential and foster care support rather than sever family ties. Wherever possible, efforts are made for family reunification (Kaplan & Girard, 1994).

The movement for family support and preservation services arose separately from developments in the field of family therapy, with little cross-fertilization until more recently. Family support programs, linked with the field of child development, have tended to focus on early mother–child relationships but have expanded to involve the family caregiving network. A multisystemic perspective is essential to integrate various program efforts with families and communities, from preventive approaches, such as family life education and psychoeducational support groups, to more intensive interventions for crises and more entrenched problems. A family life cycle orientation can guide a multigenerational framework for services with multistressed families to foster healthy pregnancy and early childrearing; child and adolescent development; strong marriages; caregiving for elders and members with disabilities; and end-of-life care. Workers in all programs for vulnerable youth and families can increase their effectiveness and reduce their risk of overload and burnout through training in strengths-oriented systemic assessment and family intervention skills (e.g. Berg, 1997; Madsen, 2003; Minuchin et al., 1998).

Evidence-Based Multisystemic Therapy Models

The development of several evidence-based, family-centered, multisystemic intervention models offers effective approaches to foster resilience with high-risk and seriously troubled youth, their families, and larger community systems (Henggeler, Schoenwald, Borduin, Rowland, & Cunningham, 1998; Liddle, Santistaban, Levant, & Bray, 2002; Sexton & Alexander, 2003; Ungar, 2004b). These family therapy approaches with adolescent conduct disorder and drug abuse yield improvements in family functioning, including increased cohesion, communication, and parenting practices, which are significantly linked to more positive youth behavioral outcomes than in standard youth services. Multisystemic interventions may take a variety of forms. Family therapists may involve school counselors, teachers, coaches, and peer groups; they may work with police officials, probation officers, and judges to address legal issues. They might help a youth and family access vocational services, youth development organizations, social support networks, and religious group resources.

With families that are often seen as unready, unwilling, or unmotivated for therapy, these approaches engage family members in a strengths-oriented, collaborative alliance. They develop a shared atmosphere of hope, expectation for change, a sense of responsibility (active agency), and a sense of empowerment. Rather than seeing troubled youths and their families as "resistant" to change, attempts are made to identify and overcome barriers to success in the therapeutic, family, and social contexts. Therapeutic contacts emphasize the positive and draw out systemic strengths and competencies for change. Clinicians maintain and clearly communicate an optimistic perspective throughout the assessment and intervention processes.

ASSESSMENT AND INTERVENTION PRIORITIES

A family resilience approach to practice is based on the conviction that even the most distressed families want to be healthy and have the potential for change and growth. That potential may be blocked by depleted resources or self-defeating survival strategies. Family members may not see other options in their situation. A strength-based reorientation begins in the first contacts with a family.

Assessing Family Stress, Vulnerabilities, Strengths, and Potential

In an assessment, many families' past experience with judgmental, deficit-based evaluation may lead them to hear even neutral questions as blame-laden. In resilience-oriented practice, it's important to be explicit that our intentions in gathering information are to understand family stresses and their impact for families, as well as family objectives and pathways for moving forward. We assess families within a positive framework, searching for resources and potential as well as vulnerabilities and constraints, all in relation to their challenges and their aims.

Most often, a request or referral for help centers on an immediate crisis focused on one family member, such as a child's behavior problems. On contact with the family, a number of problems often become evident and other family members may be in distress. When we understand how a son's vandalism, a father's disappearance, financial hardship, and a mother's depression are all connected, it's easier to focus on common concerns and aims. When presenting problems, such as child misbehavior, are reactive to family stress—and exacerbate that stress—we then engage family members to pull together to make things better. This collaborative approach helps to calm down the entire system and instill hope that other problems can be mastered.

Information gathering lays the groundwork for therapist–family collaboration in identifying strengths and prioritizing areas of concern.

What are all the significant family connections? How have family members attempted to deal with their problems or a crisis situation? What patterns of interaction escalate anxiety or conflict, increasing vulnerability and risk? Which members could be most helpful in strengthening the family? What hidden resources might be tapped to manage stresses and overcome barriers to success? How can change in the core family unit have a positive ripple effect for other members? It can be very hard to gather information when a family is in perpetual crisis and members' attention is scattered. Rather than waiting for things to calm down, it's better to make some time in early sessions to understand major stresses and identify patterns and constraints connected with members' distress.

Genograms (McGoldrick et al., 1999) are essential tools to diagram very complex family systems—for instance, those with extended kinship care; stepfamily constellations across households; families where a parent has had multiple partners and children have different fathers; those with members in and out of various living arrangements; or those involving foster care placements. A therapist might draw a large genogram interactively with a family. Children are often very interested to see how people are connected and where each one fits in the network of relationships. Seeing everyone on the same page can facilitate a sense of coherence for fragmented families that have experienced many losses, cutoffs, dislocations, and reconfigurations. Visualizing the connections can help a therapist, as well as the family, to feel less confused and overwhelmed.

Drawing a family timeline fosters a developmental perspective, as family members recall key nodal events and their impact. What organizational shifts occurred at what times, and how did a family attempt to handle traumatic events? In a multistressed family, a timeline helps to order the jumble of events and changes in family life over time. For instance, family members can better comprehend a parent's withdrawal into alcohol abuse when seen in the context of a pileup of painful losses. Both the genogram and the timeline are valuable visual and concrete tools for assembling many disconnected fragments of experience into a fuller, more coherent family narrative.

When family life has been saturated with problems, it's essential that genograms and timelines also identify particular relationships, events and periods of time that offered islands of calm, satisfaction, connection, and hope in the midst of the turbulence. These positive experiences, often invisible when assessment and therapy are problem-focused, offer resources to be drawn upon and enlarged. A woman abused by her mother's boyfriend may have found shelter in a very positive relationship with a grandmother. Even if that person is no longer nearby or alive, identifying the positive qualities in the relationship can provide a template in forming new, healthier relationships.

Diagnostic assessment can be essential in identifying serious mental illness and substance abuse, determining the risk for destructive behavior, and evaluating the need for psychotropic medication. However, labels such as "borderline personality disorder," which locate the problem in a person's character structure, tend to reinforce a sense of permanent damage and defect. It's more helpful and hopeful to identify problematic behavioral and interactional patterns that people can take steps to change. We should also be careful not to label a family by its members' problems (e.g., "an alcoholic family"). In a strength-based approach, therapists should put nothing in a case report that we would not feel comfortable sharing with family members. By encouraging clients to read and offer input in letters to agencies or courts we respect them as active partners in therapy. Similar transparency is communicated in the reflecting team approach to family therapy supervision (Nichols & Schwartz, 2005). The team first observes a family session through a one-way mirror and then exchanges places with the family so that the family can directly hear and observe their discussion and feedback.

Key Family Resilience Processes: Framework for Assessment and Intervention

The three-domain framework of key family resilience processes, presented in Chapters 3–5, was developed over many years for effective intervention with families presenting many serious and persistent problems. It facilitated my own shift from labeling families as "severely dysfunctional" to identifying particular vulnerabilities and resources that can be strengthened. In the midst of crisis and chaos, multistressed families and clinicians can be flooded. The framework keeps me mindful to search for resources and not become overwhelmed by a myriad of problems. As information emerges helter-skelter in the course of interviews, we can map it in a useful way to keep a systemic perspective and to target key elements for intervention focus to strengthen family resilience.

Belief Systems

The experience of recurrent crises, disappointments, and failure can lead families to carry the foreboding belief that something bad is bound to happen. This expectation generates collective anxiety and skews perceptions of ongoing experience and future possibilities. The pessimism of family members overwhelmed and unable to see alternatives or solutions further erodes confidence and blocks competence. All-or-none global generalizations are common, with difficulty in seeing shades of gray between extremes (e.g., always or never, all powerful or powerless, victim or villain). Catastrophic fears and destructive behavior patterns often radiate from constant exposure to community violence and a socially toxic environment (Garbarino, 1997) or ripple down from multiple traumas and losses in family history (see Chapter 11).

In poor inner-city families, the grim statistics of life chances have fostered a foreshortened sense of the life cycle. With a high proportion of young males of color lost to violence, drugs, or prison, many youths have lost a sense of future. Boyd-Franklin & Anderson (2001) contend that African American families and their communities must be all the more determined to raise their sons to overcome these challenges, following the wisdom of an Ashanti proverb, "You must act as if it is impossible to fail."

When families are buffeted by severe and persistent adverse conditions that are largely beyond their personal control, such as chronic poverty and racism, professionals need to help them counter a pervasive sense of helplessness and hopelessness. It is important not to give up on families that seem at first to resist our help. Listening to their prior experiences can shed light on their pessimism and mistrust: their many disappointments may have led them to expect to fail (and to expect us to let them down). By conveying our belief in their potential, we can help families to believe in themselves, and can thus foster pride, courage, perseverance, and hope for the future. Cornell West (1995) contends that although he is not optimistic about the immediate future of race relations, he does not give up hope of a better time to come. This hope fuels actions that increase the likelihood for success. He asserts, "As long as hope remains alive and meaning is preserved, the possibility of overcoming oppression stays alive" (p. 23).

Harry Aponte's (1994) work with poor minority inner-city families led him to recognize not only their physical hunger (for bread) but also a spiritual hunger. Despair robs them of meaning, purpose, and hope. A pervasive sense of injustice, helplessness, and rage is rooted in being denied access to opportunity, power, and privilege in society. Aponte urges therapists not to limit our work to pragmatic solutions but also to attend to spiritual needs. In the midst of despair, strong religious ties sustain a spirit of love, courage, and endurance for most families in poor communities. Aponte believes that therapists can make a difference if we recognize the power of that spirit: In addition to more jobs, better schooling, and health care, we must work to cultivate a diversity of cultural values, social structures, and spiritual practices to foster meaning and purpose in their lives. He calls on therapists to work as catalysts for community activism, to mobilize the spirit of hope to transform oppressive conditions.

Belief in the sustaining power of a relationship can fortify individuals through adversity even when they are separated and cut off from direct contact. In her novel *The Color Purple*, Alice Walker (1983) tells the life story of Celie, an African American woman who grew up in crushing poverty in the South, was sexually abused by her father, and then suffered chronic maltreatment by her husband. Throughout life's ordeals, Celie drew on her relationship with her sister for resilience. Although they were separated at adolescence, their nourishing connection was sustained over the years in imagination and in letters they were uncertain were ever received. They carried on daily conversations with each other in their heads. The meaning of their relationship was so profound that they continued to write letters over the years, despite the fact that neither's letters reached the other (because Celie's husband secretly hid them), until they were discovered much later in life.

Organizational Patterns

Most multistressed families seen in social service agencies are single-parent and reconstituted families. We must keep in mind that families of varied forms can function and raise their children well. However, chronic instability in household residence or family membership is very disruptive and heightens the risk for child maladaptation. In families with many problems and scarce resources, repeated losses and dislocations compound difficulties. If a parent repeatedly moves in and out or if multiple partners of a parent or other relatives come and go, the family organization, roles, patterns of interaction, and relationships can become fragmented and chaotic.

Therapeutic priorities are to increase the stability and cohesion of the family unit and to increase the reliability of contact and commitments to children as much as possible. If children have different fathers, or a parent has seemingly dropped out of the picture, it's important to ask specifically about the amount and dependability of contact and financial support. It's important not to write off parents who have not been reliably involved in the past without exploring their current situation (e.g., they may be gainfully employed, or no longer abusing substances). More often than expected, they care deeply about their children, have a strong desire to become more involved, and can be helped to cooperate with the custodial parent or guardian for the sake of their children. If barriers can be surmounted, and a child's safety is protected, in my experience, it is never too late for absent parents to become more involved in supporting their children's growth and success.

Family Disorganization: Building Structure, Stability, and Leadership. Unremitting stresses and multiple crises are disorganizing over time, wearing down a family's ability to function well. Roles become poorly integrated, and family members have difficulty collaborating to structure daily life and to resolve the problems that accumulate. Frustration often boils over into extreme reactivity, intense conflict, or disruptive behavior, further splintering family bonds. A lack of security and consistency ensues when family members may move in and out of households and go their separate ways. Yet amid this chaos is a deep longing for calm, security, and stability.

An all-or-none paradigm is evident in shifts between extreme rigidity and disorder. Having experienced so much upheaval, families may hold on to what they can and what is familiar. An unspoken rule might be "Don't rock the boat," because the threat of "capsizing" again is so great. When families in crisis are overwhelmed and disorganized, the therapeutic setting must provide a safe haven and solid structure. The fear of lives flying out of control is a common source of "resistance" to change in therapy. Therapists need to understand such anxiety and provide reassuring calm, order, and stability. Pushing too quickly for change may fuel fears of runaway change and loss of control. It's extremely important to work toward large changes in small, grounded incremental steps. Although we cannot control our clients' lives (nor should we), we need to be clearly in charge of sessions and interrupt runaway processes or destructive escalations to help families feel in control of the therapeutic process.

Family leadership, worn down by stress, may have become erratic and ineffective. Limit setting and discipline are often approached inconsistently or in an all-or-none fashion, without follow-through until a parent reaches a boiling point and explodes or threatens to send a misbehaving child away. A parent may be unsure of how to provide both nurturance and discipline. Framing discipline as setting caring limits and loving consequences can be very helpful.

In many families, parents or other caregivers need support in maintaining their position of authority. When a parent is overwhelmed by several unruly children, it can reinforce a sense of helplessness and incompetence if the therapist simply takes over. It's important to put parents in charge and to support them in setting rules and limits. We empower parents by joining forces with them and backing them up to bolster their authority and leadership. We may need to take charge initially, but we should always model with the aim of increasing parents' competence and confidence to take over leadership themselves.

In many cases, a child may be drawn into a parentified position to fill the void as "man of the house" or caretaker for a depleted parent. Skews of overfunctioning–underfunctioning need to be rebalanced. Older children can be encouraged to share responsibilities as long as parents do not abdicate leadership. Concrete guidelines, such as posting a chart of weekly chores and allocating them fairly among family members, can help to alleviate skews and to reinforce structure and follow-through. Weekly allowances or treats can reward children's efforts and build a sense of both personal autonomy and responsibility. Such therapeutic methods, grounded in structural family therapy and social learning models, are common to the many current family therapy approaches with multistressed families noted above.

Assessing whether overwhelmed families are motivated poses the wrong question; rather, we need to ask how we can help them keep their heads above water to take on efforts for change. We should also be careful not to pile still more demands on already overloaded parents. Inability to follow through only reinforces their sense of deficiency and failure. It's important to acknowledge how difficult their position is. After just an hour of pandemonium in a session, or hearing about the myriad of problems they are facing during the week, we can use our own sense of being overwhelmed to identify with parental challenges and applaud their efforts and perseverance.

Family Fragmentation: Building Connection and Collaboration. Many overwhelmed families become fragmented, with members left to fend for themselves. Family members rarely share mealtime or enjoy pleasurable contact. Families often become socially isolated and alienated, lacking positive supports. Disengaged family patterns are seen commonly in abuse and neglect, and with children showing serious conduct disorder. A depleted parent may be unaware of children's whereabouts or their drug or alcohol use. Overwhelmed parents may take flight from responsibility or seek escape in alcohol or drug use. Violence or threats of abandonment may come out of a sense of desperation when parents snap. It's important in such cases to help reduce the pileup of stress and frustration, to recruit kin and social supports, and to structure time and space for respite so that parents can replenish their energies.

Family Enmeshment: Strengthening Boundaries and Differentiation. In some families, members become enmeshed: boundaries blur and thoughts, feelings, and identities are fused or distorted. Parents may confuse their own needs with those of their children. Inconsistent and unclear boundaries can lead to intrusion and lack of privacy or violation in sexual abuse. Parents inappropriately draw children into their marital affairs. Jenny, age 17, was hospitalized for self-destructive behavior after carving small crosses in her arms. Family assessment revealed her overinvolvement in her parents' intense marital conflict. When asked how it made her feel, she replied, "Caught in the crossfire."

All-or-none relationship patterns often lead family members to take flight by cutting off all contact. Family relationships may oscillate between pseudoautonomous distancing and falling back into overinvolvement and helpless dependence—a pattern common in drug and alcohol abuse. When one child is embroiled in parental needs and conflicts, siblings may disengage as a survival strategy. Jenny's brother "took the geographical cure" (as he put it)—abruptly leaving home, driving 500 miles to the north woods of Wisconsin, and living in a cabin off a dirt road with no telephone. When he returned, curious to "check out" the family therapy, he sat quietly through a session with a bemused smile. Later he confessed that he had been high on drugs, in order to keep "a safe distance." Intense, ambivalent attachments and loyalties cannot simply be resolved by physical separation. Family therapy, combined with individual work, helps to untangle members and to help them move together gradually toward more autonomy. Especially in cases where a child has been pulled in as an emotional mate or caregiver, it's crucial to strengthen generational boundaries and to work on couple issues separately.

Some families have become so disorganized, fragmented, and/or enmeshed that family life is chaotic and frighteningly out of control, as in the following case:

The Washingtons were referred for family therapy after two brothers, aged 13 and 15, were arrested for vandalism. Most recently, they had set their mother's bed on fire. It was learned that the mother had given her bedroom to her oldest son, Mark, 17, and appointed him "man of the house," after throwing the father out because of recurrent drunkenness and assaultive behavior. The mother's family-of-origin experience was also complicated by alcohol abuse, mental instability, and violence. Her sister had in fact "lost all control" and beaten her small child to death.

The therapist was understandably overwhelmed by the history and unsure of where to begin. It was important to identify and alter interactional patterns that reinforced vulnerability. When clear structure is lacking, things get out of control; the catastrophic fear is that anything can happen, from violence and murder to possible incest. Although the household was calmer and safer from violence without the father, the mother, who had relied on his "law and order" authority, felt unsure of her ability to be in charge. Furthermore, she held down a demanding job and was exhausted when she got home. Their apartment was in disarray. The mother slept on the sofa, while the 12-year-old sister was sleeping in the same room with her two "wild" brothers. Their living structure reflected and reinforced their sense of chaos.

It was crucial to shore up family stability, leadership, and boundaries. The therapist framed these objectives normatively, affirming the mother's position of respect as head of the household and the healthy needs of all family members. The therapist strongly encouraged the mother, as a hard-working single parent with "two shifts" of job and family demands, to reclaim her own room, where she could close the door for some respite. The family members were encouraged to envision new ways of organizing their apartment so that everyone could claim a space of their own. At the next session, they sketched the floor plan with a magic marker and the kids cut out pieces of paper to represent the furniture to be moved around. They enjoyed this task and it gave them a sense of control in planning their living space. The therapist supported the mother's suggestion that a small storage room could be cleared out for the daughter, framing this decision normatively, in terms of a teenage girl's need for privacy from her brothers. The mother got the eldest son to move back in with his brothers, helping to calm them down. The boys pitched in together to decorate personal space around their beds with photos and posters. We can encourage families such as this one to make structural changes by facilitating their own creative solutions.

Communication Processes

Clarity. Family vulnerability is heightened when there is pervasive unclarity: Everyone may talk at once, go off on different tangents, and not listen to others. Parents may be inconsistent in words and deeds. Messages become distorted, and members think they can read minds, confusing one another's thoughts and feelings. Important issues remain murky (e.g., "Are Dad and Mom splitting up? What's going to happen to us?"), elevating anxieties, when messages are unclear and inconsistent.

It is crucial for therapists to be clear and consistent, especially in defining our relationship: what our role and commitment are to all family members, what they can expect of us, and what we will expect of them. It's important to keep sessions on a regular, predictable schedule, as much as possible, and to make every effort to follow through on expectations.

Setting communication rules helps to bring order and focus to therapy. When family members talk over one another and constantly interrupt or shift their attention, a turn-taking rule in sessions is needed: "Only one person talks at a time. That way, when it's your turn to talk, everyone will be able to listen to you." Framing the rule in terms of the positive benefit to each member is more effective than issuing a critical warning not to interrupt others. A toy microphone might be passed around, like the "talking stick" used in tribal meetings; the person holding the microphone can talk while others listen.

Open Emotional Expression. A pileup of tensions in a family heightens emotional reactivity. Repeated negative interactions corrode family members' feelings and block mutual understanding. Members stop listening and just counterattack or withdraw. As therapists, we must be active and firm to interrupt cycles of blame, shouting, or cursing, and to help family members to handle frustration, disappointment, and anger in more constructive and respectful ways. When sensitive issues can be discussed more calmly, anxieties lessen and problems are tackled more effectively. Often blaming and scapegoating are fueled by self-blame, shame, and guilt, which should be explored. It is crucial to distinguish feelings from actions: Intense anger may be understandable in a situation, but acting on feelings in destructive ways is not acceptable. When harmful actions are denied or blamed on others, we must help members take responsibility for their own behavior, even when they feel provoked.

With persistent stress, a family may burn out, emotionally exhausted from the onslaught. Some members may try to maintain control and lower anxiety by prohibiting expression of thoughts and feelings that might be upsetting or endanger the family unit. They may avoid conflict out of catastrophic fears that it will escalate out of control into violence or abandonment, as it may have in past experience. Yet when stresses mount and needs go unmet, there is a greater risk of periodic explosions: Conflict may be sealed over until it can be contained no longer and erupts like a volcano (again, in an all-or-none pattern). It's essential to understand catastrophic fears and to help family members express differences and hurts in ways that foster understanding and healing.

It is also important to help family members own and tolerate a range of feelings, while helping them to modulate the intensity of emotions (Johnson, 2002). It's essential to set ground rules in therapy, so that family members feel safe to express concerns in sessions without fear of getting clobbered when they get home. Moreover, if emotions become too intense, members may distort or remember little of what happened in a session. As therapists interrupt destructive spirals, members experience safe limits if they start to lose control. It's important to help family members gain skill in managing and repairing conflict. We can help them notice signs of mounting tensions and interrupt their part in cycles before they spiral out of control. We may note how sensitive an issue is and encourage them to talk calmly about it, or have them take time out until they can do so. We can underscore valid points on each side and acknowledge concerns of all members. We might interrupt an intense interaction to explore how other relationships are affected. We can ask a father how conflict with his son is reminiscent of interactions he had with his own father. We can keep the focus on an issue and add other dimensions to it, while defusing tensions.

When the interaction in a session is volatile, it is crucial to allow time to process and calm an upsetting exchange, and to bring feelings under control in a cooling-down time before the session ends. Family members then gain the ability to open up a sensitive issue and yet contain it, with a greater sense of control over runaway processes. Often members don't bring up a highly charged issue until just before the end of a session. It's important to acknowledge the importance or sensitive nature of the issue when discussion must be tabled until the next session, so that there will be sufficient time to give it the attention it warrants. Therapists must be alert to defuse any danger that demands immediate attention, such as a threat of harm to oneself or others. All family members should be given a card with contact phone numbers for the therapist or agency and a crisis hotline if need arises between sessions. Many times, clients have told me that just having the emergency contact numbers in their wallet eased anxiety and helped them manage a threatening situation.

In problem-saturated families, members can become so caught up in a quagmire of crisis and despair that they have no enjoyable time together. Encouraging pleasurable interaction is especially important in sessions and in giving tasks. For example, I might ask an estranged noncustodial father to plan an activity with his son they would both enjoy in the coming week. I nudge the conversation along from a father's hesitance ("I don't know what he'd like; he never seems interested in anything I suggest") or a child's self-protective indifference. I encourage dialogue between them to gain agreement on a clear, concrete plan, with approval of the custodial mother. I may also need to work with the mother on lingering anger at her ex-spouse, to facilitate change that will benefit their children and ultimately the mother herself, as well.

Collaborative Problem Solving. Action-oriented, concrete solution-oriented approaches work best with overloaded families. Clear, attainable objectives should be defined, with small, realistic steps to reach them. Families are likely to experience repeated failure if they hold vague, unrealistic expectations without taking steps to build a solid base. A first priority may be addressing a family's concrete needs, such as adequate housing, day care, or job training. Again, small, manageable tasks should be tackled first. Each success builds more confidence in the ability to solve other, more complicated problems. It also builds trust in the therapeutic relationship and in family teamwork. Tasks should be designed to reduce stress and to strengthen family structure.

Therapists, like families themselves, can become flooded by the many problems families are struggling with. We need to help family members prioritize and focus their attention. When we normalize and anticipate possible setbacks or upheaval if a new crisis hits, they are less discouraged by inevitable bumps in the road. Failure is not falling down, but staying down. Although we and our clients can't control everything, what matters is our determination to rebound and redouble our efforts.

From Problems to Possibilities. From a family resilience perspective, it is not enough to reduce current stress and conflict; it is crucial to enhance families' problem-solving skills and their resources in meeting future challenges. The focus extends from solving presenting problems to preventing future ones. For example, we can ask family members how they might prepare for a threatened crisis or avert it altogether. We might also have them imagine the possibility that *no* crisis will occur over the coming week. What would it take for that to happen, and how could they celebrate? We want to encourage them to anticipate not only how things can go wrong, but how they can help them go right.

When family members are struggling to keep afloat, therapy, like

learning to swim, empowers them by helping them develop their own resources. As therapists, our strong conviction in families' potential matters more than clever techniques. Possibilities are generated as dilemmas
are viewed in ways that expand rather than limit options. Rather than
focus on reducing negative behaviors, therapy is more successful when
we help families gain new skills, competence, and confidence. For instance, instead of trying to get a father to stop yelling, it's more effective
to help him learn more caring ways to get his message across and improve relationships. To master the art of the possible, we help families
learn from how things have gone wrong, harmful events that can't be
changed, and refocus on how they can succeed and move forward, as in
the following case:

> Crystal, age 14, was referred for individual therapy following her
> second attempt to run away from home. It was learned that she had
> been sexually abused by her grandfather when she was younger, and
> just recently by her mother's boyfriend, Rick. Her mother had
> ended this relationship after the incident, but Crystal angrily blamed
> her for not having protected her over the years. Her therapist, wish-
> ing to be supportive, joined in faulting the mother, only to find that
> after the session Crystal took a handful of pills in a suicide attempt.
>   Family therapy was begun, focused on drawing out family re-
> sources to handle the current crisis. The mother was genuinely re-
> morseful for not having been aware of any of the abuse or more
> tuned in to Crystal's distress. The therapist acknowledged both
> Crystal's pain and her mother's regret, suggesting that they could
> learn from those experiences to approach this crisis in a new way.
> She credited the mother for ending her relationship with Rick, and
> thus demonstrating that Crystal's well-being came first. They fo-
> cused on what might be done next, brainstorming about possible
> options. Crystal wanted to have Rick prosecuted. Her mother
> agreed to press charges. The therapist enlisted Crystal's two older
> brothers to support Crystal and their mother through the ordeal of
> the legal maze and the trial ahead.
>   Over the next 3 months, the therapist tracked and commended
> the family's progress in doggedly pursuing the case. She supported
> the mother in remaining firm when Rick tried to get her to back
> down. The family members experienced a new solidarity in taking
> on this challenge and in their ultimate success at winning a convic-
> tion. Crystal threw her arms around her mother in the last family
> session, and thanked her mother and brothers: "You really came
> through for me this time. I feel like we're all really family for the
> first time."

Families are empowered when they gain access to their power. While acknowledging and honoring trauma and suffering that has occurred, we can put our weight on the side of hope—the potential that things can be changed for the better. We can emphasize the positive intentions, tap underutilized strengths, and celebrate progress and success.

MASTERING PRACTICE CHALLENGES

Reaching Out to Families

Many multistressed families become frustrated, wary, and mistrustful of well-intentioned "helpers" because of repeated negative interactions and unhelpful experiences with numerous systems. Family survival strategies may lead members to guard against further involvement with professionals. Boyd-Franklin (2004) notes that many African American families have developed a healthy suspicion of social service agencies and their providers. This skepticism can take many forms, from overt anger to missed sessions or lack of follow-through with agreed-upon plans. A discouraged family may protect itself by actions that express feelings of "Why bother? Nothing ever works out, and no one really cares." As helping professionals, we need to understand such learned pessimism and respond by making every effort to connect productively. This requires—and demonstrates—our perseverance to hang in with reluctant family members in order to gain trust and acceptance.

One rule of thumb is to include in therapy all family members whose participation can strengthen relationships and contribute to lower risk and vulnerability. For example, a mother may come for help, but may say that the alcohol-abusing father is unwilling to come in. Without his involvement in therapy, problem interactions are likely to remain stuck or worsen. Individual coaching, especially with a person who is in a one-down position in a relationship, is unlikely to improve destructive patterns or a partner's problem drinking. Also, putting one partner in charge of changing the other worsens power struggles and conflict. Change may prove impossible, and separation may be for the best, but pessimistic forecasts should not deter us from reaching out to try to engage the reluctant partner.

Issues concerning blame, shame, and vulnerability are often a source of resistance for men to take part in therapy, especially in cultures where pride, authority, and invulnerability are intertwined in images of successful manhood. We can best enlist a father's active involvement in therapy as a caring parent, underscoring his potential power and pride in helping his children succeed.

In multistressed families, siblings may keep to the edge of family life and often become keen observers of the family drama. Yet they may fear that involvement will pull them into quicksand. Engaging higher-functioning siblings in family therapy can benefit them as it provides resources to more distressed members. We can help those who have distanced from embroilment in family problems gain ability to be in contact with their family and still hold their own boundaries. We can strongly encourage them to come to family sessions and invite their comments and collaboration, yet also respect their needs and limits, so that they feel in control of the extent of their involvement.

The unclear role of a live-in boyfriend in a family should be explored, assessing not only any heightened risks (e.g., substance abuse), but also his potential strengths as a partner and support in parenting. When a mother's past couple relationships have been unstable, children may express anxieties about a new relationship in problem behavior that heightens the risk of another breakup. Unclarity also results in confusion for children around such issues as attachment, authority, and boundaries. Not including a live-in partner in the structure of therapy reinforces a boundary around the single-parent family unit, making it harder for couple and informal stepparent relationships to develop. We can acknowledge the partners' uncertainty about their future relationship commitment, yet encourage them to support each other and manage relationships with the children as they resolve presenting problems. By working collaboratively, it can help to stabilize and solidify their relationship.

Crisis Intervention and Crisis Prevention

Some families seem to be in perpetual crisis, reeling from one traumatic event to the next. Family members who are overwhelmed may think of therapy as an emergency room service, a lifeline in times of crisis. Without a systemic frame and clear objectives, therapy too will cast about in all directions, reeling from crisis to crisis. Each new crisis interrupts focus on any one problem-solving effort. Therapists, like families themselves, can get caught up in a reactive mode: We all become swept up by the latest crisis and its aftermath. Yet many crises can be anticipated. It's essential to get ahead of the next wave. If we do a good systems assessment and structure family interviews sufficiently, we can better anticipate problems and increase our ability to tackle hazardous situations before they get out of control. One therapist was relieved to learn initially that a mother's abusive boyfriend was in jail and out of the picture. However, 6 weeks later, the family was in crisis after the mother was battered once again by the boyfriend. The therapist hadn't asked when he was likely to be released and how she would handle that. Thus, the opportunity was missed to plan ahead for what she would do if he returned.

Searching for Strengths amid Persistent Crises

General Aims

With families flooded by problems, it is particularly challenging to resist the pull of pathology and to search for strengths. When families come for help in crisis, the problematic aspects of their lives stand out, and helping professionals may become as overwhelmed and discouraged as they are (Waters & Lawrence, 1993). We may become frustrated and pull back from engaging fully with the family or thinking creatively about change. When our clients sense our loss of hope and commitment, they feel worse about themselves and are more likely to give up and drop out of therapy. Gaining an appreciation of their healthy strivings gives us hope, which fuels energy to work with those strengths to overcome the chaos in their lives. When we underestimate our clients, we lose sight of their potential for mastery. There may be truly impossible cases, but that has rarely been my experience, nor that of my strength-oriented colleagues.

Even in the most troubled families, areas of competence can be found and enlarged as sources of pride and accomplishment. We are most effective when we encourage family members to develop options and skills rather than dwelling on their limitations. In the unfolding process of therapy, we face constant choices about what to pick up on. If we get caught up in a family's hopelessness and helplessness, therapy bogs down. Every maladaptive response also contains the seeds of healthy striving that can be cultivated. As Waters and Lawrence (1993) observe, parents may lose control and become abusive *because* they care so much and want so badly for a child to do better. We need continually to emphasize hope, caring, and small gains, to enable the parents to hang in and act on their best intentions. Although there is most often caring alongside abuse or neglect, there are some cases (e.g., families with seriously drug-addicted parents) where caring has been extinguished over time and cannot be revived. And yet we should not write off the possibility of change, but make a determined effort to support new beginnings, as we search out other positive resources in the kin network.

The general aims of a resilience-oriented approach with vulnerable families can be summarized as follows:

- Overcoming the cycle of suspicion, rejection, failure, and withdrawal
- Forging a trusting relationship through direct, honest, respectful communication
- Encouraging families to prioritize their many needs and aims
- Believing in family members' potential; giving them hope and confidence that they can improve their situation and overcome long-standing problems
- Increasing family members' ability to solve problems, avert crises, and advocate on their own behalf

To achieve these aims, we can draw on an array of techniques from strength-based family therapy approaches. The ultimate aim is to enable family members to regain control of their lives and belief in their competence and worth.

One of the hardest challenges for us as therapists is to align empathically with family members who are slow to change. We may also be drawn in to demonize men who have been abusive or mothers who have failed to protect their children. While addressing problem behavior, we need to resist the pull to pathologize the person. We can gain empathy from seeing each person in the context of his or her relationships and life struggles: a single parent who is overwhelmed and undersupported; a wife whose trust in men has been shattered by past sexual abuse; a father who himself was abused and knows no other way to discipline children. When therapists view entrenched problems as constitutional and inevitable, it may relieve them of a sense of failure for therapeutic gridlock, but they further erode their clients' sense of worth and life chances in doing so. We can open up possibilities for change by appreciating our clients' struggles and viewing therapeutic impasses as shared challenges, requiring courage, perseverance, and renewed teamwork.

Learning and Growth from Past Trauma

Often problems in one generation are repeated in the next. When a mother is worried that her 16-year-old daughter is sexually active and will get pregnant, a genogram may reveal that she herself became pregnant at 16. Although the immediate crises and chaos presented by a family can make history taking very challenging, learning about past conflicts and traumatic events—particularly those occurring at the same nodal point in the life cycle a generation earlier—often sheds light on concerns in presenting problems.

In an integrative therapeutic approach, work is present- and future-focused, but is linked to each family's past. It is important to make connections and distinctions between past and present challenges and responses: A client may have been powerless as a child, but now as an adult, he or she can learn from the past and take charge in dealing with current situations as a partner or parent. The therapeutic task is to bring intergenerational patterns and linkages to light, and then to take lessons from painful past experience and seize the opportunity to do things differently with one's partner and children. It can be helpful for children to learn stories of their parents' struggles growing up, and it helps parents to gain empathy for their children's positions. We can ask questions such as: "What did you need that your parents were unable to provide?" "Alongside their limitations, what positive memories do you have of them and your relationship? Now that you're a parent, what can you learn from your experience to better meet your children's needs?" Parents can be commended for caring enough about their children to take steps to prevent a painful history from repeating itself. We can encourage them to act on their best intentions and their yearning to create the strong bonds longed for in the past.

Recruiting Models and Mentors

Models and mentors can be found and recruited in even the most troubled family. In cases where parents are absent or limited by serious mental illness or substance abuse, it's crucial to engage other members of the extended kin system. Older siblings can be valuable resources, drawing on their abilities and talents to teach or assist younger children who are having difficulty. For instance, older siblings can read with younger ones or help them with homework, building their relationship along with skills. Extended family members can also be valuable resources for resilience.

The life of the poet Maya Angelou is a moving story of the power of kin bonds for resilience in overcoming childhood adversity: Because her parents were heavily involved in an unsafe environment of substance abuse, gambling, and promiscuity, the father sent Maya, age 5, and her brother, Bailey, age 4, across the country to their grandmother's care. The strong sibling bond they forged gave each the courage and confidence to overcome many crises and life challenges. Their grandmother provided the stability and security they desperately needed. Living in poverty in the black part of town in the rural South, the grandmother sustained her own resilience through her deep religious faith and personal connection to God, whom she talked to like a favorite uncle. Every day after school Maya would go to the small store run by her great-uncle Willie, where he would grill her on her homework. Uncle Willie was a man of humble means with little formal schooling; he was also lame and had a severe speech disability. Yet he valued education and became her mentor and champion. He prodded her to do her best in her studies and to aim high in her life aspirations. She wrote a poem honoring him (Angelou, 1986), to encourage others to seek out their own Uncle Willies in their relationship networks and to serve as he did for others in their lives.

Creating Problem-Free Zones

Because families come to therapy and counseling to address problems, we need to be careful not to replicate a family's grim experience of life as a barrage of problems. It's important to encourage conversation about nonproblematic and positive areas of life. Faces will light up and conversation will become animated as we show interest in school and activities, highlights of the week, and pleasurable times, however fleeting. It brings welcome relief to laugh together about humorous moments. As we amplify areas of competence and success, it instills hope and encourages family members to see beyond problems. When daily life is consumed by problems, we can help family members to structure problem-free zones: plan a family outing or a "date" for parents to enjoy with problem talk "off limits"; agree on a rule of no fighting at the dinner table or in a couple's bedroom.

In particular, structuring in time and activities for parents to have respite from constant demands enables them to feel nurtured, to "refuel," and then to function more effectively. A single mother can be invited to pick times in the coming week for herself when she is "off duty," and mobilize family members to ensure that her time and space are honored. Recruiting extended family members—aunts, uncles—to pitch in periodically, even in small ways, can also relieve the constant stress.

Reformulating "Termination"

When families present multiple and recurrent problems, it is difficult to determine not only where to begin, but also how to end our work. Since family members are likely to continue to experience high stress in their lives, their success should be defined not by the absence of problems, but by the family's greater resilience to deal with them more effectively. What matters most is that members gain stronger personal and relational resources to manage and overcome the challenges that lie ahead.

When our therapeutic relationship is meaningful, ending it is likely to reactivate our clients' intense feelings of all other painful losses, especially those beyond their control. "Termination" may stir up clients' memories of past abandonment, and beliefs that they were unlovable or drove a parent or partner away. We should anticipate and explore upset and setbacks, and help families not to see them as signs of failure. When a therapist or agency must end therapy before a family is ready, it's essential to clarify that it is not their fault and does not mean that we didn't care about them. In ending, it's important to convey what we liked best about each family member, the progress they have made, and the further gains we believe they are capable of making. If the family is transferred to another therapist, it is crucial to help them make a good connection. With vulnerable families, it can be helpful to extend gradually the length of time between sessions. This enables the family to experience some control and predictability in the process and to become increasingly confident in their own abilities, with the therapist still available to help them head off more serious difficulties and sustain their gains. A last session can be marked by a celebration of all the family has accomplished.

Combined Therapeutic Modalities

Support groups are valuable adjuncts to family counseling, helping families decrease isolation and develop a mutual support system. A weekly support group for overwhelmed single mothers is immensely beneficial in building confidence and competence.

Relationship skills programs are increasingly being recommended for high-risk couple relationships. Follow-up services are especially important because the stress and unexpected challenges of their lives can easily set them back or distract them from maintaining what they have learned in the program. One promising approach is to involve trained mentor couples who either live in the community or come from similar backgrounds. Other useful approaches are monthly support groups of participants after the program has ended, or inviting participants to return for a booster session at any time, but especially during any difficult transitions in their lives.

Treatment models for substance abuse, violence, or sexual abuse, beyond the scope of this book, typically employ a multimodality approach (e.g., Sheinberg & Fraenkel, 2001). Family systems experts in abuse urge a contextual approach and strongly recommend individual or group intervention focused on social accountability and on stopping abusive behavior patterns as an immediate priority before couple or family therapy is safely begun (Almeida et al., 1998).It's important to coordinate all approaches, with good communication among the professionals involved.

Outreach and Home-Based services

When families are buffeted by stresses, therapeutic services need to be accessible and scheduled at convenient times. Therapists often need to go the extra distance to engage family members and to sustain their efforts and gains over time. When an appointment has been missed, a reminder phone call for the next session communicates our investment and promotes continuity in the therapy process. Clients may be asked to phone in and leave a message of midweek progress. One therapist was frustrated and ready to give up working with a single mother who was unreliable in taking her psychotropic medication. Without it, she became neglectful of household and parenting responsibilities, and was in danger of losing custody of her children at an upcoming hearing. The consulting team encouraged the therapist to give her a strong, clear message that she must take her medications in order to function well enough to keep her children, and that he expected her to phone his office every morning over the next week, leaving a message that she had taken her medication. The therapist, discouraged by her setback, first had to overcome his own doubts that she would follow through. However, she did so, and by the second week her improved functioning enabled her to keep on track herself with medication and parenting responsibilities.

Home visits indicate to family members that professionals are invested in them and that they are worth the effort. They can also provide a clear view of both the risks and the potential resources in the family's living arrangements, as in the following case:

Jimmy Monroe, age 12, an only child, lived with his mother, Charlayne, and her longtime boyfriend, Al Stevens. Nine months earlier, Jimmy's mother, in an acute psychotic episode, had tried to suffocate him with a pillow in the middle of the night. Jimmy had gone to live with an aunt while she was hospitalized and stabilized on medication, and was now again living at home. Charlayne failed to keep several appointments with Jimmy's new social worker, who then scheduled a home visit. As the worker approached the apartment, the front shade was suddenly pulled down and no one answered her knocking.

In group supervision, the worker was encouraged to set up another home visit. This time Charlayne, wearing a bathrobe and somewhat disheveled in appearance, opened the door. The worker showed her some of Jimmy's artwork, praising his creativity. Charlayne warmed a bit and offered some coffee. In the kitchen a man's voice could be heard. Sensing that they might presume her disapproval of a live-in boyfriend, the worker took the initiative, asking, "Oh, is that Mr. Stevens? Jimmy has told me he thinks the world of him." As Al entered the room hesitantly, the worker greeted him cordially and, with Charlayne's OK, invited him to join their conversation. She began by orienting them to Jimmy's program and her role as a counselor. She explained her reason for meeting them: The program found that kids did best when their families were actively involved in supporting their success. She would set regular meetings to update them on Jimmy's progress, to respond to any concerns they or Jimmy might have, and to work together with them as a team. She answered their questions and let them know how to reach her. They were off to a good start. Charlayne thanked the worker for coming back, and Al offered to walk her to the bus stop, saying that the neighborhood could be a little rough toward dusk. She accepted his offer and took the opportunity to get to know him better.

After each session Al continued to walk the worker to the bus stop, at times bringing up concerns about Charlayne. He worked a night shift and worried about her night terror and difficulty sleeping; she often sat up with the TV on until his return and then slept most of the day. First, Charlayne's medication was adjusted to enable her to sleep more soundly through the night. Then they explored how Al might switch to a morning shift so that he could be home at night. The worker also encouraged his interest in spending more time with Jimmy. More regular dinnertime and weekend outings increased their sense of "family."

Conversations then explored future hopes and dreams and ways of moving toward them. Charlayne and Al wished to get a larger apartment on a safer block but they were financially strapped. Though Charlayne had daydreams of getting a job, she lacked skills and transportation, and felt overwhelmed by the challenge. Together, they brainstormed about possibilities in the neighborhood. Charlayne astonished the worker only a month later by landing a part-time job in a nearby convenience store. Her functioning and sense of worth were enhanced by the job, paycheck, and social contact; as a result, she took better care of herself and Jimmy. Al and Charlayne playfully teased each other about ways to spend her new earnings. With remarkable progress by Jimmy and his family over the school year, monthly follow-up sessions were held to keep things on track. The family moved into a larger apartment, where Jimmy could play safely outside with friends.

Dogged persistence by a helping professional can be powerful in bringing about crucial structural and interactional changes in a family. In this case, the worker's supportive encouragement by her consultation team bolstered her own perseverance.

Home visits do present challenges. The first priority for productive settings is to create a workable space and quiet atmosphere, setting boundaries from intrusion. Enlisting family collaboration in this process sets the stage for therapeutic partnership. We might ask what space would work best for talking comfortably with minimal interruption; we can ask family members to take turns answering the phone or tending to a baby. Structuring a home session establishes a small island of calm in a sea of turmoil. This achievement is all the more significant because it takes place in the home unlike the artificial setting of a therapist's office, demonstrating that it is possible to gain more control over the bombardment of stresses in daily life.

Families and Foster or Kinship Care: A Collaborative Approach

Although the child welfare system is committed in theory to maintaining children in their own homes, placement is a common option taken to protect children from imminent danger. Poor minority children, especially from African American, Latino, and Native American families, are vastly overrepresented in out-of-home placement. Training of child welfare professionals in family systems concepts and methods enables them to work more effectively to strengthen family capacities. By expanding their lens beyond the limitations of a primary caregiver or the risk posed by an offender, potential resources can more readily be tapped in the extended kin and community network. By involving the family in placement decisions, they are more likely to support the best arrangement for children.

When placement is necessary, maintaining the continuity of key relationships should be a priority. Traditionally, when foster care has been viewed as a means of rescuing children from dysfunctional families. This sets up parents and foster caregivers as adversaries, the bad parents versus the good parents, when collaboration is much more beneficial for children (Minuchin et al., 1998). We can avoid further trauma for children by not abruptly severing all bonds to parents, siblings, and extended family members.

Preventing Recidivism: Easing Transitional Stresses

Recidivism in child placements has been high. The transitional challenges when children return home require a systemic lens, as in the following case:

> Eight-year-old Terrell was being seen by an agency in individual therapy for "separation anxiety" over the past 2 years, after he and three siblings were removed from their mother's custody because of cocaine dependence and neglect and were placed in custodial care with their maternal grandmother. The mother left the abusive relationship with her boyfriend as part of her recovery efforts. With the support and encouragement of a drug treatment sponsor, she kept off drugs, maintained regular participation in Cocaine Anonymous, got off public assistance and into a job, and recently regained custody of her children.
>
> Over the next month, Terrell became increasingly agitated. In regaining their mother, the children had now lost their grandmother, their caregiver for 2 years. The mother, still angry at her mother for having initiated the court-ordered transfer of the children, had cut off all contact between the children and their grandmother. Their loss and conflicted loyalties with the prohibition against contact were all the more painful and confusing since the grandmother had just moved to an apartment on the same block to be near them.
>
> In the following weeks, Terrell's therapist noticed that his mother looked haggard in the waiting room and asked how she was doing. She said she was about to quit her job because of the stress and added vaguely that she might look for some other work just to get out of the house. She seemed overwhelmed and depleted, but when asked whether she'd like to see a therapist for herself, she declined, saying that she was too busy and didn't have time.
>
> Called in as a consultant to a staff meeting at this point, I offered a family resilience perspective to the case. It was important to apply a systemic approach to guide intervention efforts through these transitional crises. First, the original presenting problem—Terrell's separation anxiety—was clearly intensified by the recent cutoff of the grandmother's contact. His siblings, who had also suffered this abrupt loss, were also cranky and difficult for mother to

handle. The emotional upheaval of the recent separation and dislocation for the children needed to be ameliorated. Family interventions were held to repair the strained relationship between the mother and grandmother and to negotiate their changing role relations. Planning and support services were essential to support the mother's efforts to meet the challenges in parenting of four young children while managing a full-time job.

The mother and grandmother were helped to shift from their competition for the children's love and loyalty, and from a struggle over authority and competence, to build a collaborative relationship. The therapist facilitated brainstorming of ways they could work together as a team across households, with the mother in charge as primary parent and the grandmother supporting her efforts. Yet, for the mother, needing help was viewed as an indication that she'd "messed up" again, loaded with attributions of failure, blame, and shame. Now having difficulty managing, she was at high risk of relapsing and losing her children once again. It was crucial to reframe the grandmother's role at this time—not rescuing the kids from a deficient mother, but supporting her daughter's best efforts to succeed with her children and her job and sustaining the vital bond the children had with their grandmother. The problems were normalized and contextualized: They were all undergoing stressful transitions, changes in attachments, households, parenting roles, and job demands. The intervention focus was redirected from repairing past damage to helping the family master current and impending challenges.

The transitional crisis also presented the opportunity to explore the father's potential contribution. He had never been contacted in the 2 years of his son's treatment, since the parents were unmarried and living apart. We learned that he was living in the community and saw the children almost weekly, although he contributed no financial support. This information surprised the staff members, who had written him off; this resource had been completely overlooked. He had a fairly steady construction job and, with ongoing investment in his children, could be brought into the picture and encouraged to contribute to the family's financial security. Here again, obtaining this help needed to be reframed from implying the mother's deficiency to making reasonable expectations of a caring father for support of his children.

As this case illustrates, in the return of children the transition period should be planned carefully, preparing children and caregivers in both households over at least several weeks. Parental visits should be well structured and gradually increased; emotional upheaval should be anticipated, troubleshooting for any potential crises. Posttransition structural changes (e.g., shifting role relations and child care arrangements) should also be planned to ensure children's safety and to buffer anticipated stresses. It is important to provide intensive intervention during the stressful transition period, followed by several monthly sessions to sustain gains. It is crucial not to dismiss the potential contributions of family members who may have been unable to provide care in the past. Images frozen in time need to be checked out and updated, recognizing the human capacity for change and growth.

A range of coordinated services may be needed to enable families to function effectively, including substance abuse counseling; education, job training, and housing referrals; parenting groups; and domestic violence counseling. The first few months is often a "honeymoon" period in family relationships while problems of basic survival predominate. Services and counseling often end within 3–6 months. However, the time of highest risk is toward the end of the first year, with substance abuse relapses, the return of abusive partners, neglecting behavior, and disillusionment about family life. Periodic sustaining contacts help to solidify gains and to prevent recurrence of serious problems.

When child placement and family reunification are being considered, a careful systems assessment is recommended to determine not only if there is clear and present danger, but also whether extended kin resources can be mobilized to provide essential protection and care. We should make every attempt to involve key family members in making decisions. In a New Zealand model program, a family council—much like a tribal council—is convened, rallying the strongest resources in the extended family, whose input could be valuable. Together with professionals, the family members weigh the various options, taking stock of kin and community resources. The collaborative process reduces the sense that children are being removed by outside forces beyond family control, as well as the likelihood of arbitrary court decisions. Involving key family members also promotes their collaboration with an unrelated foster family, their ongoing contact with children, and their investment in a successful placement experience. Any decisions for child placement should be made without robbing parents of humanity, dignity, and hope that they can turn their lives around.

Sustaining Vital Connections

We need to create a balanced service delivery system, viewing family preservation and out-of-home placement as complementary, not mutually exclusive, alternatives. We must see foster and biological families not as adversaries, but instead as collaborators sharing concern for their children's well-being (Minuchin et al., 1998). Assessment should determine not simply where children should live, but how they can be nurtured and protected from abuse *and* at the same time maintain some linkages with key family members, extended kin, and community, as well as with cultural traditions and spiritual sources of resilience. When placement is required, we should find ways for children to sustain vital bonds through monitored contact with parents, visits with other relatives, phone calls, e-mail, cards, and letters. Even when direct contact efforts aren't possible, it's important for children to have photographs of family members and to hear stories of their family history and cultural heritage. A necklace, a scarf, or a favorite shirt from a parent, older sibling, or grandparent can be a precious "belonging." Older children can be encouraged to keep journals or diaries to record their current experiences and their memories of the past, and to voice hopes and dreams for the future.

Building Therapeutic Partnerships

In work with multistressed families, we must broaden the traditional view of therapy and of our role as therapists. When families have been beaten down, it's important to take an active, mobilizing position instead of waiting for family members to become "motivated." A pragmatic approach that includes creativity, flexibility, and a variety of interventions is most effective. We may serve as facilitators, advocates, and allies, as well as models and nurturing mentors. We can draw from our own experiences and offer examples of others who have prevailed in similar straits to offer new perspectives and hope. A primary goal of all intervention is to generalize the trusting relationship that develops to the family's social world.

Today there are more families in crisis, but fewer therapists and sessions for such families, due to funding cutbacks and managed care restrictions. In agencies working with multineed families, unrealistic expectations of staff members, case overload, and insufficient resources can create an unhealthy work environment and contribute to burnout. A worker may come to feel as overloaded, undersupported, and depleted as a parent. Principles similar to those of resilience building with families apply to work systems: Provide adequate pay and resources, opportunities for professional growth, peer case consultation, staff involvement in decision making, recognition of workers' value, and opportunities to succeed. Such incentives sustain workers' personal investment and job commitment with very challenging caseloads. In a preventive approach, agencies can identify highly vulnerable families—those in precarious situations that lack resources and have been beset by numerous problems. Through outreach at moments of crisis, our job will be much easier than after serious symptoms have developed.

A collaborative approach is essential when overwhelmed family members wish for a therapist to solve their problems, or even to *become* the solution—that is, to assume the role of rescuer or to replace an absent parent. Many of us therapists have had early life training in assuming responsible roles in our families of origin to rescue or take care of other family members. Vulnerable clients may tug on our own inclinations to rescue them. Family members' distress may be so great that they wish we could move in with them and never leave. Our attempts to set limits may be misconstrued as not caring about them. We should stay mindful that their neediness may be great because their resources are drained or they are unprepared for responsibilities, especially when parents have lacked adequate parenting themselves. We may come to feel weighted down, as if we are sinking in quicksand along with them. Some warning signs we should heed include "forgetting" to return family members' calls or feeling relieved when they miss an appointment.

As therapists, we have to be clear about our own role and boundaries. While reaching out and actively engaging families, we need to model a relationship of caring and commitment with realistic limits. Therapy can become skewed, burdensome, and unproductive: As we become overresponsible, family members become even less confident of their own ability to surmount their challenges. We do not serve our clients well—or care for ourselves—if we foster long-term dependence as their only lifeline. Families are empowered when we help them mobilize potential resources in their own kin networks and communities for support with urgent needs. We all do best under duress by strengthening real-life connections.

CHAPTER 11

Recovery from Trauma, Traumatic Loss, and Major Disasters

Strengthening Family and Community Resilience

We need to help one another—that is the only thing that is keeping us alive.
　　　　　　　　　　—PAUL RUSESABAGINA, *Hotel Rwanda*

This chapter extends beyond the borders of the family to explore the value of a resilience-oriented, multisystemic family and community approach to recovery from major trauma and loss when catastrophic events occur. Case illustrations and interventions are described in response to community violence, genocide and refugee trauma, and terrorist attacks to suggest ways to foster family and community resilience in the wake of widespread natural and human-made disasters.

TRAUMA, SUFFERING, AND RESILIENCE: MULTISYSTEMIC PERSPECTIVES

The word "trauma" comes from the Latin word for *wound*. With traumatic experiences, the body, the mind, the spirit, and relationships with others can be wounded. The predominant therapeutic models used for treating survivors of trauma and major disaster have been individually focused and pathology based, centered on identifying and reducing symptoms of posttraumatic stress disorder (PTSD). The resilience-oriented approaches in this chapter draw on family and community strengths and resources for recovery and posttraumatic growth.

The trauma field grew out of recognition of the psychological impact of wartime combat and other catastrophic events. Following Grinker and Spiegel's (1945) pioneering study of soldiers under stress in World War II, studies of Vietnam War veterans (Catherall, 1992) documented the long-lasting trauma effects that many suffered. That research, along with studies of interpersonal and mass trauma, led to new classifications of acute stress disorder (ASD) and PTSD (see the DSM-IV-TR American Psychiatric Association, 2000; see also the international classification [ISCD], World Health Organization, 1972). Acute stress disorders, which are commonly experienced in the immediate aftermath of extreme trauma situations, can lead to more severe and chronic PTSD for some individuals. Defined as a mental disorder, PTSD includes a wide range of symptoms, such as intrusive thoughts and recollections, sleep disturbances and nightmares, hyperarousal, avoidance of reminders of the trauma, emotional numbing, and social withdrawal. It is often accompanied by depression, anxiety and panic disorders, substance abuse, violent outbursts, and destructive behavior toward the self and others. Treatment of PTSD has been individually oriented, with cognitive-behavioral methods widely used.

Family systems approaches to major trauma grew out of Reuben Hill's (1949) groundbreaking study of adjustment in World War II veterans and their families. In the growing field of traumatology, Charles Figley and others brought attention to the stressful impact on relational systems of war, catastrophic events, violence, and sexual abuse (Catherall, 2002; Figley & McCubbin, 1983). Families were found to be valuable resources contributing to the recovery of a member who was suffering trauma effects. However, major trauma, such as the killing and loss of lives in war, may not only haunt survivors. It also affects their closest relationships and the well-being of loved ones in secondary traumatization or in compassion fatigue (Figley, 2005). This occurs not only through learning about the trauma experienced, but even more through ongoing contact and caregiving when disruptive symptoms and harmful behaviors persist. Therefore, a family systems approach is essential in the treatment of major trauma.

Van der Kolk and colleagues have advanced a biopsychosocial understanding of trauma, its treatment, and its prevention, including attention to variables that influence vulnerability, resilience, and the course of posttraumatic reactions (van der Kolk, McFarlane, & Weisaeth, 1996). The effects of trauma depend greatly on whether those wounded can seek comfort, reassurance, and safety with others. They need strong connections, with trust that others will be there for them when needed to counteract feelings of insecurity, helplessness, and meaninglessness.

A family and community resilience framework offers a contextual and broadly inclusive practice approach. It situates the trauma in the extreme experience and taps natural strengths and potential resources in relational networks for recovery. Although major traumatic events are experiences beyond the normal range of human suffering, symptoms of PTSD are generally assessed and treated as a mental disorder in an individual. A family and community resilience approach situates the disorder and trauma in the abnormal events and their ripple effects through individuals, families, and communities. Both individual and relational symptoms often result, such as anxiety, depression, conflict, and estrangement. Family and community interventions are most helpful in recovery, fostering human connections, healing, and transformation.

A resilience-oriented approach is especially valuable in traumatic situations in its focus on rebounding from crisis events and overcoming persistent challenges. Although some individuals are more vulnerable than others, no one is immune to suffering from trauma in extreme situations. This practice approach responds compassionately to symptoms of distress and memories of pain, helplessness, and loss; it contextualizes the distress and expands focus to identify and affirm strengths and resources in active initiative, recovery, and adaptation. Strengthening resilience entails both endurance of harsh conditions and perseverance in efforts to overcome them, "struggling well" to work through emerging difficulties with indomitable spirit.

Most valuable in the concept of resilience is that, beyond coping or weathering adversity, the traumatic experience can yield remarkable transformation and growth. Posttraumatic growth has been found to be a measurable, concrete expression of resilience in action—the ability not only to survive, but even to thrive, in response to extreme conditions (Calhoun & Tedeschi, 1999; Lindley & Joseph, 2004; Tedeschi & Calhoun, 1995; Tedeschi, Park, & Calhoun, 1996). Forged in the cauldron of crisis and challenge, new strengths, untapped potential, creative expression, and innovative solutions can emerge as we reach more deeply within ourselves and reach out to connect with others. In times of great tragedy, ordinary people show extraordinary courage, compassion, and generosity in helping kin, neighbors, and strangers to recover and rebuild lives. Mental health professionals can best foster recovery by mobilizing this capacity to heal and grow stronger in families and communities.

TRAUMA AND TRAUMATIC LOSS

As we've seen throughout this volume, crisis, trauma, and loss can occur in a wide range of human experiences. Trauma situations may involve death, physical illness, bodily harm, or disability; kidnapping, torture, incarceration, or persecution; relationship dissolution, job loss, migration/relocation, violence, and sexual abuse. Much psychotherapeutic attention to trauma and recovery has focused on interpersonal violence and sexual abuse, notably, in the seminal work of Herman (1992), and in the systemic approaches of Almeida (Almeida, Woods, Messineo, & Font, 1998), Sheinberg and Fraenkel (2001), Trepper and Barrett (1989), and others. This chapter focuses on trauma and loss in extreme situations in the larger environment, in widespread violence and in natural and human-made catastrophic events.

The important interface of trauma, loss, and grief has been recognized in the fields of traumatology and bereavement (Figley, 1998; Neimeyer, 2001). Tragic (e.g., untimely, sudden, and/or violent) death is the most common source of trauma (Norris, 2002). Traumatic loss situations that pose high risk for complicated recovery and require careful assessment and intervention focus are summarized in Table 11.1 (see also Chapter 8).

Various forms of trauma experienced in catastrophic events can involve multiple losses, such as loss of sense of physical or psychological wholeness (e.g., with disfigurement, dismemberment, or other serious bodily harm or torture); loss of significant persons, roles, and relationships; and loss of the intact family unit, homes, and communities. The loss of the head of the family or the leader of the community is especially difficult. With the loss of children there is the tragic sense of loss of the future. Shattered assumptions in our basic world view can occur, such as a loss of security, predictability, and trust (Kauffman, 2002). The loss of hopes and dreams for all that might have been is often the hardest to bear. Thus, approaches to treating complicated loss are useful in recovery from trauma.

In traumatic loss, symptoms such as depression, anxiety, substance abuse, and relational conflict or withdrawal are common. Survivors who

TABLE 11.1. Assessment of Traumatic Loss Situations

The meaning and impact of traumatic deaths are influenced by a number of variables in the loss situation that require careful assessment and attention.

Violent death

A violent death is devastating for loved ones and especially for those who witnessed it or narrowly survived themselves. Preoccupation with causal accusations, guilt, or wishes for revenge is common. The senseless tragedy in the loss of innocent lives is especially hard to bear, particularly in deliberate acts of violence, as in school or workplace shootings. War zones pose a constant threat of injury and death for civilians as well as those in combat; such deaths can haunt survivors and those involved.

Untimely death

Untimely losses are hardest to bear. The deaths of children and young spouses seem unjust and rob future hopes and dreams of the family. The loss of parents with young children requires reorganization of the family system.

Sudden death

With sudden losses, such as due to a shooting, an accident, or an earthquake, loved ones lack time even to say their good-byes. Like a bolt out of the blue, a sense of normalcy and predictability is shattered. Shock and intense emotions, as well as disorganization and confusion, are expectable in the immediate crisis period. Family members may need help with painful regrets or guilt over what they wish they had done differently, had they anticipated the event.

Prolonged suffering

With prolonged physical or emotional suffering before death (e.g., with assault, torture, or lack of medical assistance), the agony for family members can be great, coupled with guilt, anger, or remorse.

Ambiguous loss

Ambiguity as to whether a loved one is alive or dead (e.g., a missing family member) can immobilize families and block mourning. A family may be torn apart, hoping for the best while fearing the worst. Survivors often cannot begin mourning until the body, some remains, or personal effects are recovered. Some hold on to any hope or a miracle for return. Some hold a funeral without a body; others wait. Families need help in pressing for whatever information they can gain, and in resuming lives in the face of remaining uncertainty.

Unacknowledged, stigmatized losses

Mourning is complicated when losses or their cause are unacknowledged or hidden due to social stigma. The stigma surrounding the HIV/AIDS epidemic has contributed to secrecy, misinformation, and estrangement, impairing family and social support, as well as critical health care. It also furthers the spread of disease to women, children, and communities worldwide.

Pileup of effects

Families can be overwhelmed by the emotional, relational, and functional impact of multiple deaths, prolonged or recurrent trauma, and other losses (persons, homes, jobs, communities) and disruptive transitions (e.g., separations, migration).

Past traumatic experience

Past trauma and losses can be reactivated in life-threatening or loss situations, intensifying the impact of current events and complicating recovery.

are blocked from healing may perpetuate suffering through self-destructive behavior or revenge and harm toward others. Massive trauma or the loss of hope and positive vision can fuel transmission of negative intergenerational patterns (Danieli, 1985), with consequences for those not yet born.

When traumatic loss is suffered, we should not expect resolution in the sense of some complete, "once-and-for-all" getting over it. Traumatic losses may never fully be resolved. Thus, resilience in the wake of trauma and loss should not be seen as readily getting "closure" on the emotional experience, bouncing back, and moving on. Recovery is a gradual process over time. Various facets of grief may alternate and reemerge with unexpected intensity, particularly at anniversaries and other nodal events. Attention commonly oscillates between preoccupation with grief and reengagement in a world forever transformed by the loss (Stroebe & Schut, 2001).

Mourning was thought to require detachment, or letting go, in traditional psychiatric approaches. Instead, adaptive mourning is best facilitated through transformation of all that was lost to continuing bonds through spiritual connections, memories, deeds, and stories that are passed on across the generations. Coming to terms with traumatic loss involves finding ways to make meaning of the trauma experience, put it in perspective, and weave the experience into the fabric of one's individual and relational identity and life passage.

FACILITATING FAMILY AND COMMUNITY ADAPTATION TO TRAUMA AND LOSS

In fostering recovery from major traumatic events, we can usefully apply the four tasks in adaptation to loss identified in Chapter 8, where they are discussed more fully (see also Walsh & McGoldrick, 2004; Worden, 2002). Helping professionals can facilitate healing and resilience by encouraging individuals, families, and communities to actively engage in these adaptational tasks.

1. Shared acknowledgment of reality of traumatic event, losses
   • Clarification of facts, circumstances, ambiguities
2. Shared experience of loss and survivorship
   • Active participation in memorial rituals, tributes, rites of passage
   • Shared meaning making; emotional expression; spirituality

3. Reorganization of family and community; planning for survivors' well-being
   - Restabilization to foster continuity and change
   - Realignment of relationships, reallocation of roles, functions
   - Rebuilding of lives, homes, livelihood, kinship, and community
4. Reinvestment in other relationships and life pursuits
   - Constructing new hopes and dreams; revising life plans

Ways of coping and mourning vary with family, cultural, and religious preferences. Families may need help to develop tolerance for different coping styles, decisions, and pacing of grief processes among members. In community and multifamily interventions, there needs to be openness and respect for cultural differences, as well.

FAMILY AND SOCIAL PROCESSES IN RISK AND RESILIENCE

In response to traumatic events, attention to the following family and social belief systems, organizational patterns, and communication processes can reduce vulnerability and risk and can foster resilience.

Belief Systems

It is important to understand each family's belief system, rooted in their cultural and religious traditions, which influence their perceptions and response in traumatic experiences.

Making Meaning of Traumatic Events and Loss

Resilience is fostered as we help family members gain a sense of coherence, rendering their crisis experience more comprehensible, manageable, and meaningful as a shared challenge. After a tornado ripped through their neighborhood and destroyed their home and business, the father in one family recounted, "At first we were in a state of shock and disoriented, at a total loss what to do. Then we dusted ourselves off, took stock of our predicament, and then took charge to clear out the debris. We just kept hugging each other and taking it step by step."

Family members may struggle over time to make sense of trauma and loss, to put it in perspective and make it more bearable (Nadeau, 2001). Shattered assumptions are a profound symbolic loss with catastrophic events (Kauffman, 2002). These core beliefs ground, secure, and orient people, providing a sense of reality, meaning, or purpose to life. The assumption may be that I will grow old with my partner; that God is just; that others may be trusted; that things will happen in a certain, predictable way; that there is a future. When such assumptions are shattered by a sudden, unexpected catastrophic event, there is a deep need to restore order, meaning, and purpose. Meaning reconstruction in response to trauma and loss is a central process in healing (Neimeyer, 2001). It can reflect a new kind of wisdom born of experience and a testament to survivors' strengths. In recovery work, we may need to help people reconstruct a new sense of normality, identity, and relation to others to adapt to altered conditions.

Commonly families grapple with painful questions such as: Why us? Why my child and not me? How could this have happened? Who is to blame? Was it accidental or deliberate? Could it have been prevented? Such concerns remain salient when the cause, for instance, of a plane crash or explosion, remains unclear. Clinicians need to explore factual information and beliefs that foster blame, shame, and guilt surrounding a traumatic loss. Such causal attributions are especially strong where questions of responsibility, negligence, or prevention arise. It is important to help members share such concerns and come to terms with both accountability and limits of control in the situation.

Hope: A Positive Outlook

In times of deepest despair hope is most essential. Resilience involves coming to accept what has been lost and directing efforts to master the possible. In the wake of devastating trauma, we can help families regain hope and investment to rebuild their lives, revise lost hopes and dreams, make new and renewed attachments, and create positive legacies to pass on to future generations.

Transcendence and Spirituality

With traumatic loss, transcendent cultural and spiritual values and practices provide meaning and purpose. For some, faith beliefs open up a pathway of forgiveness (see Chapter 12). Many find solace in the belief that a traumatic event and loss may be beyond human comprehension but part of God's larger plan, or a test of our faith. Prayer, meditative practices, and faith communities offer solace and support. Spiritual connection, memories, stories, and deeds can honor the best aspects of those who died and all that was lost. Participation in memorial rituals, vigils, anniversary remembrances, rites of passage, and celebrations of milestones in recovery all facilitate healing and growth. They also provide opportunities to reaffirm identity, relatedness, and core social values of goodness and compassion (Imber-Black et al., 2003). Finding ways to celebrate holidays and birthdays, which often go unmarked in times of turmoil, can boost spirits and reconnect all with the rhythms of life that continue beyond loss.

Suffering can be transcended through creative and symbolic expression, as in writing, music, and the arts. Music, such as participation in community and congregational singing, can be uplifting and joyful, restoring spirits and energies to carry on. Finding ways to express the trauma experience through journals and artwork can be important in healing and resilience, especially for children. Healing is aided by memorial dedications to honor those who were lost. Many find transformation through community activism or advocacy to benefit others and prevent future suffering. Recovery is a journey of the heart and spirit, bringing survivors back to the fullness of life.

Organizational Patterns

Flexible Structure

Families and communities must effectively organize to respond to a traumatic event. Flexibility is needed to adapt to unforeseen challenges and changing conditions. At the same time, to reduce the sense of chaos and disorientation that occurs with disruption and transitional upheaval, it is crucial to restore order and stability as well as possible. Children, in particular, find reassurance as daily routines can be resumed or new arrangements put in place Strong leadership and coordination of response efforts is essential, with collaboration between families and social networks. In major disasters, community groups, agencies, and all government levels involved in rescue, recovery, and reconstruction efforts must have clear plans, lines of authority, and reliable communication. With the loss of basic infrastructure, family and social systems must reorganize, recalibrate, and reallocate roles and functions. Clear rules and guidelines must be established and followed through consistently.

Connectedness

With traumatic experiences, helplessness and terror are common. We have an urgent need to know that we can count on others for support, comfort, and safety. While high cohesion is essential, family members need tolerance and respect for individual differences in crisis response. Some may show anxious clinging or need to be in constant contact with loved ones; others may avoid the pain or loss by distancing. In chaotic situations or evacuations, every effort should be made to keep family members together, so they are not left to fend for themselves, isolated in their suffering, and worried about others. When separations occur or are forced, contact information and communication are essential to ease worries and facilitate reunion. The persistence of ambiguous loss is agonizing for family members. When trauma has involved a violation in human connection, for instance, in harm by a family member, friend, coworker, or neighbor, trust and security are very difficult to restore. If relationships were troubled or estranged at the time of a loss, distress is intensified by unresolved conflicts. Counseling can be helpful in fostering healing, reconnection, and reconciliation (see Chapter 12).

Extended Kin, Social, and Economic Resources

With major trauma and loss, it is most important to mobilize kin, social, and community networks for emotional and practical support (Speck, 2003). Involvement of extended social systems might include friends, neighbors, and health care providers; clergy and congregational support; schoolteachers and counselors; employers and coworkers; and neighborhood or community organizations. Multifamily community support groups are ideal contexts for exchanging information, sharing painful memories and feelings, providing mutual support, and encouraging hope and efforts for recovery. Financial assistance is also crucial with the loss of homes and jobs, medical expenses, or rebuilding costs.

Communication and Problem Solving

Clear, Helpful Information

Families may need help to clarify facts and circumstances of a traumatic event and steps they can take to improve their situation. To reduce suffering, those in charge of emergency and recovery plans must provide clear, consistent, and accurate information. When errors or changes occur, information should be updated swiftly to reduce confusion and frustration. Internet resources can be lifelines for information and connection. After the failure of government response to Hurricane Katrina, one resident in the stricken area remarked, "If Fed Ex can track packages worldwide how come the government can't even track the delivery of ice" (which melted in trucks awaiting communication on their destination.)

Emotional Sharing and Support

A traumatic event can trigger feelings of anger, fear, anxiety, guilt, and blame among the survivors, with ripple effects throughout kin and community networks. It is important to foster a climate of mutual trust, empathic response, and tolerance for a wide and fluctuating range of emotions over time. One boy said the upheaval in his family was like "a roller coaster ride that wouldn't stop." When differences are viewed as disloyal or threatening, members may submerge feelings, which may then be expressed in somatic, emotional, or behavioral symptoms or in substance abuse.

Collaborative Problem Solving

Practical assistance to fill immediate needs is essential. Turn goals for recovery into realistic steps, tasks, and projects. Over time, with the slow pace of recovery and rebuilding, it is important to rally family and community collaborative efforts to experience even small gains and progress. Above all, it's crucial to learn from a disaster experience—both the event and the response—to be proactive in disaster preparedness to lower future risk and to have response plans in place that will build connection, reduce suffering, and strengthen resilience.

PATHWAYS IN RECOVERY AND RESILIENCE

Early intervention is important for those who have suffered trauma and traumatic loss (Litz, 2004). Reducing acute distress and mobilizing resources for recovery can be crucial in preventing more serious and chronic symptoms of PTSD. However, we should be wary of a "quick fix" out of traumatic experience. Crisis intervention can be immensely helpful. However, some debriefing programs designed for crisis workers (e.g., CISD; see Emmerik, Kamphuis, Hulsbosch, & Emmelkamp, 2002) have been misapplied in a one-session format with survivors of mass trauma immediately after the event. Suffering can be exacerbated by a narrow focus on individual trauma symptoms; by heightened concern that common trauma reactions could be a sign of PTSD, a psychiatric disorder; and by opening up intense and painful memories and feelings, including helplessness, rage, and feeling overwhelmed. It is crucial (1) to normalize and contextualize distress, (2) to draw out strengths and active coping strategies for empowerment, (3) to offer follow-up sessions, as well as mental health services for those in severe distress, and (4) to mobilize family and social support for ongoing recovery.

The following facilitator guidelines are useful for early intervention in family or group sessions with those affected by trauma:

- Start with grounding in members' personal identity, family, community, cultural, and spiritual connections.
- Invite them to share their crisis experiences. Offer acknowledgment and compassionate witnessing of recent (and ongoing) crises, losses, hardships, or injustices they have suffered.
- Draw out and affirm strengths and resources they've witnessed, or tapped in endurance and coping efforts.
- Facilitate meaning making and mastery. Shift focus from what has happened to them to what they can do about their situation (from helplessness and victimization to active initiative and empowerment). Shift from global feelings of being overwhelmed to manageable steps they can take in progress toward recovery and rebuilding lives.
- Identify sources of resilience to tap in important connections in their lives (link to those noted above) as lifelines in the recovery process.
- Identify personal, relational, and spiritual resources they, or their families of origin, drew upon in past times of adversity and how they might be helpful now.

Families, teachers, counselors, shelter workers, and other caregivers can find journals and artwork especially helpful with children. One program designed for use in many disaster situations to facilitate meaning making, emotional expression, and active coping uses activity books to help children express in drawings and words the experience they have been through. For instance, drawing, coloring, and word activities in "My Hurricane Katrina Story," helped children to remember, document, and integrate not only the sad, bad, and scary parts, but also the helpful, brave, and good things people did. Older children, in journal format, were asked to describe what they learned, what would be helpful now, and things they and their families and community could do to prepare for another hurricane (Kliman, Oklan, Wolfe, & Kliman, 2005).

The long and varied pathways in healing and rebuilding lives require a longitudinal approach (Litz, 2004) with the flexible availability of professionals and the support of kin and social networks over many months, and often much longer. To prevent and treat long-term posttraumatic stress complications, it is crucial to attend to the traumatic deaths and other losses suffered and to facilitate the four tasks of adaptation to loss, as described in the sections above. This will require pacing over time and weaving back and forth of attention to emotional griefwork and immediate practical challenges. Survivors frequently note that there were times when they suffered so deeply they didn't know if they could face another day, or felt that life no longer had meaning, but then rallied to carry on. As studies of resilience amply document, in struggling through hardship, in reaching out to others, and in active coping efforts, people tap resources they may not have drawn on otherwise and gain new abilities and perspective on life.

Each survivor's experience is unique. It is particularly traumatic for those who could not save loved ones. One man was in anguish that he had been unable to hold on to his disabled wife as they tried to escape a burning building. Still, her last words kept him going: "Take care of the kids and grandkids." He said, "It's hard every minute, every day, but I can do it; her voice and her spirit give me the courage and determination."

A disaster can reactivate past trauma but also offer opportunities for further healing. Families of the victims of a terrorist-caused plane crash at Lockerbie, Scotland, found their pain revived by the TWA crash 8 years later—as one father described it, "like a scab torn off a deep wound." Yet many of those families came forward and offered support to the surviving families, finding that their assistance furthered their own long-term recovery as well.

TRAUMATIC LOSS IN COMMUNITY VIOLENCE

When serious harm or murder is committed by relatives or close acquaintances, such relational traumas can be devastating because they are inflicted by loved ones and those who are trusted and depended upon. Posttraumatic difficulties commonly persist for survivors in fears of trust, commitment, and intimacy, particularly in couple relationships

(Johnson, 2002). Yet every day, violence also takes place in our communities and in our larger social world. As Kaethe Weingarten (2003) notes, it can become a common shock, affecting us yet barely arousing us until our lives or the lives of those we know are directly affected. The tragic killing of Ennis Cosby, as he changed a tire at the side of the road, evoked a compassionate response nationwide. The loss of the only son of Bill Cosby, an American father figure who transcended racial barriers, underscored the vulnerability of all families to human tragedy beyond their control.

One shooting death, near my own neighborhood, began with an escalation of taunts between white and Latino youths, which turned lethal. With the catalyzing influence of a parish priest and his congregation, and with the courage and resilience of the parents of the boy who was murdered, a remarkable journey of recovery, transcendence, and transformation occurred over the following year (Shefsky, 2000; Terkel, 2000, 2002).

When Mario Ramos, an 18-year-old Latino gang member, shot and killed another boy in the community, the pastor of his church, Father Oldershaw, told the congregation, "He is a son of our parish; we must reach out to him and his family and offer our prayers and assistance." He visited Mario's family, hardworking, caring immigrants who were in deep pain and struggling to comprehend their son's act of violence. The priest then visited Mario in detention, ministered to him, and encouraged parishioners to write to him and to pray for the family whose son he had killed. Although the parents, Maureen and Steve Young, were not members of his parish, Father Oldershaw extended himself, going to their home to offer his condolences and to say he simply wanted them to know he was there for them if there was any way he could be of assistance. Steve, who wasn't home at the time, was at first angered by the visit: "This was his kid who killed our son!" But a few nights later, unable to sleep, he called the priest after midnight and they talked for over an hour. The priest's outreach and compassion led the parents to attend services at the church, where they found solace in the caring community.

Over several months, the outreach to Mario by the priest and parishioners began to foster a genuine transformation in Mario; he left the gang, affiliated with a Christian group for support, and wrote a letter to Mrs. Young to express his deep remorse for the killing and to ask for her forgiveness. "There's no way I can bring back your son; I only hope that something good can come out of this."

Before his letter reached her, Mrs. Young's own deep faith led her to write to Mario, to offer compassion and forgiveness. Their letters crossed in the mail. As she later explained, she came to this decision to help herself to heal from the tragedy and to be better able to help her family in their unbearable suffering. Her husband hadn't been able to work for months, her surviving children were devastated, and the youngest son had run into traffic hoping to be hit so he could join his big brother in heaven. She understood her husband's deep anger, and the common human impulse for revenge that many around her were expressing, but she spoke out against any revenge. She said she felt she would lose her mind if she didn't try to draw something positive out of the tragedy. She found inspiration from her childhood Catholic upbringing, recalling from the Bible that unforgiveness corrodes the mind, the body, and the spirit. In offering forgiveness, she also clearly conveyed the devastating impact his actions had had on her entire family.

Mrs. Young continued contact with Mario and urged him to take responsibility to make something good of his life, investing herself in his rehabilitation. As she later said, "He came into our life through an act of violence, but now he's in my heart. . . . There's no way to bring back my son, but here's a life with potential that I don't want to waste." Although her husband owned that he was initially too angry to share her feelings, he respected her decision and both were able to tolerate and honor each other's positions and join together to help their surviving children with their grief.

At Mario's sentencing hearing, Father Oldershaw sat with Mario's mother to give her courage. When Mr. Young arrived, the priest introduced them. Although Mrs. Ramos spoke no English, Steve saw the sorrow in her eyes for his loss and he tearfully embraced her, realizing that they both had lost their sons: his to a grave and hers to prison.

Mr. Young did not take the path of forgiveness to the extent his wife had. Yet, crucially for their relationship, he respected her way of healing. He found his own transcendent path through community activism. He took leadership in a local chapter of a national organization to stop gun violence and worked tirelessly so that other families would not suffer such a tragedy. His wife later joined him in those efforts. Both found that their outreach for others furthered their own healing, yielding more energy to devote to their children's recovery over time.

Families of victims of violence are in need of ongoing support and advocacy, because all too frequently they experience further trauma and strain in lengthy, convoluted legal processes and all-consuming efforts to seek justice. Most are better able to go on with their lives when they feel that justice has been served. One father, who was drinking himself to death after his daughter's sexual assault and murder, was helped to realize that she would not want him to be consumed with grief and rage nor to give up on life. Also, in family sessions, his wife and surviving children helped him to see that they needed him more than ever. With our encouragement, many survivors find strength and new purpose in joining with others to prevent similar tragedies from happening.

An entire community can be traumatized by persistent violence, blighted conditions, and discrimination. Racial tensions and violence are often fueled by repeated experiences of denigration and disrespect toward ethnic minorities and others who live on the margins of society and who lack social acceptance and economic advancement. For poor families in blighted neighborhoods, daily life is much like living in a war zone (Garbarino, 1997). Catastrophic fears and destructive behavior patterns are often grounded in multiple traumas and losses in the family and community. With a brother in prison and a son recently killed in a drive-by shooting, one mother sadly observed, "We never know who will be with us or lost tomorrow." Many parents and youths try to numb the recurrent pain, terror, and helplessness with alcohol or drugs, or by shutting off emotions and concern about themselves or others, in the belief that "If I don't care, then it won't hurt."

Neighborhood-based programs such as Take Back the Streets build family and community resilience, as they combat violent crime by bringing together residents, police, and social agencies to work collaboratively and build a sense of pride and empowerment. In many programs, older men form mentoring relationships with gang members and preteen recruits, in efforts to stem the tide of violence and encourage school and job pursuits toward a better life.

MAJOR DISASTERS

Major disasters produce severe disruption, trauma, and loss for individuals, families, and communities. Whether by natural disasters, such as earthquakes, hurricanes, and drought, or by human-caused disasters, as in war and terrorism, there is widespread suffering. The pileup effect of multiple losses, dislocations, and adaptational challenges can be overwhelming. As one mother put it, "It's a cascade of sorrows."

Counselors and other professionals can help to heal emotional wounds by understanding the particular impact and meaning of a trauma situation and reknitting fractured relationships, as in the following case:

> Many months after floodwaters inundated a coastal community, a teacher in a nearby town found a 12-year-old boy sleeping in the streets, alone in his suffering. When asked to describe what had happened that day, he told her he was with his father, approaching their house, when they saw his mother carried off in the flood surge. His father yelled at him to swim out and save her, but he stood frozen in place as his father berated him. Afterward he ran away and had not seen his family since. He was too ashamed to tell his father he didn't know how to swim. He couldn't forgive himself for not saving his mother's life. He was still reluctant to visit his father, only a town away, but agreed to go with the counselor to see his uncle. Upon hearing the account, his uncle reassured him that the floodwaters that day were too strong for even a good swimmer to save the many lives that were lost. He added that he knew that the father himself could not swim, which was why, in his own helplessness, he turned to his son with such desperation. The uncle took the boy in and arranged a reunion of father and son, beginning their healing from that tragic day.

The sadness of all that was lost is compounded when former lives can't be rebuilt. Meaning making and recovery involve a struggle to understand what has been shattered, how to build new lives, and how to prevent future tragedy. As in an earthquake, we need to learn what defects in structures contributed to their collapse, but we can learn even more from the construction of structures that withstood such damage.

In a major disaster with widespread trauma, multisystemic approaches, with the active participation of local residents, facilitate both family and community resilience (Landau & Saul, 2004). Community-based coordinated efforts, involving local and national agencies and, where needed, international humanitarian assistance, are essential to meet the challenges. Major disasters that disrupt family systems, work organizations, and communal structures and services are often the most debilitating because they may lead to community fragmentation, conflict, and destabilization. Unresponsiveness to catastrophic events can compound the traumatic impact.

Multisystemic approaches can capitalize on the richness of individual, family, and community resources that are the critical components of healing from devastating widespread trauma and loss. Judith Landau's conceptual framework, grounded in experience in disaster recovery in many parts of the world, underscores the vital importance in identifying and linking with these natural resources to create a matrix of healing throughout the community (Landau, 2005). This approach can be highly effective in ensuring long-term viability and hope for the future. By tapping the inherent resilience of communities, professionals can best foster their healing. Natural leaders and change agents within the community can be encouraged, with professionals taking a consultative role. Family and community members with diverse skills, talents, and ages can contribute in different ways to the resilience of the community. The elderly can bring memories and lessons of coping with previous adversity, while the young renew the capacity for play and creativity.

With massive psychosocial trauma in major disasters, whether natural or human-caused, Landau and Saul (2004) have found that community resilience encompasses the following four themes:

1. *Building community and enhancing social connectedness as a foundation for recovery.* This includes strengthening the system of social support, coalition building, and information and resource sharing.
2. *Collective storytelling and validation of the trauma experience and response.* The emerging story needs to be broad enough to encompass the many varying experiences.
3. *Reestablishing the rhythms and routines of life and engaging in collective healing rituals.*
4. *Arriving at a positive vision of the future with renewed hope.*

These themes fit closely with the key processes in resilience described above in terms of belief systems, organizational patterns, and communication processes.

In the aftermath of the devastation caused by Hurricanes Katrina and Rita on the coasts of Louisiana and Mississippi, the abysmal failure of government rescue and recovery efforts compounded the trauma, suffering, and chaotic displacement of residents. As too often occurs in a major disaster (Norris & Alegria, 2005), those most affected—and most neglected—were those most vulnerable, especially people of color, those with limited means, the elderly, and those with serious health problems. Shockingly, many bodies remained unattended over many months, prolonging the agony of families waiting to claim their loved ones and bury them with dignity. For disaster preparedness and recovery, the utmost importance of federal, state, and local emergency planning, coordination, communication, and follow-through cannot be overemphasized.

THE TRAUMA OF WAR, GENOCIDE, AND REFUGEE EXPERIENCE

In our times we've seen the vast human toll and devastation wrought by warfare, including violent ethnic, tribal, religious, and political conflicts and genocidal campaigns in many parts of the world. Family members may be forceably separated, kidnapped, or made to witness killing and brutal abuses of loved ones. Young boys may be pressed into combat and young girls sold in sex trafficking. Violence, in all its forms, can have severe, lasting, multigenerational effects (Weingarten, 2004). Even when civil war was averted at the end of apartheid in South Africa, the dislocations in societal transition and the trauma of past losses and atrocities heightened the value of relationships. In *Nomathemba*, (Shange & Shabalala, 1995), a drama about those turbulent times, the group Ladysmith Black Mambazo chants throughout: "Sorrow felt alone leaves a deep crater in the soul; sorrow shared yields new life."

The comfort and security provided by warm, caring relationships is especially critical in withstanding the trauma suffered in war and genocide, which induce social and personal uprooting, family disruption, separation and loss, mental and physical suffering, and vast social change (Weine, 1999). The security provided by families in war zones is found to be crucial in buffering such stresses as bombings, air raids, and the horrors of witnessing atrocities and violent death (Garmezy & Rutter, 1983). When evacuation is necessary, children fare best when able to stay together or at least keep close contact with other family members.

A Community-Based, Resilience-Oriented Approach with Refugee Families

Refugee families face a myriad of challenges: overcoming experiences of physical and psychosocial trauma and loss, navigating disruptive transitions and further losses in migration, and adapting to a new culture and way of life. Many are forced to leave their homeland and seek asylum to escape ethnic, racial, religious, or political persecution. Many are involuntarily displaced, fleeing from harsh conditions wrought by war or ethnic conflict or by drought, famine, or other environmental disasters over which they had little or no control. Many are forced to move from place to place or live in refugee camps, where they may be trapped for years or even decades. Many have experienced starvation, torture, rape, imprisonment, and dehumanizing treatment or conditions; many have suffered multiple traumatic losses of loved ones, homes, and communities and have witnessed brutal atrocities (Kamya, 2004; Mollica, 2004; Weine, 2006). When they migrate to a safe haven, such as North American or European countries, they often experience a profound loss of their social network (Sluzki, 1998) and a sense of homelessness and rootlessness, caught between two worlds and belonging to neither (Falicov, 2003). Ongoing stressors in adaptation to a new culture—finding living quarters, jobs, health care, and schools for children; surmounting language barriers; navigating immigration laws; learning social rules and customs; experiencing discrimination and the loss of identity and status—compound the difficulty, with pileup effects over time. Survivor guilt and worries about loved ones left behind can add to suffering. Marital and intergenerational tensions common in migration can be intensified by past trauma.

Community-Based, Resilience-Oriented Groups with Bosnian and Kosovar Refugee Families

A project developed by the Chicago Center for Family Health in collaboration with the Center on Genocide, Psychiatry, and Witnessing at the University of Illinois demonstrates the value of a community-based family resilience approach. In 1998, we were called upon to develop resilience-based multifamily groups for Bosnian refugees, and the following year, for ethnic Albanians arriving from Kosovo. As a result of the Serbian genocidal campaign of "ethnic cleansing," families in both regions experienced the devastating bombing and destruction of homes and communities; they suffered and witnessed widespread atrocities, including brutal torture, rape, murder, and the disappearance of loved ones.

Our family resilience approach was sought out because many of the refugees were suffering posttraumatic stress symptoms but were not utilizing mental health services, which were viewed in the refugee community as unhelpful and pathologizing, particularly in the deficit-based approach to PTSD as a mental illness and the narrow focus on treating individual symptoms (Weine et al., 2004). Traditional social services for immigrants were seen as helpful in assimilation and adaptation to the United States, but refugees tended not to discuss experiences of trauma and loss or their needs for connection to their cultural roots. Our resilience approach attends to suffering and losses contextually, as understandable in recovering from an abnormal and deeply traumatizing experience while, at the same time, facing the challenges of adaptation to a new culture. It counteracts the deep sense of shame that people often feel in revealing their vulnerabilities and suffering. This approach locates the trauma not in the individuals but in the extreme situation they have experienced and views the family as central in efforts to foster recovery and adaptation.

The program, called CAFES for Bosnian families and TAFES for Kosovar families (Coffee/Tea And Family Education and Support), utilized a 9-week multifamily group format. Families readily came, because it tapped into the strong family-centered values in their culture. It was located in a neighborhood storefront, where residents felt comfortable and could easily access services. It offered a compassionate setting to encourage families to share their stories of suffering and struggle. It also drew out and affirmed family strengths and resources, such as their courage, endurance, and faith; their strong kinship networks and deep concern for loved ones; and their determination to rise above their tragedies to forge a new life. The focus of sessions oscillated; at times family members shared stories and strengthened positive connections with distant kin, and with cultural and spiritual roots, and at other times, they tackled practical demands and challenging situations in their new lives. Resilience was strengthened by encouraging efforts to bridge cultures and to gain a sense of belonging in both old and new worlds (Falicov, 2003). This approach with the refugee families was experienced as respectful, healing, and empowering. To foster a spirit of collaboration and to develop resources within their community, paraprofessional facilitators from their community were trained to co-lead groups and remained available as needs might arise.

Resilience-Oriented Family and Community Services in War-Torn Regions

The positive response to the Bosnian and Kosovar refugee services led to a request to develop community-based, resilience-oriented, family-centered services in Kosovo. The aim of this project was to provide training to enhance the capacities of Kosovar mental health professionals and paraprofessionals to address the overwhelming service needs in their war-torn region by strengthening family capacities for coping and recovery in the wake of trauma and loss. The Kosovar Family Professional Educational Collaborative (KFPEC) was developed as an ongoing partnership between mental health professionals in Kosovo, through the University of Pristina, and teams of American family therapists, through the auspices of the American Family Therapy Academy, the Chicago Center for Family Health, and the University of Illinois. In describing the value of this approach, Rolland and Weine (2000) noted:

> The family, with its strengths, is central to Kosovar life, but health and mental health services are generally not oriented to families. Although "family" is a professed part of the value system of international organizations, most programs do not define, conceptualize, or operationalize a family approach to mental health services in any substantial or meaningful ways. Recognizing that the psychosocial needs of refugees, other trauma survivors, and vulnerable persons in societies in transition far exceed the individual and psychopathological focus that conventional trauma mental health approaches provide, this project aims to begin a collaborative program of family focused education and training that is resilience-based and emphasizes family strengths. (p. 35)

In many NGO programs, experts arrive with enthusiasm, dispense advice, and leave without sufficient ongoing efforts or collaboration to address long-term challenges. In contrast, this project was carefully planned and implemented collaboratively with Kosovar professionals, headed by Dr. Farid Agami, with sustained contact and periodic return training sessions, each geared to emerging local needs and priorities. Over an initial 12-month period (2000–2001), five teams of American family therapists conducted weeklong training sessions in Pristina. Bringing varied orientations to family therapy, such as structural and narrative approaches, they all emphasized a family resilience–based perspective, recognizing that Kosovar professionals would adapt the framework and develop their own practice models to best fit their culture and service needs. Readings found to be valuable (including chapters from the first edition of this book) were translated into Albanian. Between visits, contact was sustained through e-mail and collaborative writing. One piece told of a family in which the mother had listened to the gunshots as her husband, two sons, and two grandsons were murdered in the yard of their farmhouse. Team members talked with her and her surviving family members in their home and asked about what has kept them strong:

> The surviving son in the family responded, "We are all believers. One of the strengths in our family is from God. . . . Having something to believe has helped very much."

"What do you do to keep faith strong?" the interviewer asked.
"I see my mother as the 'spring of strength' . . . to see someone who has lost five family members—it gives us strength just to see her. We must think about the future and what we can accomplish. This is what keeps us strong. What will happen to him [pointing to his five-year-old nephew] if I am not here? If he sees me strong, he will be strong. If I am weak, he will become weaker than me."
"What do you hope your nephew will learn about the family as he grows up?" asked the interviewer.
"The moment when he will be independent and helping others and the family—for him, it will be like seeing his father and grandfather and uncles alive again." (Becker, Sargent, & Rolland, 2000, p. 29)

In this family, the positive influence of belief systems was striking, in particular, the power of religious faith and the inspiration of strong models and mentors, including the deceased.

Many families saw their resilience as strengthened by their cohesiveness and adaptive role flexibility:

"Everyone belongs to the family and to our homeland, alive or dead, here or abroad. Everyone matters and everyone is counted and counted upon." . . . When cooking or planting everyone moves together fluidly, in a complementary pattern, each person picking up what the previous person left off. . . . A hidden treasure in the family is their adaptability to who fills in each of the absented roles. Although the grief about loss is immeasurable, the ability to fill in the roles . . . [is] remarkable. (Becker et al., 2000, p. 29)

Currently, other collaborative projects are continuing, with an emphasis on treatment and prevention of substance abuse, AIDS, and human rights violations that tend to increase with the chaos and breakdown of social systems and economies in postconflict regions of the world. And yet, the spirit of resilience emerges in creative efforts to build a new community-based family-centered health care system (see Chapter 9).

MAJOR DISASTER AND TRAUMATIC LOSS IN TERRORISM

In this age of widespread terrorism, we are living in a more volatile and uncertain world in which our basic sense of security is threatened. Terror has become a destabilizing force in the world order, threatening the integrity of our experienced world as predictable and orderly. With the terrorist attacks of September 11, 2001, Americans experienced what others in the world have gradually come to cope with (Malkinson, Rubin, & Witztum, 2005). The trauma in the United States was intensified by the unpredictability and utter incomprehensibility of the event. In this loss of our assumptive world, illusions of invulnerability were shattered and a palpable sense of the precariousness of life and death was widely experienced (Walsh, 2002b).

Lessons from the Oklahoma City Bombing: Community Response and Resilience

A remarkable demonstration of community resilience emerged in the 1995 Oklahoma City bombing of the Murrah Federal Building, which killed 168 people and injured 842, including children in day care (Sitterle & Gurwitch, 1999). Although foreign terrorists were immediately suspected, it shocked the nation to learn that the bomber was a young, white American, who plotted the attack with his friend. Although the bombing had a devastating impact on the community, local people came together in recovery efforts. Amid the immediate chaos and suffering, people collaborated in efforts to aid and support those severely impacted. Outreach and organizational efforts included thousands of professionals, volunteers, and rescue workers who joined forces in creating effective crisis intervention for those in need and a strong support system for responders.

Of the many well-organized and effective programs, most notable was the creation of the Compassion Center within a local church, where hundreds of families gathered awaiting information about their loved ones. Although things were chaotic at the outset, a multiagency effort was quickly organized to provide accurate information about the rescue effort, to facilitate the efforts of the medical examiner's office, and to provide emotional support and assistance. The Center coordinated multiple emergency and community organizations that worked together to respond to the many needs of the survivors' physical and psychological traumas.

Mental health services were also organized within the Compassion Center, following with three core aims (closely fitting organizational and communication keys to resilience, described above): (1) to provide a safe and protective environment for families to share their suffering; (2) to provide a sense of order, predictability, and structure; and (3) to provide information to the families in a respectful way. The mental health operations served four basic functions: support services, family services, death notification, and stress management.

Rituals were important in fostering unity and healing for survivors, families of the deceased, and the wider community. They facilitated the channeling of grief and terror into meaningful and life-affirming activities, and they instilled faith in the long healing process. Informal memorials and offerings were created at the bombing site, as well as an official memorial and a "survivor tree." In addition, remembrance events, such as the 1-year anniversary commemoration, paid tribute to all those whose lives were taken.

Resilience is especially challenging if an entire community is affected. In their study of that recovery, *When a Community Weeps*, Zinner and Williams (1999) note that the grief a community experiences may become either a developmental crisis or opportunity for that community. Catastrophe, tragedy, and suffering can often lead to a breakdown in community morale and stagnate future development. In Oklahoma City, it strengthened resolve to rebound and propelled the community into new areas of growth. Learned resourcefulness—rather than helplessness—marked their recovery. Community members stepped forward to fill many roles, providing a mutually beneficial arrangement of helping others in need while equipping volunteers with an empowering sense of control and efficacy. It was precisely this process of working together, making meaning, and mastering at least *some* part of the traumatic experience that promoted the community resilience.

Resilience in the wake of the September 11 World Trade Center Attacks

The terrorist attacks on September 11, 2001 caused shocking devastation and massive ripple effects for families and communities near and far. In the small space of this chapter, only a few vignettes and two notable projects in New York recovery can be described, but they reveal the resilience possible when survivors, families, and communities come together.

In New York, thousands of people gathered at the site of the attacks to organize support services, aid in the recovery of bodies and cleanup of the site, or simply to lend a helping hand wherever it may have been needed. Numerous remembrance events took place in the following days, weeks, months, and anniversaries, in candlelight vigils, community gatherings, and the opening and outreach of places of worship. Again, a community showed that it could endure the worst forms of suffering and grief, and with time and great efforts, turn them into an opportunity for growth and community empowerment.

Sparks of this resilience kindled many positive developments (Walsh, 2002b). Two months later, a plane crashed after takeoff in a neighborhood of Queens, a working-class Irish and Italian-American community that had lost many firefighters at the World Trade Center. On that flight headed for the Dominican Republic, most of the casualties were from the Dominican community in Washington Heights, a poor neighborhood in upper Manhattan at the other end of the subway line. As all New Yorkers reeled from yet another plane crash and fear of more terrorism, a leader of the Dominican community and Mayor Giuliani were moved by the intertwined suffering of these two communities and together seized the opportunity to plan a joint memorial service, bridging a long-standing racial divide and bringing together communities that had never before had contact. Family members remarked that they had always assumed they were so different and had nothing in common. In coming together in sorrow, they discovered that they shared deep religious faith and valued strong families and hard work. Perhaps the greater challenge lies in sustaining the strong spirit and connection that emerge in times of crisis after people return to their everyday lives.

Over time, families of the victims organized into advocacy groups, such as "the Jersey Moms," speaking out in public arenas to press for an independent commission that could bring all the facts to light for a clearer understanding how the terrorist attacks came about and how they might have been prevented; and to draw up recommendations to prevent and prepare for any future attacks. Their concerted efforts to make meaning of the crisis event, draw lessons from it, and take action for the future are core processes in relational resilience.

The Lower Manhattan Community Recovery Project

As Landau and Saul (2004) note, community members, who make up the natural support system, have many advantages over outside providers in effecting change after a crisis. They have greater access to the local knowledge of existing resources and to vulnerable populations, and have relationship networks that have developed over time. They are often already engaged in positive social processes that build community solidarity, such as community association meetings and voluntary work. Because these efforts are driven by the community members' priorities and preferences, they are generally more successful than programs imported into the community by outsiders. Community members also have a greater investment in the development of their neighborhoods and are more likely to maintain activities long after the funding for an immediate crisis dries up or attention shifts to a new crisis elsewhere.

In the Lower Manhattan school communities directly affected by the September 11 terrorist attacks, attention focused on potential pathology in children, with little place for parents to discuss their concerns. Schools were closed and families were displaced from their homes and neighborhoods for 3–4 months. In January 2002, with the plan to return displaced children to their home schools, many parents were feeling distress about returning to the place where they had experienced the horror. A community-based coordinated effort, involving local agencies and residents, was organized by Jack Saul and colleagues to facilitate child, family, and community resilience (Landau & Saul, 2003). In this model program, multifamily groups and parent–teacher networks were set up, serving as a valuable resource for families to share their experiences, respond to concerns of their children, provide mutual support, and mobilize concerted action in recovery efforts. Parents, teachers, school counselors, and staff established family support groups that made connections across school communities, enabling the sharing of ideas about how to address emotional issues.

These support groups developed into a series of community forums, expanding the notion of healing beyond a focus on individual stress reactions to community-wide recovery. In this context, many varied reactions were normalized and a framework was offered, identifying common phases through which a community might pass following a disaster:

1. "United we Stand": Initially, people experienced shock and then came together, sharing and letting down their guard.
2. "Molasses and Minefields": With growing fatigue and irritability, stresses accumulated, tempers flared, and people retreated into groups where they felt safer. At this stage, the focus was on ways to reduce stress and tensions in the community.
3. "A Positive Vision of Recovery": At this stage, the community came together to build hope for the future, gaining understanding that recovery is not a passive process, but on active collaboration for a common purpose.

At each meeting, small subgroups, by children's grade level, discussed their concerns and ways parents and teachers could best help the children, care for themselves, and support each other. During this process, when individuals became overly irritable or markedly distressed by overestimating future threats, they received constructive feedback, helping them to modulate their reactions and assessment of their situation.

Through this process, the community connectedness provided a matrix of healing and support along with sound reality testing. A videotape of the forums was made for distribution to parents.

A community-needs assessment was conducted with 100 forum participants. This led to the creation of the Downtown Community Resource Center for Lower Manhattan, a public space where community members could come together and share ideas, projects, resources, and their combined creativity. They formed a community-based disaster preparedness and response initiative that produced a published manual. They developed such projects as a video narrative archive; a theater of witness project; a community website; a computer education program for senior citizens; peer support programs; various art projects; and a Samba school. The ripple effects of these programs have been long-lasting.

Family Meetings as Community Intervention for Ambiguous Loss

In another project, co-led by Pauline Boss (Boss, Beaulieu, Wieling, Turner, & LaCruz, 2003), a team of systems-oriented therapists worked with families of World Trade Center labor union workers who were missing after the terrorist attacks. Community-based, multiple family group meetings were organized, with additional counseling services available. To be responsive to the cultural diversity of these families, most of whom were immigrants, intervention teams were multilingual, multiracial, and of differing cultural belief systems. Group leaders helped families share their experiences and feelings concerning ambiguous loss, where no bodies or remains were found. A basic premise was that when a loved one remains missing, it is the situation of ambiguous loss that is abnormal, not the distressed family members. Even the healthiest ones, who showed strong resilience in migration and other life experiences, felt distressed and powerless.

The group interactions and mutual support were healing and empowering. One daughter, devastated by the loss of her father, was helped enormously when a coworker of his, a survivor attending the group, spoke up. He informed her that he saw her father in the tower and that he had saved 1,000 lives before he perished. He told her that when she goes to football games and sees all the people in the stands, she can be proud of her father's courage in saving so many lives (Boss et al., 2003).

The families came from cultures that valued community and favored the family group meetings over individual therapy approaches. Meetings were held in a union hall, where they felt more comfortable than in a mental health setting. The families voted to extend the sessions over many months, with several widows taking on leadership roles, and they prepared a memorial tribute for the 1-year anniversary.

Challenges and Opportunities

In the wake of the terrorist attacks, national surveys revealed that most Americans found strength, comfort, and solace by turning to their families and loved ones and by turning to their faith. These troubled times can awaken us to what really matters in life and inspire us to reorder our priorities and take initiative in caring actions to benefit others. In the face of continuing terrorist threats worldwide, we must redefine normality and carry on lives in the face of continuing uncertainty and new threats. The rush to demonize enemies and seek revenge has led, as it has all too many times, to war and further suffering. Many citizens have suffered additional indignity in the profiling of suspected terrorists and outright racism, discrimination, and mistreatment. The greater challenge is to better understand the many roots of terrorism and seek to address inequities and injustices that fuel it. We must question old assumptions, learn more about our world, gain understanding of the suffering of others, and engage in shared reflection and positive actions for meaning making, healing, and transformation.

FORGING RESILIENCE IN THE WAKE OF TRAGEDY

Communities have shown that they could endure the worst forms of suffering and grief, and with time and great efforts, rebuild and grow stronger. After a fire destroyed the city of Chicago in 1871, forward-looking community leaders gathered the world's greatest city planners and architects to rebuild it, literally out of the ashes. That resilient response to tragedy made possible the transformation of the skyline and lakefront with innovative skyscrapers and vast public parks. In our times, we will need strong leadership, investment, and collaborative efforts to rebuild communities devastated by major disaster.

As clinicians, our own resilience is tested in work with major trauma and loss. It is helpful to draw strength from our families, friends, communities, and spiritual resources, just as it is for those we are assisting. We may suffer compassion fatigue (Figley, 2005) in witnessing the many stories of trauma and in experiencing our clients' ongoing distressing symptoms. It is especially challenging for rescue workers and professionals when they and their own families have been affected by the crisis event. Support groups can be valuable resources, as they are for trauma survivors and families. Yet, we can also reap benefits as we draw inspiration and insights from the remarkable resilience that many families demonstrate as they rise to meet their challenges. It can inform our other therapeutic work and strengthen our own capacity to meet difficult human challenges.

As therapists and counselors, we cannot heal all the wounds suffered in major trauma and humanitarian crises. We can create a safe haven where family and community members are able to open up and share deep pain and intense emotions We can offer compassionate witnessing (Weingarten, 2004) for their suffering and struggle and admiration for the strengths they have shown in the midst of crisis and the efforts they are making for recovery. When we shift focus from symptoms to strengths, people find they have many unexpected competencies and resources they can draw upon. We can rekindle their hopes and dreams for a better future, support their best efforts and actions, and facilitate relational resources toward those aims. We can encourage their mutual support and active strategies to overcome the many challenges that may lie ahead. The aim of resilience-oriented practice is to help families and communities draw on strengths through troubled times and expand their vision of what is possible through shared efforts. Thus recovery becomes a creative process arising from the synergy of members coming together to work toward a common purpose. The goal of courageous engagement with life guides our work: our encouragement fosters courage, confidence, and perseverance in rebuilding and transforming lives. The worst of times can, indeed, bring out the best in the human spirit. In building resilience, we are helping families and communities not only to survive but to regain their spirit to thrive.

In the wake of tragic events, what is most remarkable is the resilience that emerges in the many stories of recovery, heroism, and courage. In the midst of crisis and trauma, extraordinary compassion, generosity, and wisdom also can emerge. Over time, with shared reflection, we must all strive to integrate the fullness of traumatic events into the fabric of our individual and collective identity. Our response to tragedy can embody the humanity that binds us all together. We are, despite our differences, one human family.

CHAPTER 12

Reconnection
and Reconciliation
Bridge over Troubled Waters

> History, despite its wrenching pain,
> Cannot be unlived, and if faced
> With courage, need not be lived again.
> —MAYA ANGELOU, "On the Pulse of Morning"

I was often viewed as a resilient person, and came to see myself that way as well. I accepted the common belief that because I was inherently resilient, I was able to "raise myself up" despite my family adversities. Like the resilient individuals from dysfunctional families in many case studies (Higgins, 1994; Wolin & Wolin, 1993), I followed the conventional wisdom and avoided contact with my family after leaving home. After college, I took the "geographical cure"—traveling halfway around the world, and returning to settle just halfway back, only going home for brief visits. Weekly phone calls were easier, since my father, who never quite got over the Great Depression, kept an egg timer next to the phone. At 3 minutes he'd announce, "Well, time's up!" and, in midsentence, our conversation was over.

Like many of my peers in young adulthood, I went into psychotherapy and focused on painful childhood experiences and my parents' shortcomings, which were catalogued and embroidered upon by the therapy. I increasingly thought of myself as resilient despite my family influence. It was only later that I came to realize that I'm resilient because of those challenges and because of the hidden strengths in my family that were not in my therapy story. Through those difficult childhood experiences, I emerged hardier than I might have if I had grown up in a placid, "ideal" environment.

Yet the dogma of family dysfunction and the linkage of resilience with disconnection from one's family continue to be dominant themes in U.S. culture and the field of mental health. In her book *The Transcendent Child*, Lillian Rubin (1996) attempts to understand how she herself managed to triumph over childhood adversity in a "dysfunctional family," by selecting and interviewing several other resilient individuals, whose stories she tells along with her own. As she notes, they all followed a similar pathway, distancing from their families of origin as a survival strategy. None have reconnected or reconciled over the years; their families have been left behind, cast in stone as damaged, pathetic, and destructive characters in their early life dramas, as they have moved on into other relationships. Such cutoffs are certainly understandable in cases of persistent strife and abuse, and may be the only option in extreme situations.

Yet in most cases, disconnection is neither the necessary nor the optimal pathway for individual resilience. A causal inference is too often made—that is, the leap from description of common patterns of estrangement to the prescription that disconnection is essential for resilience. Individuals are encouraged by the recovery movement and by traditional clinical theory to push away from contact and to assume fixed views of their families as hopelessly dysfunctional and their relationships as beyond repair. In the same fashion, many individuals leave marriages and other significant relationships by casting off old partners, maintaining negative views of them, and plunging into new relationships with the hope of starting afresh. Like our culture's mistaken view of resilience as simply putting our troubles behind us and moving on, these cut-and-run solutions may bring short-term relief, but leave long-term unresolved issues and a pessimism about resolving relational problems that is carried on life journeys and transmitted to the next generation. These disconnections leave a hole in our heart and in the fabric of our lives. We can best achieve a sense of inner wholeness and a compassionate connectedness with the human community through reconciliation.

In my early research with families of seriously disturbed young adults, I was surprised by the strengths many so-called "dysfunctional" families showed in the midst of their adversities. Moreover, my experiences as a family therapist have convinced me that positive changes can occur even in the most troubled relationships and at any time in life. My encouragement of relational repair is based on the conviction (expressed throughout this book) that our resilience is strengthened as we gain new perspective on past adversity; appreciate the challenges and strengths, as well as the limitations, of those who may have hurt or failed us; and integrate the whole of this experience into our lives and relationships. This closing chapter offers guiding principles and case examples demonstrating the possibilities for reconnection and reconciliation. These processes are described, with applications to the healing of family-of-origin wounds, couples on the brink of separation, and postdivorce family relationships. Difficult dilemmas in forgiveness for past grievances are considered. Although forgiveness is not always possible, the opportunities for personal healing and growth are most often greater than anticipated. Throughout this discussion, I've chosen to speak with a personal voice as well as a professional one, and from an inclusive "we" position, bridging therapists and clients as human beings struggling to come to terms with painful experiences from our past as we leave our legacies for the future.

HEALING RELATIONAL WOUNDS

When most clinicians consider family influences, the pathological bent remains strong, focused on uncovering sources of dysfunction in childhood parenting and family-of-origin relationships. In traditional psychodynamically oriented therapies, intergenerational dynamics have been approached as negative introjects to be contained or resolved through corrective transference relationships with a therapist. Intergenerational family therapists developed therapeutic approaches to facilitate awareness of transactional patterns and change directly with family members, either within or between sessions, to update past relationships and work through unresolved conflicts and losses (Framo, 1992). The contextual family therapy approach of Boszormenyi-Nagy (1987) has focused on the reconstruction and reunion of current extended family relationships through the resolution of grievances involving multigenerational legacies of accountability and loyalty. The Bowen approach (Bowen, 1978; Carter & McGoldrick, 2001) fosters personal growth and relational healing through coaching methods that help clients gain more differentiated, genuine relationships by reducing anxiety and emotional reactivity. Bringing a resilience perspective to this work, efforts to heal relational wounds are facilitated by gaining a contextual view of life challenges, gaining appreciation of unrecognized strengths, and seizing opportunities to overcome barriers to reconciliation.

THERAPIST, HEAL THY OWN RELATIONSHIPS: PERSONAL JOURNEYS AND REFLECTIONS

If therapists are to help clients overcome pessimism and anxiety about change in long-standing patterns, we must have a strong conviction that some change is possible in most cases. Such a conviction is difficult if we ourselves have given up on change in our own family relationships. Similarly, it may be difficult to help partners repair their couple relationship while a therapist is currently going through a painful separation and unable to overcome similar impasses. However, therapists who have reached a good understanding and reasonable reconciliation following relational breakdown can draw on their experience in helpful ways. Curiously, research has not attended to this link between a therapist's own current state of relational resolution and the outcome of therapy with couples and families seeking reconciliation. In the hope that my own personal efforts at reconciliation may inspire others, I offer some of these experiences in coming to know my parents better and transform our relationships. As Imber-Black affirms (1995), opening family histories and secrets to the light, despite the anxieties it can raise, can be powerfully healing.

Reconnecting with My Father: Learning His Adversities, Struggles, and Resilience

Although my early experiences as a family therapist and researcher convinced me that positive changes could occur in even the most troubled relationships, there was one nagging exception: my own relationship with my father, which I had given up on. I felt an uneasy dissonance between the professional and the personal—touting the strengths and possibilities for change in other families, but writing off my father as a hopeless case. For many years I carried disappointment, anger, and embarrassment about my father. He was a shy, unassuming man who walked with a limp. His adage was "Don't get your hopes up too high; then you'll never be disappointed." He made do with little and was looked down upon as a failure by others in our family and community who were impressed by social status and financial success. I received this view of him and felt his shame. Clearly, it was time to work on my own family relationships.

I was fortunate to be able to consult with Murray Bowen, and doubly blessed for the opportunity to process much of my work with my close friend and colleague Monica McGoldrick, who was also working on her family relationships at that time. We shored each other up, encouraging each other to stay hopeful and to persevere; our own bond was a source of resilience for us both in our change efforts.

I had many opportunities to practice Bowen reconnection skills as I reengaged with my father. I had not seen him since my mother's death, 4 years earlier. When I phoned to tell him I wanted to fly out to visit him, instead of sounding pleased, he gruffly replied, "Well, don't expect me to pay for your airfare." I took a deep breath and assured him I didn't. Indicating no pleasure at the thought of my visit, he replied, "Well, I have a lot of work; I won't have much time to spend with you. And the apartment's a mess." I took a deeper breath and said, "That's OK; I thought I'd stay with a friend. [This was a break with the norm of a home stay.] I could meet you for dinner after work, if you're free." He retorted, "Oh, you mean you're really coming to see your friends." At this point, with my anger mounting, it would have been easy to chalk up another failed attempt and quit. Here I was, making this great effort, and there he was, unappreciative and hopeless. However, I tried not to get defensive or annoyed, and reasserted that my main wish was to see him. The call ended without an inkling of encouragement from him, but I went ahead with my plan. When my flight arrived at midday, my dad surprised me by being at the gate; he had taken a sick day so that we could spend time together.

It's very important to keep in mind that in efforts to reconnect, we must take the initiative and not get reactive if the immediate response is disappointing. And, I had to try to understand my father's position. I had been working toward reconnection for some time unbeknownst to him. My call came to him out of the blue and he reacted defensively, to protect his feelings. As I now came to realize, he had missed me terribly. I tried to put myself in his place: Why was I calling now? Did I want something from him? Was I just being "polite" and really motivated to visit my friends? He was aware of my discomfort with him over the years, and had lost hope that I genuinely cared about him and might actually want to see him.

My efforts to reconnect with my father reaped benefits far beyond my expectations. Over the next few years, our relationship deepened with each contact, yet not without occasional friction. He was a quiet man who didn't like to talk about problems or painful subjects. He and his family never spoke about their past. It took my genuine interest in hearing more about his life, and my doggedly persistent urging over many visits, for him to share stories of his childhood and reveal the suffering he had endured and his remarkable comebacks.

My father never wanted to talk about his limp; my mother gathered it was caused by a sports injury in adolescence. I seized an opportunity to learn more at a family wedding, cornering my uncle, who had had enough champagne to open up. I was astonished to learn that my father had fallen from his high chair as an infant, breaking his hip. This was in 1909, before the advances in modern medicine. He had undergone surgery three times by the age of 10; each time, he was encased for many months in a plaster cast from waist to foot. Each time, when the cast was removed, his hip had slipped out of place again. This ordeal forced him to spend his childhood at home, unable to walk freely or play with his brothers or peers. With tremendous perseverance by his parents (who used up their entire modest savings), his leg was finally repaired, although by then it was shorter than the other. He started school at the age of 11, where, although he was bright, the young children in his first-grade class made fun of him. Awkward and embarrassed, he left school at 14 and completed his GED on his own. He later enrolled in a local college, working for a pharmacist to put himself through school. After 3 years, the college went bankrupt and closed, an early casualty of the Great Depression. His boss praised my father's hard work and promised to give him the pharmacy at retirement, if he would continue to work for very little pay through those hard times. When my parents married, they were struggling financially, yet hopeful for the future. Despite their best efforts, the pharmacy folded in 1939 and my father's dreams were once again dashed. My parents then started over, moving to a new community where my uncles gave my father a small, failed business to try his hand at. They both worked hard; I was born; and just as they seemed to be doing well, a fire in our apartment building wiped out everything they had. It could be said that I was born into adversity, but we also had good fortune: The day of the fire, I was in the hospital having my tonsils out, which saved all our lives.

I pieced together much of this story as my father and I continued our journey of reconciliation. Putting his life into perspective fundamentally altered my view of him and my feelings toward him. My anger and disappointment melted as a compassionate understanding of his life emerged. He was no longer a failure in my eyes, but instead a hero, who had struggled valiantly to overcome the many hardships and cruel disappointments in his life. He was a loner, a misfit, never quite comfortable in social situations or in the company of more financially successful relatives. Yet in many ways he was the strongest, most resilient one in his family. He met his life's adversities with courage. Tested repeatedly, he always rose to meet the challenge. His mother's care through childhood and his loving bond with my mother encouraged his resilience.

While I was growing up, my father worked 7 days a week, 12 hours a day—except for the occasional Sunday drive we took, when he put up a sign: "Open every day but not today." He managed to build our small house himself, along with a neighboring carpenter, plumber, and electrician, who traded services with him. My mother also worked very hard as a music teacher, yet always made time for community service projects. My father worked until, at 70, he could no longer stand on his feet all day. Then, living only on Social Security, he got up each day and did full-time volunteer office work for his men's organization to raise money for hospitals serving children with disabilities. In clearing out his apartment at his death, I found many service awards, which in his modesty he had never mentioned.

I had never understood my father until I was able to put the fragments of his life together and gain a sense of coherence. In the early phase of reconciliation, I experienced tremendous sadness at "time lost," as I regretted all those years when my disappointment and shame at my father's deficits had blinded me to his strengths and blocked our relationship. Those last precious years of discovery and reconnection until his death are a continual wellspring of love and inspiration in my life.

As Monica McGoldrick (1995) reminds us, there are few pure saints or sinners in real families. If we look for redeeming qualities in family members who are seen only as villains or failures, we will begin to see them. Following the wisdom of Native Americans, we may have to believe in those possibilities in order to see them. In the same way, if we can believe that even the most troubled or estranged relationships have the potential for change and growth, we are more likely to act in ways that indeed foster reconnection and reconciliation.

Seizing Opportunities to Reconnect: Understanding My Mother's Secrets, Sorrows, and Strengths

My mother had been cut off from her family after leaving the Catholic Church and then converting to Judaism when she married my father. Although we received annual Christmas cards from her brother, I had only met him once briefly, as a child; he had turned a cold shoulder when my mother sought his support during hard times. Shortly before my mother's death, when I was 27 and eager to know her better in what little time we had, she shared a secret she had kept even from my father: She had been a nun for 17 years. She died before I could ask the many questions I was left with.

Several years later, in the usual holiday card from my uncle, he mentioned that he was looking forward to a family reunion. However, he offered no details or invitation. Overcoming my initial anger and identification with my mother's painful exclusion, I decided to take a risk and write back to express my interest and ask if I might attend. He replied immediately with a gracious invitation. I learned that the reunion was in honor of the retirement of Sister Honoria as Mother Superior of her order. She was my mother's cousin and had been her closest confidante through her teen years and early adulthood: as best friends, they had entered the convent together at the age of 16. This was an opportunity I couldn't miss.

I also learned that there were other relatives going to the reunion from Chicago—relatives I didn't even know lived in my city. As we flew to the reunion together, I found myself more anxious than I had anticipated; these newfound cousins were friendly, yet conversation was superficial and awkward, with no mention of my mother. At the reunion, everyone greeted me warmly, but still no one spoke of my mother. I felt strangely as if I had somehow landed in this family all by myself. And I felt a pang of disloyalty to my mother for wanting to reunite with those who had rejected her.

My family therapy tools of the trade saved the day, relieving my anxiety and making connections. I first pored over old photographs, eager to hear about the whole cast of characters. Then I sat down at the kitchen table with paper and pencil and began to sketch a genogram, asking questions as I drew. Soon family members gathered around, curious and eager to add their pieces or make corrections, and stories began to flow. As I brought up my desire to hear stories of my mother, they dug out photos of her in her nun's habit; they too had been carrying the secret, unsure whether I knew. Over the next 2 days, relatives kept coming up to me with more stories. I encouraged them to talk with one another, to put together partial accounts, and to contact others who couldn't be there to "fill in the blanks" and send me any more recollections that might come to them. I promised to draw up a complete family genogram and send it to everyone, which I did several months later with a New Year's greeting.

At the reunion, I invited Sister Honoria to go for a walk. She too had hoped for a chance for us to talk. My first question concerned my desire to comprehend how my mother had become a nun. I learned that my maternal grandmother, a deeply religious French Canadian Catholic, had hoped that my mother's brother, whom she favored, would become a priest. When he left the seminary after a year to marry his sweetheart, my mother seized the opportunity to gain her mother's favor by entering the convent.

As I learned about this hidden phase in my mother's life, the discordant parts in my understanding of my mother as a person became more coherent. A gifted musician, she became a highly admired teacher, organist, and choir director. But she experienced her deep personal spirituality, humanity, and love of life as increasingly at odds with her hierarchical, ascetic, and cloistered environment. With great anguish, she came to the courageous decision to leave the order for the real world. In that time (the 1930s) such a decision was shame-laden and unforgivable. After she left the convent, her mother refused to see her; she died within the year, and my mother was not informed of it until after the funeral. This loss of reconciliation was a deep sadness my mother carried secretly all her life. I now understood the sorrow I had seen in her eyes, the sadness that could find no comfort.

Reaching Out to Widen the Circle

At the family reunion, I felt particularly anxious when I saw my mother's cousin Alma. I had a dark memory of her from childhood, the only time my mother and I visited her. Having married well, she lived in luxury. She received us coldly; my mother said afterward that she thought she was too good for us. Picking up my mother's embarrassment, I took this to mean that it was my father's fault for being the wrong religion and not a financial success. Seeing her again, I felt intimidated and wary, although she warmed up to me and invited me to visit her.

After the reunion, I kept meaning to visit Alma, but I found myself putting it off. When many months had passed, I finally pushed myself to call and visit. I felt trepidation as I approached the house, which looked just as I remembered from childhood. Alma greeted me warmly and had a large box of old photographs waiting for me. As she shared memories over the photos, her tears came. She confessed that she had been very jealous of my mother as a child. Her own father, a lumberjack, had disappeared on a logging job and was presumed dead, although his body was never found. Her mother, left penniless, was forced to work long hours in a laundry and sent Alma to live with my mother's family. Sealing over her losses and grief, she became aloof and resentful of the loving bond she saw daily between my mother and her father. It was the reactivation of that old pain that had triggered her defensive coldness when my mother and I had visited her. I hugged her with a new affection when this visit ended, treasuring the many photos and new perspectives she gave me.

Three weeks later, another relative called to tell me that Alma had died in her sleep. I realized that because of my busy schedule and my procrastination, we had nearly missed this transforming connection. Learning from this experience, I now urge my clients and students not to put off acting on good intentions to transform painful experiences and heal wounded relationships. This is especially urgent with elders and those with life-threatening illness. Yet all of our lives are unpredictable, and we should never take time for granted in any relationship. A key to relational resilience is active initiative—seizing the opportunities before us and persevering to create the new relational possibilities we yearn for.

Naming: Bridging the Divide

Naming is often a way of making connections across the generations and in joining families by marriage. In my own family, naming became a way for my mother to weave together the disparate threads of her life and identity. Her mother, a devout Catholic, named my mother and her brother Mary and Joseph. After Joe left the seminary, my mother not only took his place by entering the convent; she even took his name, becoming Sister Josephine. When she eventually left the religious order to lead a "normal" life, she held on to that part of her identity by changing her name to Mary Jo, preferring to be called simply Jo. (Interestingly, the same year my mother came out into the world, Katharine Hepburn portrayed Jo in a film version of *Little Women*.) When she married my father and converted to Judaism, everyone called her Jo. To bridge the cultural and religious divide and to win the approval of her new mother-in-law, she named me after my father's maternal grandmother, Frimid. (My middle name, Carolyn, is her own mother's name.) Only when I reached adulthood did I learn that Froma (Frimid) is derived from the Jewish name Fruma, meaning "pious" or "spiritual." My name would thus have had special meaning for my mother. Although she chose a secular life, she embraced Judaism—even becoming temple organist and later, B'nai B'rith president—and remained a deeply spiritual person.

THE PROCESS OF RECONCILIATION

All family relationships are bound to have occasional conflict, mixed feelings, or shifting alliances. When conflict has been intense and persistent, when ambivalence is strong, or when relationships have become estranged, family therapy offers possibilities for reconciliation.

The potential for reconciliation is determined not so much by the severity of the grievances as by the depth of the will to be reconciled (Anderson, Hogue, & McCarthy, 1995). Reconciliation is not a hasty peace. Rather, it's a process of mutual reengagement, requiring a readiness on the part of each person to take the other(s) seriously, to acknowledge violations to the relationship, and to experience the associated pain. Reconciliation is more than righting wrongs; it brings us to a deeper place of trust and commitment.

Seeing Others with Different Eyes; Changing Ourselves in Relationships

We tend to see things not as they are, but as we are.

> Roscoe, who grew up in a very troubled family (his mother was chronically depressed and his father was an alcoholic), came to think of his family as toxic and his well-being as dependent on keeping as much distance as possible. He avoided all contact, especially with his mother. Still, thoughts of her triggered inner turmoil. Altering this fixed view was the key to change: "I began to understand that the only way my relationship with my mother could change was for me to see her with different eyes." With the support of his therapist, Roscoe began to develop new relationships with his parents on a different basis; all have grown and changed. They still have occasional problems, but are able to talk about them and move through them.

In the work of reconnection and reconciliation, we need to see and hear in new ways. The most important element is respectful, genuine curiosity about the lives and perspectives of others. One of my psychology professors, Neil Postman, offered a valuable lesson: Once you have learned to ask questions—relevant, appropriate, and substantial questions—you have learned how to learn, and no one can keep you from learning whatever you want or need to know.

In family-of-origin work toward reconciliation, we first survey the entire extended-family field in the family evaluation process. A genogram and timeline (McGoldrick et al., 1999) are essential tools to diagram the network of relationships and to note important information and the timing of nodal events. This map guides discussion to explore the meaning and significance of connections. Whereas traditional individual therapy relies on the internalized images and perspectives of the client, which are inherently partial and subjective, family therapists encourage clients to contact extended-family members and others in order to clarify obscured information and to gain multiple perspectives on key family members and relationships.

Opportunities can be seized to reconnect with families at holiday gatherings and at events marking transitions, such as weddings, bar mitzvahs, graduations, and funerals. We can encourage clients to actively plan and shape family gatherings, and to invite family members to bring photos and memorabilia. One client, wishing to repair estranged relationships in her family network, decided to organize a "No-Excuses Family Reunion." On the invitation, she drew message bubbles filled with possible excuses people might give for not attending: "I'm running in a marathon that weekend," "My cat is scheduled for surgery," "Nobody wants to see me anyway." Humor can work wonders.

Setting out to change others is usually doomed. Such failed attempts reinforce the frustration and hopelessness commonly experienced. As Bowen (1978) has advised, therapeutic efforts are most fruitfully directed at changing oneself in relation to other family members. Follow-through is essential to handle the anxiety generated by the process and by the system's initial self-correcting attempts that undermine change. To achieve success, we must deal with our own anxiety, keep from becoming reactive if initial responses are disappointing, and persist in our best efforts. Because of the recursive nature of human systems, if we change our own part in transactions, change by others is more likely to follow over time. Whatever the response, as the process enlarges our own perspective, we gain a more compassionate acceptance of others' strengths and limitations. As Monica McGoldrick (1995) observes, we would all like to be ourselves with our family members—to have them accept us as who we are. But we lose sight of the prerequisite: that we accept them for who they really are, and get past the anger, resentments, and regrets of not being an ideal family.

I once worked with Lydia, whose daughter, Amber, age 22, had run off with her boyfriend and cut herself off from the family 4 years earlier, after the death of her father in an auto accident. The harder Lydia pursued Amber, the more she distanced, refusing any visit or phone contact. We considered the vicious cycle that had ensued: The mother's pain and frustration at Amber's estrangement had fueled guilt-inducing complaints that were self-defeating. Amber, further alienated, accused her mother of only needing her to meet her own needs, adding that her therapist agreed (although having never met the mother).

I worked with Lydia's long-standing pain at the double loss of her husband and daughter, and encouraged her own efforts to move on with her life. I supported her efforts to make meaning of Amber's flight—to see it less as a rejection of her mother, and to consider other possibilities from a normative, developmental perspective, such as an adolescent's survival strategy at the devastating loss of her father. I helped Lydia sustain hope in the possibility of eventual reconciliation with her daughter, even in the face of repeated rebuffs. I encouraged her to write occasional letters and cards, sending news and photos. It was important to convey the caring yet undemanding message that she loved Amber and was keeping their connection alive and her door open. Lydia called me a year later to tell me that Amber had finally called and then come home for a visit; the healing of their relationship was progressing.

The process of reconnection is advanced by redeveloping personal relationships with important family members, repairing cutoffs, detriangling from conflicts, and changing one's own part in emotionally charged vicious cycles. Humor can detoxify emotional situations. In attempting change, Bowen (1978) advised: Don't attack; don't withdraw; and don't defend. Clients often ask, "What else is there to do?" The "what else" lies at the heart of effective change: the ability to hold an assertive, centered position, and to express one's own thoughts, feelings, needs, and concerns with respectful consideration of others. This must be accompanied by a genuine effort to understand their positions and to strive for a better relationship (Carter & McGoldrick, 2001).

The use of photographs can help to connect those estranged, as they trigger storytelling about family members and their past. Letters can be another effective aid in reconnecting. Therapists can offer feedback for clients to express their pain and their aims without attack or defensiveness. Letters also allow an entire message to be conveyed and considered without an immediate defensive reply and counterreaction. When a relationship has been strained for a long time, it's wise to proceed slowly, step by step, not expecting too much too soon. We can actively pursue a relationship, but cannot force one. At times, we may need to step back and renew efforts more gradually or take a different tack. Keeping a systemic perspective helps us to anticipate possible setbacks, understand them, and rebound undeterred.

Learning Family Stories of Adversity and Resilience

When people have a fixed negative view of parental deficits, it's helpful to look back more broadly in family history to gain a contextual, evolutionary perspective and to search for nuggets of resilience at times of past challenges. I encourage many clients (and my students) to explore their families' migration experiences, attending in particular to the trauma and losses suffered, their struggles and triumphs, and the resilience they forged to endure hardship and make their way in a new life.

Some have little or no sense of their families' history. Many have learned, for the first time, how family members came to the United States or made other disruptive life transitions. In many ethnic minority families, relatives have shared long-buried painful stories: accounts of forced migration and cutoff in Native American families; accounts of slavery and racism endured by African American families; stories of Holocaust survivors; experience of trauma and privation by Southeast Asians. Some family members came as political refugees; others fled their native lands to escape religious persecution or impoverished conditions. In all cases, it's important to search for resilience in the midst of trauma, loss, and dislocation. As we ask questions about the strengths that enabled our families to reorient and prevail, the stories themselves are enlarged. Reconnecting with the strengths of our ancestors can be empowering as we realize the courage, perseverance, and inventiveness that enabled them to endure and surmount adversity.

Respectful Confrontation

In seeking reconciliation, ways must be found to express anger and disappointment and yet to be respectful and considerate toward others, as the following case illustrates:

> In one Mexican American family, three young adult sons had all become estranged from their parents, but the mother's heart attack led them to come to their priest to seek help in mending their relationships. The sons carried considerable anger toward their father for his long-standing harsh and abusive treatment when they failed to meet his expectations. However, they were reluctant at first to accept the recommendation of family counseling; they hesitated to

confront him because they had been brought up never to show disrespect to their father. They also feared an explosive reaction. Distancing from the family had been their adaptive strategy. The family counselor, who was also Mexican American, acknowledged his own hesitation in opening up these wounds, since respect toward elders is such a strong value in Mexican culture. The therapeutic challenge was to face these sensitive issues in a respectful rather than an attacking way, with the goal of reconciliation.

The father, José, pained by his sons' estrangement, was quite open to family sessions to heal the wounds. With the counselor's facilitation, the sons talked about how it had felt to receive his harsh treatment and about their belief that they could never please him. The father hung his head, remaining silent. The therapist asked what was going through his mind. He said that he himself had suffered beatings and humiliation by his father, whom he had fled through immigration. José had never before talked about this experience and became tearful in realizing how he had turned into his father, driving his sons away. This acknowledgment led him to make a heartfelt apology. The sons were deeply moved by their father's account and his genuine remorse. Still, at the following session there was uneasiness about how to move forward and what to do with lingering feelings about the past. The counselor noted that the family members had mentioned the importance of their Catholic faith but hadn't gone to church all together in years. He asked whether this might be a resource. The mother suggested that they all go to mass the next Sunday and pray for guidance in healing their relationships. After the mass, the oldest son invited them all to his house for tamales (an old family tradition on Sundays), where José met his grandchildren for the first time. The healing had begun.

Weaving Disparate Parts into a Larger Whole

The process of reconciliation involves attempts to weave together two or more disparate views or experiences into a larger whole that holds and respects each in its place. The juxtaposition of elements of the traditional and the modern was one of the most startling images striking me in some Arab societies, where women cloaked from head to toe ride around town on motorbikes. These incongruous behaviors may not be synthesized in their lives, and may even remain jarring in their contrast; yet they come to be seen as part of the larger whole of their history and their ongoing experience, incorporating traditional and modern aspects. In our own family and social world, we may not be as aware of such incongruities. Yet as we struggle to know ourselves and our loved ones better, this bridging perspective can span ethnic or religious differences, can encompass both suffering and triumph, and can find joy in the midst of sorrow.

The acceptance of diverse aspects of a relationship as parts of a larger whole offers a path out of irreconcilable polarities (e.g., "How could my father have loved me if he hurt me so badly?" "Was it a loving or destructive romance?"). It requires a shift in our perspective from a split view to a larger, holistic perspective—from an "either–or" stance to a "both–and" position. A father may be both loving and harsh; a romantic relationship may be both passionate and destructive. We can then weigh and balance the various elements to make decisions about the whole experience of such relationships.

The Courage to Reach Out

Our families build our physical, emotional, and relational resilience through love and trust. I was most fortunate; despite my parents' persistent hardships and the toll these took on our lives, I never doubted their love and trustworthiness. In many families those resources have been depleted by hurtful actions, such as neglect, long-standing addictions, or physical, emotional, or sexual abuse. When an individual is harmed or violated by another family member, family transactions—powerful beliefs, patterns of organization, and communication processes—may allow the abuse to be denied or perpetuated. Individuals often distance and cut themselves off altogether from the family, finding that contact reactivates destructive transactional patterns and pain. Yet they carry disappointment, anger, and mistrust with them on their life journeys. Self-doubt and blame can permeate other relationships with partners and children.

Attempting reconciliation takes enormous courage because we may reenter relationships and reach out to others, only to find that they rebuff our efforts or still cannot be trusted. The work involves both risk and opportunity: the risk of reexperiencing hurt and no change; the opportunity to experience new relational possibilities. The challenge is to reconcile grievances and forgive injuries to the fullest extent possible. When others are unable to respond as we would wish, we have still gained in generosity, and gained a sense that we've done all we could. This facilitates greater acceptance and enables us to embrace life with fuller integrity.

Even in cases of serious past injury or injustice, relationships can be reconciled and past emotional damage healed through work toward reconciliation, as Terry Hargrave (1994) has found in helping people achieve forgiveness by building love, justice, and trust. His approach involves four intertwined "stations" focused on insight, understanding, giving the opportunity for compensation, and the overt act of forgiving. This work can be painful and difficult. In the course of seeking understanding, we may get in touch with rage and sorrow, or a threatening image of an abuser. Yet when this work is carefully guided, it can be unexpectedly successful because it deals with a powerful vortex where past and future relationships can be changed simultaneously.

Creating Rituals for Healing and Reconciliation

Active involvement in meaningful rituals can be valuable in healing strained relationships after family trauma, as in the following case:

> Raymundo, a trainee in our program, told of his powerful experience of a "family healing ceremony" held by a pastoral counselor for him and members of his family of origin. With the family seated around a table, the pastoral counselor first helped them to construct a large genogram and place it in the center of the table. Family members were invited to tell their own stories of suffering—from drinking problems to intense conflict and abuse. The counselor then asked for accounts of strength and resilience, to rebalance their stories, identify potential resources, and generate hope for positive change. He asked each to specify the relationship impasses they most hoped to heal, and to point out the relevant parts of the genogram. All family members were encouraged to contribute to this healing conversation from their own positions, expressing both their worries and their hopes. As each spoke in turn, the others were asked to listen attentively. Then they were each asked three questions: Did they desire reconciliation? Would they be willing to own accountability for their part in problems? Would they share in responsibility for improving relations? Each in turn affirmed a commitment to these vows and to working together in family therapy to achieve them. In conclusion, the priest led a silent meditation for the success of family reconciliation, with all holding hands. For Raymundo and his family, this experience was quite profound and marked a turning point in healing their relationships.

It is never too late for rituals that honor loved ones and foster connection. On the 20th anniversary of my mother's death, I wanted to mark the event in a meaningful way with my husband and small daughter, who had never known her. Inspired by her love of music, I arranged a short memorial concert of carillon bells at my university. We climbed to the roof of the tower and, as the bells peeled, we looked out at the evening stars in the sky, knowing her light was among them.

Time Can Heal Old Wounds: Reconciliation between Aging Parents and Adult Children

Fitting the popular belief that "you can't teach an old dog new tricks," Americans carry the expectation that relationships between adults and their parents are cast in stone and unalterable. In my clinical work, I am grateful for my doctoral studies in human development and the abundant research revealing the potential for growth and change throughout middle and later life (Walsh, 1999a). As Bateson (1994) observes, in response to new circumstances, individuals can (and may be forced to) reinvent themselves many times over. With life experience and the wisdom that comes with aging, people can and do change their ways, even after many years of destructive behavior. Moreover, as older adults seek to bring meaning and coherence to their lives, they attempt to come to terms with problematic and regrettable aspects of their relationships, and look for new opportunities to repair frayed bonds. This involves accepting what cannot be changed in the past, developing new perspectives on experiences, putting regrets in their place, and celebrating the successes.

At various phases in the life course, different issues come to the fore and others recede. As we change and grow through our experiences, our remembrance of the past and current feelings about past events and relationships are altered. A conflict over autonomy and control that flared with burning intensity between an adolescent son and his father may no longer be relevant when the son is more secure in his identity in midlife and the father has mellowed with age. Likewise, the impact of past traumatic events may be altered with subsequent experience. A woman's mothering of a newborn is influenced less by her own early relationship with her mother than by the degree of resolution she has achieved in that relationship over time.

Adult development thus presents new possibilities for healing of old intergenerational wounds. In early and middle adulthood, such relationships continue to be renegotiated on an adult-to-adult basis. Rapprochement commonly occurs with such transitions as parenthood, when the younger generation directly experiences the challenges involved in child rearing and begins to gain empathy for their own parents. As we age, we may find an increasing number of things we need to learn from and can appreciate in our elders. We may discover that our parents, like Mark Twain's father, become wiser every year.

Yet time alone is not sufficient. Many relationships become frozen at an earlier point of conflict or cutoff, as if time stood still (McGoldrick, 1995). I was struck in my research interviews of troubled families that a traumatic loss 20 years earlier could still be as painful as if it had happened yesterday when it had not been dealt with. Caregiving for an aging parent can be complicated by an adult child's lingering anger and pain at not having received good care from that parent in childhood. Unresolved issues from the past can block the ability to see and respond to aging parents as persons facing their own ongoing challenges.

> Charleen, a 35-year-old single parent, was furious with her father. He left a message on her answering machine to say that he would not come for Easter dinner at her home, because she wasn't planning to serve ham, and Easter was not the same without the traditional ham dinner her mother had always prepared. Charleen was incensed; he knew full well that she was a vegetarian and that she was going to great lengths to prepare a no-meat feast for their extended family. Charleen heard his refusal to attend as a ploy to control her, just as she had always felt controlled by him as a child. She would not give in to him and serve ham!
>
> Charleen's therapist helped to calm her reactivity and, after hearing more about their past interactions, sought to help Charleen separate this incident from her childhood experience and to understand it in a more immediate context—particularly in light of her mother's death a year earlier. Charleen knew that her father had recently retired, but, busy with her own life, she knew little else about it. Her therapist encouraged her to call her brother, who was close to their father, and get his ideas on what might have triggered the father's abrupt behavior. She was surprised to learn that her father had been forced to retire. Just before his call to her, he had gone in to work for the last day and found that his name was already removed from the door, his office was cleared out, and his belongings were piled in the hallway.

This new information shifted Charleen's perspective. She had framed the incident, as she usually saw their interactions, in the context of their old parent–child hierarchy—her father's need to wield power and authority over her. Each time her childhood drama was reactivated, she rebelled angrily against feeling controlled and manipulated by him. Now she saw his recent actions in a new light: He was an aging man, recently widowed, in a life crisis of forced retirement. She went to see him and found him jolted by the cruel way in which he was let go and by the feeling that he had lost control over his own fate. His work world, his identity, his future security, and his dignity were suddenly shattered—and he was alone, missing his wife more than ever. For the first time, Charleen felt truly like an adult in relation to an elder parent, who was facing losses all around him. She could appreciate her father's urgent need to maintain continuity with his past. She lovingly included her mother's recipe for ham in the Easter dinner preparations.

Healing Sibling Rivalries

Sibling bonds become increasingly valued over the life course. Those relationships can be blocked by old rivalries and grievances from childhood, as in the following case:

Jimmy, age 34, sought therapy to improve his relationships with his sisters. They had been estranged since the sudden death of both parents in a car crash 2 years earlier. Old sibling rivalries had pitted them against one another since childhood. Their father had been remote and their mother chronically depressed, with the siblings competing fiercely for the little attention they received. In an attempt at reconnection, Jimmy invited his siblings for dinner, but it was disastrous. His sister Carmen saw a treasured photo of their mother on the mantel and became furious with him for failing to make a copy for her, which he had promised to do at their parents' funeral. Becoming defensive, Jimmy told her to get off his case. Carmen lashed out at him for being a "self-centered mama's boy." He called her a "spiteful old nag." Enraged, she grabbed the photo and tore it up; beside himself, he struck her, causing a nosebleed. The escalation continued in ensuing weeks as Carmen hired a lawyer to sue Jimmy for damages, and he refused to apologize, blamed the incident on her, and consulted a lawyer to countersue. His other sister sided with Carmen against him. Jimmy's wife was also becoming furious at his "childish" plans for revenge.
    Old family triangles now entangled Jimmy's therapist. When she questioned Jimmy's proposed counterattack, he accused her of siding with his sister and wife against him, and threatened to stop therapy. The therapist clarified her position: She was not colluding with them against him; rather, she was trying to align with his better self. She knew him to be a decent and generous man, and she believed that deep down, he knew he had played a part in the conflict and might have some regrets. He put his head in his hands, sighed

deeply, and nodded. They now more calmly reflected on the chain of events and the relational significance of the incident: holding on to for himself (or, from his sister's perspective, withholding from her) the photo of their deceased mother, who hadn't been available when they had most needed her as children. Jimmy agreed that he needed to take responsibility for his own procrastination, since he knew how much the photo meant to Carmen. The therapist also helped him to see that no matter what his sister had done that had provoked him, he was accountable for his own violent reaction and harm to her. His therapist appealed to his better nature, encouraging him to apologize for his actions and to cease litigation, which would be self-defeating to his goal of improving his relationships with his siblings. She affirmed his idea to have enlarged copies made and framed for himself and all his siblings. A later session with all siblings allowed each one to be heard and better understood. The therapist offered the idea that, in the spirit of reconciliation, they might plan a potluck dinner together, each contributing a favorite dish. At a follow-up session, Jimmy brought photos taken of them all together, celebrating their reunion.

Terminal Illness and Threatened Loss: Opportunity for Relational Recovery

Terminal illness and threatened loss can heighten the sense of preciousness of one's relationships, and can spark an urgent desire to make amends before it is too late.

> Diane came to see me in crisis. She recounted that her 16-year-old son, Jason, had been fathered by a former boyfriend, Ron; Ron had left town when told of her pregnancy, saying that he wasn't ready for marriage or parenthood. In despair, she'd married Dwayne, a good friend who knew the child wasn't his but gladly accepted paternity. Her son had grown up believing that Dwayne was his biological father. Now, out of the blue, Ron had called her from Arizona, saying that he had terminal cancer and wanted to see Jason before he died. She wanted me to advise her on what she should do.
>   A wise therapist doesn't solve such dilemmas for clients, but helps them survey the situation and options as fully as possible to come to their best decision. First we explored the case for not telling: She worried that the news would be too upsetting for Jason, who was doing well. Her catastrophic fear was that his psychological adjustment and school achievements would plummet. Further, she worried that it could be devastating for her husband, who was

such a kind and loving father to Jason, and would risk shattering their stable family unit. She also feared that Jason would hate her for keeping the truth from him and living a lie all his life. We also explored Diane's own complex feelings in weighing her decision. She was enraged that Ron had abandoned her and their son and that over the years he had never expressed the slightest interest in Jason or contributed to his support. What right did he have to disrupt their lives now? Yet, on the other hand, she didn't want Jason to learn the truth somehow later on, for instance if Ron's other children, his half-siblings, ever contacted him. He would hate her for denying him his only chance to know his birth father. After deep soul searching, she decided that Jason had a right to know about Ron and to meet him if he chose to do so. She also believed she needed to be courageous and trust in her son and in the strong relationships she and her husband had forged with him over the years. We discussed how this secret might best be opened. She decided she should first discuss it with her husband, and they agreed to tell Jason together and to support each other through any upheaval. To prepare them, I asked how they anticipated Jason might react. They thought he might run off, but wouldn't do something self-destructive, and would likely return. I encouraged her to keep an understanding and supportive openness to "hang in" with him through a period of initial upset.

Jason was initially disbelieving, then furious at everyone. As predicted, he did storm out of the house; they called his best friend and were reassured that he was there for the night. The next day he returned and asked for Ron's phone number. As Diane and Dwayne talked things through with him, Jason decided to go to meet his father. The visit was short but meaningful. Ron showed sincere remorse for having been so scared and immature to have run out on Jason and his mother. He revealed, tearfully, that a day had not passed without his thoughts of Jason. He was also ashamed that he had not sent money for Jason's support. He wanted Jason to know that he had just signed over half of his pension to Jason to help him through college; he knew that this wouldn't make up for the lost years, but wanted to do what he could now. After returning home, Jason was very grateful for his parents' trust in him. I applauded Diane and Dwayne for being generous in giving Jason and his father this opportunity. Eight months later, Jason learned his father had died and went to his funeral, where he began to connect with his half-siblings. Through this process, contrary to Diane's fear of losing their "intact" family, they gained a fuller, truer family "intactness" in their incorporation of all significant relationships in Jason's life.

Healing and Reconciliation after a Death

"Death ends a life, but not a relationship, which struggles on in the survivor's mind, seeking some resolution which it may never find." This opening line in Robert Anderson's (1968) play *I Never Sang for My Father* conveys the protracted anguish often experienced when relational wounds were not reconciled before a death. Much of my clinical work is involved in helping individuals find healing, as I did, even many years after a loss.

> Lenore, age 43, came for therapy to explore unresolved issues around the loss of her mother when she was 9. She had just reached the age at which her mother had died, and she was experiencing a pervasive sense of emptiness in her life. Lenore had few memories of her mother, and had always believed that her mother had been cold and distant and had never loved her. I asked her to bring in old family photos; she had very few. Because her mother's health had slowly deteriorated over several years, she hadn't wanted to be photographed frail and in a wheelchair. In one photo, Lenore and several friends were in costumes for a school musical, with her mother to the side. I commented on how struck I was by her mother's fond gaze at her in the photo. She had never noticed that before, but could see it at once. She reported at our next session that she'd kept the photo with her all week, looking at it over and over, each time her eyes brimming with tears. She recalled that the photo was taken less than a year before her mother's death, when she was in great pain and limited in what she could do. Nevertheless, she had volunteered to make costumes for Lenore and her classmates. Now that Lenore could see evidence of her mother's caring, new memories flowed out of the past darkness, and she began to revise her beliefs and stories to incorporate her mother's love. She came to realize that she, too, had withdrawn as her mother's illness progressed, protecting herself from unbearable sadness in her loss.
>
> Lenore also realized that because of the long illness, she'd barely known her mother. I urged her to contact her mother's only surviving sister, still living in their hometown in the South, to learn more about her mother as a child and a young woman. Her aunt sent photos of her mother growing up and invited her to visit. It was several months before Lenore overcame scheduling obstacles and anxieties to make the trip. There she saw her mother's childhood home, heard both poignant and funny stories about her mother's life, and learned how high-spirited she had been before her illness. Her aunt gave her a letter written by her mother shortly before her death, confiding that the hardest part about dying was not

being able to be there for Lenore, and expressing her regret that the illness had robbed her of the strength to do all she might have for her. Lenore's enlarged view of her mother and their relationship, along with the new connection with her aunt and their hometown, were enormously healing. She felt more "full of life" and became more engaged in other relationships. Single with no children of her own, she was a talented schoolteacher, but she had a reputation for being cool and aloof. She brought her new "spiritedness" to her work and to more meaningful connections with her students.

Through memory and inspiration, we carry on connections with loved ones who have died. Alice Walker (1983), describing her adult relationship with her own grown daughter, once said, "This great friendship of ours is pretty eternal. I often tell her that no matter what, I will always be with her. It's my sense that the real incarnation is not necessarily coming back as someone else but, just as you inherit your mother's brown eyes, you inherit part of her soul."

RECONCILIATION IN MARRIAGE AND DIVORCE

Couples on the Brink of Divorce

In every couple relationship, there are times of trouble and tensions that can lead to disconnection. For couples today there is a greater need to reconcile differences that heighten the risk for conflict. Partners from different cultures, races, and religions bring different values and expectations to their relationship. Stresses of job and family demands and changing gender role relations add to the challenges. We expect more from committed partnerships than ever before, leading to greater frustration and disappointment when unrealistic dreams and incompatibilities collide. If we can help each partner to value the uniqueness of the other and honor the differences, these can add to the richness of the relationship.

Couple therapists, for all our experience, cannot reliably predict which couples will stay together and which will ultimately split up. Often couples come to therapy hoping that we will tell them what they should do or confirm their belief that their situation is hopeless. Often individuals consider leaving as their only option when they feel powerless in the relationship. Therapists can understand their pessimism about change, and yet encourage them not to walk away without assessing conjointly the possibilities for relational healing. Spouses often ruminate over whether to stay or to go, viewing their situation in a "stick with it or leave it" manner; staying means accepting the status quo, which may be intolerable. Couple consultations can help both partners identify and communicate changes needed for them to reinvest in the relationship and work toward shared aims in therapy. Partners can be helped to reframe accusations and complaints in terms of their own needs for a satisfying relationship, and to clarify positive aims to work toward. The possibility of reconciliation for a couple, as for a family-of-origin relationship, depends most on the depth of the will to reconcile. It requires a readiness to take the other person seriously, acknowledge violations, and make amends for the pain suffered.

A strong relationship is a loving collaboration that requires flexibility, mutual accommodation, and shared commitment. Because partners and circumstances inevitably change, all enduring relationships require regeneration, updating, and renegotiation of vows and mutual expectations (the relational "quid pro quo"). Herbert Anderson proposes the ritual of "promising again," an intentional, mutual renewal of vows requiring that each partner actively choose the other again for a committed relationship (Anderson et al., 1995). Such a ritual can occur at a transition or crisis when the customary ways of being together no longer work. Recommitment—including vows of needed change—is necessary when promises have been broken or can't be kept in the form in which they were made. The act of "promising again" expresses the choice of hope over despair. The renewal promotes new life in the bond—a vital reconnection to sustain and strengthen a relationship over its life course. Reconciliation, catalyzing needed change, brings partners to a deeper place of trust and commitment.

Healing and Reconciliation after Divorce

When a marriage is irreparably broken, how families handle adaptational processes over time can make all the difference for recovery and resilience of all members and their relationships. Divorce is rarely a quick and easy decision. It involves a complicated web of feelings and transactional processes from the first consideration of separation, through failed attempts to reconcile, tangled legal proceedings, painful losses and transitional upheavals, reorganization of households, revision of life plans, and further alterations with remarriage.

However, studies show that divorce need not shatter relationships and children's lives, so it's crucial to challenge pessimistic assumptions and labels of "children of divorce" (Bernstein, in press). Children's functioning and relationships with divorced parents often improve when no longer embedded in ongoing marital strife. In nearly half of postdivorce families, parents are able to work out amicable coparenting relationships, and many former spouses are able to sustain an informal kinship connection (Ahrons, 2004). This involves reconfiguration of family structural patterns and renegotiation of relationships.

Unfortunately, our society's ethos—just put troubles behind you and move on (a mistaken view of resilience)—leads many to cut off from troubled relationships and plunge into a new ones, as in the following case:

> Gary, age 45, requested help "to get my wife—I mean my life—in order." He explained that his prior individual therapy had helped him realize that his 18-year marriage was hopelessly dysfunctional (even though the therapist had never met his wife or suggested couple therapy). That had freed him to leave his marriage for a new, energizing affair. He remarried immediately on the heels of a bitter divorce; the new couple had a baby within the year. His teenage kids refused to see him and sent back his birthday presents unopened. Gary blamed his "ex" for turning them against him. Their continuing stormy relationships, with constant sniping and disputes over visitation and support, were now seriously straining his current marriage. Why, he wondered, couldn't they just get on with their lives and accept the new realities?
>
> A session with Gary's older children and their mother, Cindy, revealed their rage that he could just cast them off and instantly create a new family to replace them. The oldest daughter was particularly upset that Gary was so doting on his new son—much more involved than he had ever been with her. Cindy was furious for having sidelined her own needs over the years while Gary was building his career. With his abrupt departure, the whole family felt suddenly ripped apart. Gary's refusal to talk about the past left the reasons for the breakup ambiguous. Cindy tried in vain to make sense of it all—first blaming the other woman and then blaming herself. If he could be so loving with a new wife and child, maybe it was all her fault. The daughters doubted their own lovability and their ability to trust men. It was crucial to heal the wounds of the breakup and to strive to reconcile grievances and transform relationships rather than cut them off.

Overcoming Barriers to Postdivorce Reconciliation

Reconciliation is distinct from reunion. It involves coming to terms with difficult and painful aspects of a relationship in order to integrate the experience and move ahead in life. Intense, mixed emotions are common in relationship endings. As Ahrons (2004) has found, many former partners are able to put old grievances in perspective and reconcile hurts and hostilities to the extent that they can collaborate in raising their children and can maintain cordial, respectful relations. It's crucial to clarify ambiguities that may fuel children's reunion fantasies: They will not be getting back together as a couple or a family unit, but they will always do their best to be there for the children.

Counseling and mediation can be useful in overcoming barriers to such reconciliation (Bernstein, in press; Gorell Barnes, 1999). With divorce, a devaluing of the relationship and the other person commonly occurs; this loosens attachments, eases the pain of loss, and diminishes the sense of shame and guilt. The adversarial legal system intensifies conflict and polarization. Divorce holds stigmatizing implications of failure and inadequacy. As each partner grapples to make meaning of the painful loss, "divorce stories" take shape. Each partner's narrative construction of the marriage and its breakdown can influence relationships for years to come. Hetherington and colleagues (Hetherington & Kelly, 2002) found that postdivorce accounts given by ex-spouses were so different that "blind" raters could not match individuals who had been in the same marriage. Stories that demonize the ex-spouse can keep individuals trapped in a helpless, victimized position or an angry, accusatory stance. Those who feel depressed, enraged, or powerless over an undesired breakup or unforgivable actions by a former partner often try to punish the other. After fighting over possessions, men commonly withhold child support payments as women withhold visitation in a vicious cycle of reactivity and mutual retaliation. Therapists and mediators can lay important groundwork at the time of divorce to prevent such avoidable fallout.

Long-term follow-up studies show that most children's successful postdivorce adaptation is enhanced when both parents can remain involved with their children and collaborate as much as possible in their rearing and financial support. Joint legal custody facilitates continuing involvement but requires a high degree of mutual trust, cooperation, and communication. Without such collaboration, children tend to fare better in sole custody and a primary residence, while maintaining reliable contact with the nonresidential parent. An arrangement of "parallel parenting" is often most realistic. Parents each assume authority and responsibility for their own parenting, with an agreement not to interfere with the other's parental rights or to involve children in coalitions against the other. Yet, strong differences in household rules and expectations can burden children shuttling between two residences. Clinicians can help to minimize hostilities, to increase mutual respect between parents, and to agree on common guidelines so that children can be assured of reliable, nonconflictual relationships with both parents.

In cases where serious mental illness, addiction, abuse, or neglect precludes regular visits with a nonresidential parent, children can fare quite well with a sole parent or guardian who has strong executive functioning and adequate financial support. Phone calls, letters, and carefully supervised visits can be arranged whenever possible with the other parent, as well as contact with significant extended-family members.

There are many losses with divorce. Even if the partner or relationship was deeply disappointing or hurtful, divorce also involves the loss of the intact family unit and the hopes and dreams for the future of the relationships. The emotional divorce often lags behind the legal divorce, especially when continuing involvement with children restimulates old attachments and conflicts. Ambiguous loss complicates griefwork (Boss, 1999). Unlike widowhood, in divorce the marriage and intact family unit are lost, but the former partner and each parent live on, moving into separate lives and new relationships. The ex-partners are no longer a couple, and yet they remain coparents to children for the rest of their lives. The reigniting of painful, complicated feelings on contact fuels much postdivorce conflict and cutoff. One divorced man found it so upsetting to have to ring the doorbell of his former home to take his children out that he moved away and stopped seeing his children. Arranging pickups and drop-offs at school or other neutral places can ease such tensions. Internet services now facilitate such ongoing negotiations.

The tendency to vilify an ex-spouse is as strong as the tendency to overromanticize a new partner. The blame, shame, and guilt surrounding divorce, further inflamed by our adversarial legal system, often fuel brutal character assassinations that rationalize the divorce or a desired settlement. Many individuals are so hurt or bitter in the aftermath of divorce that they lose sight of the positive aspects of their former partners and their relationships, which connected them in the first place and may have yielded many good years. It takes maturity and generosity to resist joining in blaming indictments by well-intentioned family or friends. The actress Ingrid Bergman, in response to an interviewer's putdown of her ex-husbands, replied, "Please don't speak badly of them; they were wonderful men or I never would have married them."

For postdivorce resilience, it is vital to understand the hopes and dreams, the energies and efforts that were invested in a couple and in family relationships alongside disappointments and losses. It's also important to consider the contribution of each family of origin to marital expectations. I asked Joel, recently divorced, when troubles had begun. He replied, "Even before the honeymoon!" At the wedding, his father had congratulated him on finding a woman just like his mother—whom the father had constantly berated throughout their marriage. Joel noted, "That was the kiss of death for my marriage."

A client who is stuck in destructive, stereotypical victim–villain scenarios can be helped to revise such stories to include the many dimensions of the former partner and relationship, or shared pride in their children. A therapist can encourage review of the history of the relationship, from courtship through the high and low points, noting the stressors that contributed to tensions. It's also useful for clients to gain clarifying information and perspectives from the ex-spouse, other important family members, and close friends, to comprehend more clearly how the marriage dissolved. One woman, feeling inadequate for not having met her ex-husband's sexual needs, was encouraged, a year after their divorce, to ask him to meet with her and her therapist to better understand his decision to leave. He revealed that he had come to acknowledge that he was gay and could no longer live a lie. Yet, because of social stigma, he had not been able to reveal it openly at the time.

Adaptation is facilitated when both ex-partners can own their parts in the breakdown of a relationship over time. A therapist can pose questions that encourage a rebalance of negative views to include positive aspects of each other and the relationship. Helping ex-partners to make meaning of their relationship and acknowledge their part in its ending can greatly facilitate the emotional resolution of the divorce, in order to move on with life without rancor or bitterness. A sense of dislocation, loss of security, and uncertainty about the future can all fuel anxiety. With a breakup, core beliefs and assumptions about oneself and the relationship are all reexamined (e.g., "Who am I if not in relation to you? How will we manage financially?"). A therapist's questions can also encourage future-oriented possibilities: "What strengths do you see the two of you having that could help to reduce conflict? How might you set aside differences in order to collaborate in raising your children?" It's important to help the ex-partners accept what can't be changed and consider their possible options to do their best for their children's future. With time and effort, many former spouses can transform a ruptured partnership into caring kinship. One man, visiting his seriously ill ex-wife in the hospital, was unsure how to introduce himself when the doctor stopped by. His former wife said simply, "This is Sam; he's my children's father. We were together for many years, and now he's my good friend for life."

Reweaving Extended Family Ties after Divorce

In conflictual divorces, the families of origin commonly choose sides or are pushed to the margins. They often risk losing precious contact with grandchildren. Active efforts can be made to avoid triangulations and to sustain extended family ties. We can strongly encourage clients to facilitate strong connections for their children and to consider the kinds of relationships they themselves would like to maintain with former in-laws and extended family members.

One source of discomfort concerns our language and categories to define these relations, other than jokingly referring to former in-laws as "outlaws." Many years after my own divorce and remarriage, I was pleasantly surprised to hear my daughter's cousin on her father's side (my careful construction) still call me simply "Aunt Froma." I was delighted that she felt comfortable staying at our home for an overnight visit, yet I was unsure whether I could still think of her as "my niece." And what should she call my husband? "Step-uncle" seemed as absurd as "ex-aunt." Many cultures don't have our problems with language and formality in regard to family reconfigurations; they value a wide variety and continuity of informal kin ties, recognizing that children's lives are nourished by having many brothers, sisters, aunts, uncles, cousins, grandparents, and godparents—whether "step" or otherwise. In turn, the lives of elders are enriched by these dense and overlapping connections. Resilience is strengthened by forging many varied kinship bonds.

Bridging the Old and the New in Remarriage

Over two-thirds of divorced individuals go on to remarry, and many bring unresolved issues into the new relationships that contribute to the higher risk of divorce in remarriage. Researchers find that the biggest mistake in remarriage is the misguided attempt to cut ties to the past, to seal a border around the new family unit, and to emulate an intact nuclear family model (Visher, Visher, & Pasley, 2003). Children are at higher risk of dysfunction when they are drawn into loyalty conflicts, cut off from caring biological parents, or expected to form an instant replacement bond with a stepparent. Fathers who are estranged from their children in previous marriages often become blocked from developing relationships with stepchildren. Working through feelings of loss, guilt,

and fears of attachment can facilitate both reconnection and new connections. We can also help new partners understand children's need to
maintain bonds with both biological parents, in most cases. Where they
feel jealous of or threatened by a good relationship between the ex-partners,
it's helpful to frame relationships as a collaborative parenting team
across households. Children will more readily form positive step-relations
when they are not forced to take sides. The resilience of stepfamilies and
long-term adaptation of children are strongest, in most cases, when open
boundaries and kin connections across households are encouraged.

WHAT CAN BE LEARNED?: LESSONS FOR THE FUTURE

Resilience can be forged out of the cauldron of past trauma as we integrate those painful experiences into the fabric of our lives and our relationships. We can seize opportunities for transformation and growth in
our personal lives, our wider communities, and our global connections.

Transcending Trauma

In one of the most painful and enduring photo images of the Vietnam
War, 9-year-old Phan Thi Kim Phuc was running naked, her arms out-
stretched, screaming in agony and terror as napalm seared her body. She
endured a score of surgical procedures and became a political symbol of
the horror of war. By her mid-30s, she felt she was finally living a "normal, happy life" with her husband and small son in an Asian neighborhood in Toronto. In an act of reconciliation nearly 25 years after her
ordeal, she went to Washington, DC, to lay a wreath at the Vietnam
Veterans' Memorial on Veterans' Day 1996. Speaking before a large audience who greeted her with standing ovations, she told them:

> "I have suffered a lot from both physical and emotional pain. Sometimes
> I could not breathe. But God saved my life and gave me faith and hope.
> Even if I could talk face to face with the pilot who dropped the bombs, I
> would tell him, 'We cannot change history, but we should try to do good
> things for the present and for the future to promote peace.' " (Quoted in
> Sciolino, 1996, p. A1)

As PhanThi Kim Phuc chose, we can suffer brutal atrocities and yet not
be locked into a perpetual identity as victims. The first victimization may

be beyond our control; avoiding the trap of a victimized life stance is within our power. Instead, we can forge resilience by rising above the trauma, transforming the experience to galvanize our determination to make significant changes for the better.

Expanding Possibilities for Forgiveness

In fostering healing and resilience, traumatic events in the past are not erased, but perceptions and feelings concerning them, as well as their implications for our lives, can be fundamentally altered. When there has been serious harm and injustice the question of forgiveness arises. In exploring possibilities for forgiveness, we can encourage clients to shift from endless condemnation of the offender to learn how patterns of harm or injustice evolved, viewing them in social and historical context.

When a relational injustice has occurred in a couple, a family, a community, or between ethnic groups or nations, it's reasonable and just to expect the offender to be held accountable. Forgiveness and reconciliation are facilitated when wrongdoers accept responsibility for the injustice and resulting harm and vow never again to repeat it. Forgiveness is also fostered by meaningful compensation for past injustices and by trustworthy actions in the future.

In many cultural and religious traditions, forgiveness does not require acknowledgment or compensatory efforts by the offender. In the Hindu religion, such as in the Bhagavad Gita, it is said: If you want to see the brave, look at those who can forgive. It involves taking a courageous position that frees those who forgive from hatred and bitterness and opens pathways for healing and transcendence. Recent theory and research on forgiveness view it as an emotion-focused coping strategy that can reduce health risks and promote resilience in those who forgive (Worthington & Scherer, 2004). As we saw in Chapter 11, in the case of the murder of a teenager the mother's journey of forgiveness was begun primarily for her own and her family's healing, but also contributed to remarkable transformation for the bereaved family and for the offender. He rose above his initial lack of concern to take accountability, had genuine remorse, and devoted his full efforts to turning his life around. The compassion shown between the victim's parents and the offender's parents brought mutual healing.

Essentially, forgiving involves relationship transformation. The process balances personal needs to maintain integrity and protection with efforts to tap family resources of love and trust that will strengthen the individual and bear fruit in other relationships. Reconciliation may—or may not—involve forgiveness for the part of the relationship that was a violation. In many cases, one may not forgive that part, but can forgive the person and heal the relationship. In doing so, one honors the hurtful experience while keeping it in its place so that it doesn't destroy the whole.

Forgive and Remember

Contrary to the popular saying "Forgive and forget," forgiveness does not mean that the slate is wiped clean or that harmful actions should be forgotten. The pain attached to past injustices does tend to fade with time if reconciliation and forgiveness are achieved, especially when love and trust are rebuilt. However, if we forget the damage that occurred, we may not learn from it to take the steps necessary to prevent such actions from happening again in the future. Trust is best restored not when family members (or a society) act as if no violation ever occurred, but rather when they remain mindful of the past and strive to relate differently. New terms for the relationship must be set to ensure that such damage never again occurs.

Forgiveness is often confused with forgetting. Forgiving the person is confused with forgiving the offense. Understanding how past traumas contributed to parental vulnerabilities and limitations does not excuse violations. Family members must be held accountable for their motives, actions, and consequences. To explore possibilities, as therapists we might ask clients: "Are there any parts of the experience that can be forgiven? What might make it possible for you to forgive the person, if not the actions? Would it be possible to forgive the person if he or she made an effort to change and were able to acknowledge and apologize with genuine remorse? To demonstrate genuine interest in you and your well-being?"

Can or should the wounded forgive those who abused or were destructive? It is not up to therapists or other well-intended advisors to make that decision for any individual or family. Although it can be enormously fruitful, it is a decision that is up to each person who has been offended. Forgiveness is extremely complex; different paths may be taken in varied situations. When a priest has sexually abused parishioners he has also betrayed his religious vows and the trust of the faith community. When a person abuses power, seriously harms another, and violates trust, it must be weighed quite seriously. Intrafamilial relational violations are among the most devastating. One woman felt that she could never forgive her father for killing her mother. If some form of abuse continues to be a threat, the abused person might run an unwise risk to pursue a forgiving relationship with the offender. Some individuals may decide that forgiveness is not possible for them. In each case, emotional, relational, and ethical dilemmas must be grappled with. As therapists we can try to help clients to gather information and weigh various perspectives to make events, relationships, and actions more comprehensible as they come to their own decisions.

In families where there has been abuse, neglect, or other destructive behavior, therapists can strive to help clients reach a position of holding those family members accountable for their behavior, yet without blaming indictment. Therapy can attempt to increase understanding of formative experiences that shaped the vulnerabilities and limitations of those individuals. In doing so, it can generate empathy for the offender's experiences of suffering. We can encourage clients' refusal to spend their own lives immersed in accusation and bitterness. Above all, this entails our compassionate response to those who have suffered, and yet also extends compassion to parents or other offenders for their hardship and suffering. In many cases, offenders also need therapists' help in forgiving themselves for past wrongs or shameful actions.

The ability of resilient individuals and families to emerge from traumatic situations strong and healthy should not imply that they are weak and deficient if they are more deeply wounded and less hardy in recovery. Judith Herman (1992) has stressed the importance of "moral solidarity," with respect for those struggling with trauma, because they are most in need of hope and least in need of another reason to feel bad about themselves.

Truth Telling and Justice

In rebalancing stories and legacies of our history to highlight heroes and positive models, we must be careful not to tilt to the other extreme. We have to face the unpleasant as well as the affirmative side of the human story, including our own story as a nation and our own stories of our peoples. Our history as a society, like history in families, is too easily written in the voice of its dominant members, with the experiences of the marginalized and vulnerable silenced (Hernandez, 2002). In many cases, we must have the ugly facts in order to challenge the official view of reality.

W. E. B. DuBois (1935/1964) wrote of his astonishment in the study of history at the recurrence of the idea that evil must be forgotten, distorted, skimmed over. We are taught to forget that George Washington was a slave owner and simply remember the things we regard as creditable and inspiring. "The difficulty, of course, with this philosophy is that history loses its value as an incentive and example; it paints perfect men and noble nations, but does not tell the truth" (p. 722). Sadly, great nations, like our own, too often have difficulty acknowledging and repairing past injustices and harm, from slavery and genocide of native peoples to the destruction and dehumanization of wars.

Truth is at least half of justice when human rights have been violated, whether in a family, a community, or a nation. A unique experiment, the Truth and Reconciliation Commission, was formed in South Africa to gather facts and publish historical records about past atrocities during apartheid. Those who committed crimes were obliged, at the very least, to acknowledge their deeds publicly as a necessary condition of a plan for amnesty. Amnesty was then considered and offered on a case-by-case basis. In one situation, for instance, a police captain who had killed 13 women and children admitted and apologized for his actions to the victims' families, asking them "to consider" forgiving him. It was then the families' decision as to whether their forgiveness was possible (Gobodo-Madikizela, 2002).

Compensation can often further a sense of justice. Yet in some cases, survivors may feel that horrific crimes are beyond compensation. Even when survivors are unable to forgive, telling and learning the truth about past atrocities is important for a brutalized individual, group, or society to bind up wounds. It offers details about what happened and more catharsis for those who have suffered. Making sense of the senseless helps to render the horrific intelligible. The ambitious experiment in South Africa was fraught with dilemmas, as many perpetrators seeking amnesty were accused of distorting or covering up facts to deny or minimize their role. For a fully just account, the entire truth must be told. Yet in an imperfect world, such societal efforts to resist revenge and retribution and instead to seek a healing justice can foster vital transformation.

Reviving trauma can initially increase pain and conflict, especially if the cold facts are brutal or shameful. Yet the ability to integrate painful experience and move on with life is furthered by the whole truth, including its comprehension within the context of its time and place. In the words of Martin Luther King, "the truth will set you free."

Learning from History: Informing and Inspiring our Best

History is essential to our ongoing understanding of ourselves, our families, and our culture. All of us have a deep need to be connected to the larger society and to our own history, as Susan Griffin (1993) asserts:

All history, including the histories of our families, is part of us, such that
when we hear any secret revealed, a secret about a grandfather or an uncle, or a secret about the Battle of Dresden in 1945, our lives are made
suddenly clearer to us, as the unnatural heaviness of unspoken truth is
dispersed. For perhaps we are like stones—our own history and the history of the world embedded in us; we hold the sorrow deep within and
cannot weep until that history is sung.

Lifting the "heaviness of unspoken truth" is part of the process of opening communication across the generations and in our social world.

History tends to be written by the most powerful, to support their
privilege and legitimize their actions. We need to expand the power of
history to people who have been unjustly or brutally treated and
marginalized, either within their families or by societies, so that all of us
are empowered to use our understanding of the past to inform and inspire our best actions in the present and the future.

Spirit with a Broken Heart

In the powerful video documentary *The West* (Ives, Abramson, &
Kantor, 1996), Albert White Hat, a Lakota Indian teacher and mentor,
tells of his struggle to come to terms with the genocidal atrocities committed against his tribe over more than 150 years, which churned inside
his entire being:

> I grew up with a lot of the older people, listened to the stories. The sto-
> ries were inside of me. I went into a boarding school system and they
> killed those stories in that system. I came to be ashamed of who I am,
> what I am.
>
> In the late '60s I returned to the culture, let my hair grow, and
> started speaking the language. I did the Vision Quest for 5 years; I
> fasted. . . . One of those times, it was a beautiful night, the stars were
> out, it was calm, and around midnight I got up and I prayed and sat
> there a while. Then all of a sudden I had these flashbacks—of Sand
> Creek, Wounded Knee—and every policy, every law that was imposed
> on us by the churches hit me one at a time and how it affected my life.
> And as I sat there I got angrier and angrier, till it turned to hatred. And
> I looked at this whole situation, the whole history, and there was
> nothing I could do. It was too much. The only thing I could do, to me,
> was: When I come off that hill I'm going to grab a gun and I'm going
> to start shooting; and then maybe my grandfathers will honor me if I
> go that route.
>
> I got up and I turned around and faced the East and it was beau-

tiful; there was dawn light. Right above that blue light in the darkness was the sliver of the moon in the morning. And I wanted to live. I wanted to live and be happy. I feel I deserve it. But the only way I was going to do that was if I forgive. And I cried that morning because I had to forgive.

Since then I work every day on that commitment. Now, I don't know how many people feel that way, but every one of us, if you're a Lakota, you have to deal with this at some point in your life. You have to address that and you have to make a decision. If you don't, you're going to die on the road someplace, either from being too drunk or from putting a bullet in your head. So this isn't history; it's still with us. What has happened in the past will never leave us. The next 100 years it will be with us. And we have to deal with it every day.

As Albert White Hat came to realize, if we are consumed by rage, however justified, it can enslave our present and our future to past horrors, and preclude our having a decent life.

We may be drawn to the wish-fulfilling fantasy of a time machine that will allow us to go back to the past, so that we can change it. Although we can't revise the past in that way, we can revise and enlarge our perspectives on that past, learn from it, and vow to live and relate differently. This involves mastering the art of the possible, a core process in resilience.

We can strive to make meaning of past hurt and injustice, and then draw upon our inner resources and bonds with loved ones, our larger communities, and transcendent values, in order to live and love to our fullest potential and to leave positive legacies for the future. As children in our families of origin, we had little control over traumatic events; as adults and parents, we have the power and opportunity to do better— with our own children and with all others in our lives. Our shared future will be promising if we can come to understand our lives, gain compassion for the struggles of others, and take up our responsibilities to all living things.

References

Ahrons, C. (2004). *We're still family.* New York: HarperCollins.

Almeida, R., Woods, R., Messineo, T., & Font, R. (1998). The cultural context model: An overview. In M. McGoldrick (Ed.), *Re-visioning family therapy: Race, culture, and gender in clinical practice* (pp. 414–431). New York: Guilord Press.

Amato, P. R., & Fowler, F. (2002). Parenting practices, child adjustment, and family diversity. *Journal of Marriage and the Family, 64,* 708–716.

American Psychiatric Association. (2000). *Diagnostic and statistical manual of mental disorders* (4th ed., text rev.). Washington, DC: Author.

Anderson, C. M. (2003). The diversity, strengths, and challenges of single-parent households. In F. Walsh (Ed.), *Normal family processes: Growing diversity and complexity* (3rd ed., pp. 121–152). New York: Guilford Press.

Anderson, C. M., Reiss, D., & Hogarty, G. (1986). *Schizophrenia and the family.* New York: Guilford Press.

Anderson, C. M., & Stewart, S. (1994). *Flying solo: Women at midlife and beyond.* New York: Norton.

Anderson, H. (1997). *Conversation, language, and possibilities: A postmodern approach to therapy.* New York: Basic Books.

Anderson, H., Hogue, D., & McCarthy, M. (1995). *Promising again.* Louisville, KY: Westminster Press.

Anderson, R. (1968). *I never sang for my father.* New York: Random House.

Angelou, M. (1986). *Poems: Maya Angelou.* New York: Bantam Books.

Angelou, M. (1993, January 19). *On the pulse of morning.* Inaugural poem, Washington, DC.

Anthony, E. J. (1987). Risk, vulnerability, and resilience: An overview. In E. J. Anthony & B. Cohler (Eds.), *The invulnerable child* (pp. 3–48). New York: Guilford Press.

Antonovsky, A. (1987). *Unraveling the mystery of health.* San Francisco: Jossey-Bass.

Antonovsky, A. (1993). The structure and properties of the Sense of Coherence Scale. *Social Science and Medicine, 36*(6), 725–733.

Antonovsky, A. (1998). The sense of coherence: An historical and future perspective. In

H. McCubbin, E. Thompson, A. Thompson, & J. Fromer (Eds.), *Stress, coping and health in families: Sense of coherence and resiliency* (pp. 3–20). Thousand Oaks, CA: Sage.

Antonovsky, A., & Sourani, T. (1988). Family sense of coherence and family adaptation. *Journal of Marriage and the Family, 50,* 79–92.

Aponte, H. (1994). *Bread and spirit: Therapy with the new poor.* New York: Norton.

Barnes, G. G. (1999). Divorce transitions: Identifying risk and promoting resilience for children and their parental relationships. *Journal of Marital and Family Therapy, 25*(4), 425–444.

Barnett, R. C., & Hyde, J. (2001). Women, men, work, and family. *American Psychologist, 56,* 781–796.

Bateson, G. (1979). *Mind and nature: A necessary unity.* New York: Dutton.

Bateson, M. C. (1989). *Composing a life.* New York: Atlantic Monthly Press.

Bateson, M. C. (1994). *Peripheral visions.* New York: HarperCollins.

Beavers, W. R., & Hampson, R. B. (1990). *Successful families: Assessment and intervention.* New York: Norton.

Beavers, W. R., & Hampson, R. B. (2003). Measuring family competence: The Beavers Systems model. In F. Walsh (Ed.), *Normal family processes* (3rd ed., pp. 549–580). New York: Guilford Press.

Beck, A., Rush, A., Shaw, B. F., & Emory, G. (1987). *Cognitive therapy of depression.* New York: Guilford Press.

Becker, C., Sargent, J., & Rolland, J. (2000). Kosovar Family Professional Education Collaborative. *American Family Therapy Academy Newsletter, 80,* 26–30.

Becker, E. (1973). *The denial of death.* New York: Free Press.

Becvar, D. (2001). *In the presence of grief: Helping family members resolve death, dying, and bereavement issues.* New York: Guilford Press.

Bellah, R., Madsen, R., Sullivan, W., Swidler, A., & Tipton, S. (1985). *Habits of the heart: Individualism and commitment in American life.* Berkeley: University of California Press.

Bengston, V. G. (2001). Beyond the nuclear family: The increasing importance of multigenerational bonds. *Journal of Marriage and the Family, 63,* 1–16.

Berg, I. (1997). *Family-based services: A solution-focused approach.* New York: Norton.

Bernstein, A. (in press). Re-visioning, restructuring, and reconciliation: Clinical practice with complex post-divorce families. *Family Process, 45*(1).

Billingsley, A. (1992). *Climbing Jacob's ladder: The enduring legacy of African American families.* New York: Simon & Schuster.

Bonanno, G. (2004). Loss, trauma, and human resilience. *American Psychologist, 59*(1), 20–28.

Boss, P. (1999). *Ambiguous loss: Learning to live with unresolved grief.* Cambridge, MA: Harvard University Press.

Boss, P. (2001). *Family stress management: A contextual approach* (2nd ed.). Newbury Park, CA: Sage.

Boss, P., Beaulieu, L., Weiling, E., & Turner, W. (2003). Healing loss, ambiguity, and trauma: A community-based intervention with families of union workers missing after the 9/11 attack in New York City. *Journal of Marital and Family Therapy, 29*(4), 455–467.

Boszormenyi-Nagy, I. (1987). *Foundations of contextual family therapy.* New York: Brunner/Mazel.

Bowen, M. (1978). *Family therapy in clinical practice*. New York: Jason Aronson.

Bowlby, J. (1988). *A secure base: Parent–child attachment and healthy human development*. New York: Basic Books.

Boyd-Franklin, N. (2004). *Black families in therapy: A multi-systems approach* (2nd ed.). New York: Guilford Press.

Boyd-Franklin, N., & Franklin, A. J. (2001). *Boys into men: Raising our African-American teenage sons*. New York: Plume.

Braverman, L. (1989). The myths of motherhood. In M. McGoldrick, C. Anderson, & F. Walsh (Eds.), *Women in families: A framework for family therapy* (pp. 227–243). New York: Norton.

Bronfenbrenner, U. (1979). *The ecology of human development*. Cambridge, MA: Harvard University Press.

Brooks, R. B. (1994). Children at risk: Fostering resilience and hope. *American Journal of Orthopsychiatry, 64*, 545–553.

Bruner, J. (1986). *Actual minds, possible worlds*. Cambridge, MA: Harvard University Press.

Brunner, E. (1984). *Revelation and reason*. Raleigh, NC: Stevens Book Press.

Butler, K. (1997, March–April). The anatomy of resilience. *Family Therapy Networker*, pp. 22–31.

Byng-Hall, J. (1995a). *Rewriting family scripts: Improvisation and systems change*. New York: Guilford Press.

Byng-Hall, J. (1995b). Creating a secure family base: Some implications of attachment theory for family therapy. *Family Process, 34*(1), 45–58.

Calhoun, L. G., & Tedeschi, R. G. (1999). *Facilitating post-traumatic growth: A clinician's guide*. Mahwah, NJ: Erlbaum.

Campbell, J. (1988). *The power of myth*. New York: Doubleday.

Campbell, T. (2003). The effectiveness of family interventions for physical disorders. *Journal of Marital and Family Therapy, 29*(2), 263–281.

Carter, B., & McGoldrick, M. (Eds.). (2004). *The expanded life cycle: Individual, family, and social perspectives* (3rd ed.). Needham Heights, MA: Allyn & Bacon. (Original edition published 1999)

Carter, B., & McGoldrick, M. (2001). Advances in coaching: Family therapy with one person. *Journal of Marital and Family Therapy, 27*, 281–300.

Catherall, D. R. (1992). *Back from the brink: A family guide to overcoming traumatic stress*. New York: Bantam Books.

Catherall, D. R. (Ed.). (2004). *Handbook of stress, trauma, and the family*. New York: Brunner-Routledge.

Cederblad, M., & Hansson, K. (1996). Sense of coherence—A concept influencing health and quality of life in a Swedish psychiatric at-risk group. *Israel Journal of Medical Science, 32*, 194–199.

Center for Research on Child Well-being. (2003). *Barriers to marriage among fragile families*. (Fragile Families Research Brief No. 16). Washington, DC: Author.

Central Conference of American Rabbis. (1992). *Gates of prayer for weekdays and at a house of mourning: A gender-sensitive prayerbook*. New York: Author.

Children's Defense Fund. (1992). *Helping children by strengthening families: A look at family support programs*. Chicago: Family Resource Coalition.

Clinton, H. R. (1996). *It takes a village*. New York: Simon & Schuster.

Cohen, O., Slonim, I., Finzi, R., & Leichtentritt, R. (2002). Family resilience: Israeli mothers' perspectives. *American Journal of Family Therapy, 30*, 173–187.

Cohler, B. (1987). Adversity, resilience, and the study of lives. In E. J. Anthony & B. Cohler (Eds.), *The invulnerable child* (pp. 363–424). New York: Guilford Press.

Cohler, B. (1991). The life story and the study of resilience and response to adversity. *Journal of Narrative and Life History, 1*, 169–200.

Coles, R. (1967). *Children of crisis: A study of courage and fear.* Boston: Little, Brown.

Coles, R. (1997). *The moral intelligence of children.* New York: Random House.

Combrinck-Graham, L. (Ed.). (1995). *Children in families at risk: Maintaining the connections.* New York: Guilford Press.

Conger, R. D., & Conger, K. J. (2002). Resilience in Midwestern families: Selected findings from the first decade of a prospective, longitudinal study. *Journal of Marriage and the Family, 64*(2), 361–373.

Coontz, S. (1997). *The way we really are: Coming to terms with America's changing families.* New York: Basic Books.

Coontz, S. (2005). *The history of marriage.* New York: Viking.

Cousins, N. (1989). *Head first: The biology of hope.* New York: Dutton.

Csikszentmihalyi, M. (1996). *Creativity: Flow and the psychology of discovery and invention.* New York: HarperCollins.

Danieli, Y. (1985). The treatment and prevention of long-term effects and intergenerational transmission of victimization: A lesson from Holocaust survivors and their children. In C. R. Figley (Ed.), *Trauma and its wake* (pp. 295–313). New York: Brunner/Mazel.

DeFrain, J. (1991). Learning about grief from normal families: SIDS, stillbirth, and miscarriage. *Journal of Marital and Family Therapy, 18*, 215–323.

Deloria, V., Jr. (1994). *God is red: A native view of religion* (2nd ed.). Golden, CO: Fulcrum.

de Shazer, S. (1985). *Keys to solution in brief therapy.* New York: Norton.

DeSilva, C. (Ed.). (1996). *In memory's kitchen: A legacy from the women of Terezin.* New York: Jason Aronson.

Doherty, W. (1996). *The intentional family.* New York: HarperCollins.

Doka, K. (1996). *Living with grief after sudden loss.* Washington, DC: Taylor & Francis.

Doka, K. (2002). *Disenfranchised grief.* Champaign, IL: Research Press.

Dossey, D. (1993). *Healing words: The power of prayer and the practice of medicine.* New York: Harper.

Driver, J., Tabares, A., Shapiro, A., Nahm, E. Y., & Gottman, J. (2003). Interactional patterns in marital success or failure: Gottman Laboratory Studies. In F. Walsh (Ed.), *Normal family processes* (3rd ed., pp. 493–513). New York: Guilford Press.

Dugan, T., & Coles, R. (Eds.). (1989). *The child in our times: Studies in the development of resiliency.* New York: Brunner/Mazel.

Dunst, C. (1995). *Key characteristics and features of community-based family support programs.* Chicago: Family Resource Coalition.

Ehrle, J., & Green, R. (2002). *Children cared for by relatives: Identifying service needs.* Washington, DC: Urban Institute, National Survey of American Families.

Emmerik, A., Kamphuis, A., Hulsbosch, P., & Emmelkamp, P. (2002). Single-session debriefing after psychological trauma: A meta-analysis. *Lancet, 360*, 766–771.

Epstein, N., Ryan, C., Bishop, D., Miller, I., & Keitner, G. (2003). The McMaster model: A view of healthy family functioning. In F. Walsh (Ed.), *Normal family processes* (3rd ed., pp. 581–607). New York: Guilford Press.

Erikson, K. T. (1976). *Everything in its path: Destruction of community in the Buffalo Creek flood.* New York: Simon & Schuster.

Fadiman, A. (1997). *The spirit catches you and you fall down*. San Francisco: Ferrer.

Falicov, C. J. (Ed.). (1988). *Family transitions: Continuity and change over the life cycle*. New York: Guilford Press.

Falicov, C. J. (1995). Training to think culturally: A multidimensional comparative framework. *Family Process, 34*, 373–388.

Falicov, C. J. (1998). *Latino families in therapy: A guide to multicultural practice*. New York: Guilford Press.

Falicov, C. J. (2003). Immigrant family process. In F. Walsh (Ed.), *Normal family processes* (3rd ed., pp. 280–300). New York: Guilford Press.

Family Resource Coalition. (1996). *Guidelines for family support practice*. Chicago: Author.

Felsman, J. K., & Vaillant, G. (1987). Resilient children as adults: A 40-year study. In E. J. Anthony & B. Cohler (Eds.), *The invulnerable child* (pp. 289–314). New York: Guilford Press.

Figley, C., & McCubbin, H. (Eds.). (1983). *Stress and the family: Coping with catastrophe*. New York: Brunner-Mazel.

Figley, C. (1998). *The traumatology of grieving*. San Francisco: Jossey-Bass.

Figley, C. R. (Ed.). (2002). *Treating compassion fatigue*. New York: Brunner-Routledge.

Fine, M., & Harvey, J. (2005). *Handbook of divorce and relationship dissolution*. Mahwah, NJ: Erlbaum.

Fowers, B., Lyons, E. M., & Montel, K. H. (1996). Positive illusions about marriage: Self-enhancement or relationship enhancement? *Journal of Family Psychology, 10*, 192–208.

Fraenkel, P. (2003). Contemporary two-parent families: Navigating work and family challenges. In F. Walsh (Ed.), *Normal family processes* (3rd ed., pp. 61–95). New York: Guilford Press.

Frankl, V. (1984). *Man's search for meaning*. New York: Simon & Schuster. (Original work published 1946)

Framo, J. (1992). *Family-of-origin therapy: An intergenerational approach*. New York: Brunner/Mazel.

Freedman, J., & Combs, G. (1996). *Narrative therapy*. New York: Norton.

Gallup, G., Jr., & Lindsey, D. M. (1999). *Surveying the religious landscape: Trends in U.S. beliefs*. Harrisburg, PA: Morehouse.

Ganong, L., & Coleman, M. (2002). Family resilience in multiple contexts. *Journal of Marriage and the Family, 64*, 346–348.

Garbarino, J. (1997). *Raising children in a socially toxic environment*. San Francisco: Jossey-Bass.

Garbarino, J., Kostelny, K., & Dubrow, N. (1991). *No place to be a child: Growing up in a war zone*. Lexington, MA: Lexington Books.

Garmezy, N. (1974). Vulnerability research and the issue of primary prevention. *American Journal of Orthopsychiatry, 44*, 101–116.

Garmezy, N. (1987). Stress, competence, and development: Continuities in the study of schizophrenic adults, children vulnerable to psychopathology, and the search for stress-resistant children. *American Journal of Orthopsychiatry, 57*, 159–174.

Garmezy, N. (1991). Resiliency and vulnerability to adverse developmental outcomes associated with poverty. *American Behavioral Scientist, 34*, 416–430.

Garmezy, N., & Rutter, M. (Eds.). (1983). *Stress, coping, and development in children*. New York: McGraw-Hill.

Geertz, C. (1986). Making experiences, authoring selves. In V. Turner & E. Bruner

(Eds.), *The anthropology of experience* (pp. 373–380). Chicago: University of Chicago Press.

Gergen, K. (1991). *The saturated self: Dilemmas of identity in contemporary life*. New York: Basic Books.

Gilgun, J. (1999). Mapping resilience as process among adults with childhood adversities. In H. I. McCubbin & E. A. Thompson (Eds.), *The dynamics of resilient families* (pp. 41–70). Thousand Oaks, CA: Sage.

Gitterman, A. (Ed.). (2001). *Handbook of social work practice with vulnerable and resilient populations*. New York: Columbia University Press.

Gobodo-Madikizela, P. (2002). Remorse, forgiveness, and rehumanization: Stories from South Africa. *Journal of Humanistic Psychology, 42*, 7–32.

Goldner, V. (1988). Gender and generation: Normative and covert hierarchies. *Family Process, 27*, 17–31.

Goleman, D. (1995). *EQ: Emotional intelligence*. New York: Bantam Books.

Gonzalez, S., & Steinglass, P. (2002). Application of multifamily groups in chronic medical disorders. In W. F. McFarlane (Ed.), *Multifamily groups in the treatment of severe psychiatric disorders* (pp. 315–340). New York: Guilford Press.

Gorell Barnes, G. (1999). Divorce transitions: Identifying risk and promoting resilience for children and their parental relationships. *Journal of Marital and Family Therapy, 25*(4), 425–441.

Gottman, J., & Silver, N. (1999). *The seven principles for making marriage work*. New York: Crown.

Gourevitch, P. (1998). *We wish to inform you that tomorrow we will be killed with our families: Stories from Rwanda*. New York: Picador.

Grandin, T., & Johnson, C. (2004). *Animals in translation: Using the mysteries of autism to decode animal behavior*. New York: Scribner.

Greeff, A. P., & Human, B. (2004). Resilience in families in which a parent has died. *American Journal of Family Therapy, 32*(1), 27–42.

Greeff, A. P., & Van der Merwe, S. (2004). Variables associated with resilience in divorced families. *Social Indicators Research, 68*(1), 59–75.

Green, R.-J. (2004). Risk and resilience in lesbian and gay couples. *Journal of Family Psychology, 18*(2), 290–292.

Green, R.-J., & Werner, P. D. (1996). Intrusiveness and closeness–caregiving: Rethinking the concept of family enmeshment. *Family Process, 35*, 115–136.

Greene, S., Anderson, E., Hetherington, E. M., Forgatch, M. S., & DeGarmo, D. S. (2003). Risk and resilience after divorce. In F. Walsh (Ed.), *Normal family processes* (3rd ed., pp. 96–120). New York: Guilford Press.

Griffin, S. (1993). *A chorus of stones*. New York: Anchor.

Griffith, J., & Griffith, M. (2002). *Encountering the sacred in psychotherapy*. New York: Guilford Press.

Grinker, R. R., & Spiegel, J. (1945). *Men under stress*. Philadelphia: Blakiston.

Haddock, S., Zimmerman, T., & Lyness, K. (2003). Changing gender norms: Transitional dilemmas. In F. Walsh (Ed.), *Normal family processes* (3rd ed., pp. 301–336). New York: Guilford Press.

Haley, J. (1976). *Problem-solving therapy*. San Francisco: Jossey-Bass.

Hansson, K., & Cederblad, M. (2004). Sense of coherence as a meta-theory for salutogenic family therapy. *Journal of Family Psychotherapy, 15*, 39–54.

Hansson, K., Olsson, M., & Cederblad, M. (2004). A salutogenic investigation and treatment of conduct disorder (CD). *Nordic Journal of Psychiatry, 58*(1), 5–16.

Hargrave, T. (1994). *Families and forgiveness.* New York: Brunner/Mazel.

Harris, I. B. (1996). *Children in jeopardy: Can we break the cycle of poverty?* New Haven, CT: Yale Child Study Center.

Harvey, A. R., & Hill, R. B. (2004). Africentric youth and family rites of passage program: Promoting resilience among at-risk African-American youths. *Social Work, 49*(1), 65–74.

Hauser, S. T. (1999). Understanding resilient outcomes: Adolescent lives across time and generations. *Journal of Research on Adolescence, 9*(1), 1–24.

Hauser, S., Vierya, M., Jacobson, A., & Wertlieb, D. (1985). Vulnerability and resilience in adolescence: Views from the family. *Journal of Adolescence, 5,* 81–100.

Hawley, D. R. (2000). Clinical implications of family resilience. *American Journal of Family Therapy, 28*(2), 101–116.

Hawley, D. R., & DeHaan, L. (1996). Toward a definition of family resilience: Integrating life-span and family perspectives. *Family Process, 35,* 283–298.

Helmreich, W. B. (1992). *Against all odds: Holocaust survivors and the successful lives they made in America.* New York: Simon & Schuster.

Henggeler, S. W., Schoenwald, S. K., Borduin, C. M., Rowland, M. D., & Cunningham, P. B. (1998). *Multisystemic treatment of antisocial behavior in children and adolescents.* New York: Guilford Press.

Herdt, G., & Koff, B. (2000). *Something to tell you: The road families travel when a child is gay.* New York: Columbia University Press.

Herman, J. (1992). *Trauma and recovery.* New York: Basic Books.

Hernandez, P. (2002). Resilience in families and communities: Latin American contributions from the psychology of liberation. *Journal of Counseling and Therapy for Couples and Families, 10*(3), 334–343.

Hess, G., & Handel, G. (1959). *Family worlds: A psychological approach to family life.* Chicago: University of Chicago Press.

Hetherington, E. M., & Kelly, J. (2002). *For better or for worse: Divorce reconsidered.* New York: Norton.

Higgins, G. O. (1994). *Resilient adults: Overcoming a cruel past.* San Francisco: Jossey-Bass.

Hill, R. (1949). *Families under stress.* New York: Harper.

Hines, P. M. (1998). Climbing up the rough side of the mountain: Hope, culture and therapy. In M. McGoldrick (Ed.), *Re-visioning family therapy: Race, culture, and gender in clinical practice* (pp. 78–89). New York: Guilford Press.

Hochschild, A. (1997). *Time bind.* New York: Holt.

Hoffman, L. (1990). Constructing realities: An art of lenses. *Family Process, 29,* 1–12.

Holtzworth-Monroe, A., & Jacobson, N. (1991). Behavioral marital therapy. In A. Gurman & D. Kniskern (Eds.), *Handbook of family therapy* (Vol. 2). New York: Brunner/Mazel.

Imber-Black, E. (1988). *Families and larger systems.* New York: Guilford Press.

Imber-Black, E. (1995). *Secrets in families and family therapy.* New York: Norton.

Imber-Black, E., Roberts, J., & Whiting, R. (Eds.). (2003). *Rituals in families and family therapy* (2nd ed.). New York: Norton.

Institute for Health and Aging. (1996). *Chronic care in America: A 21st-century challenge.* Princeton, NJ: Robert Wood Johnson Foundation.

Ives, S., Abramson, J., & Kantor, M. (Producers). (1996). *The West* [Videocassettes, 9 vols.]. Alexandria, VA: PBS Home Video.

Jackson, D. D. (1977). Family rules: Marital quid pro quo. In P. Watzlawick & J. Weakland (Eds.), *The interactional view*. New York: Norton.

Johnson, S. (2002). *Emotionally focused couples therapy for trauma survivors*. New York: Guilford Press.

Johnson-Garner, M. Y., & Meyers, S. A. (2003). What factors contribute to the resilience of African-American children within kinship care? *Child and Youth Care Forum*, 32(5), 255–269.

Jordan, D. (1996). *Family first: Winning the parenting game*. New York: HarperCollins.

Jordan, J. (1992, April). *Relational resilience*. Paper presented at Stone Center Colloquium Series, Wellesley College, Wellesley, MA.

Jordan, J., Kaplan, J. A., Miller, J., Stiver, I., & Surrey, J. (1991). *Women's growth in connection: Writings from the Stone Center*. New York: Guilford Press.

Joshi, P. T., & Lewin, S. M. (2004). Disaster, terrorism, and children. *Psychiatric Annals*, 34(9), 710–716.

Kabat-Zinn, J. (2003). Mindfulness-based interventions in context: Past, present, and future. *Clinical Psychology: Science and Practice*, 10(2), 144–156.

Kagan, J. (1984). *The nature of the child*. New York: Basic Books.

Kagan, S., & Weissbourd, B. (1994). *Putting families first*. San Francisco: Jossey-Bass.

Kamya, H. (2004). The impact of war on children and families: Their stories, my stories. *AFTA Monograph Series*, 1, 29–32.

Kaplan, L., & Girard, J. (1994). *Strengthening high-risk families*. New York: Lexington Books.

Karpel, M. (1986). *Family resources: The hidden partner in family therapy*. New York: Guilford Press.

Kauffman, J. (Ed.). (2002). *Loss of the assumptive world: A theory of traumatic loss*. New York: Brunner-Routledge.

Kauffman, R., & Briski, Z. (2004). *Born into Brothels* [Documentary film]. United States: HBO/Cinemax.

Kaufman, J., & Zigler, E. (1987). Do abused children become abusive parents? *American Journal of Orthopsychiatry*, 57, 186–192.

Kazak, A., Simms, S., & Rourke, M. (2002). Family systems practice in pediatric psychology. *Journal of Pediatric Psychology*, 27, 133–143.

Keller, H. (1968). *Midstream: My later life*. New York: Greenwood. (Original work published 1929)

King, D. A., & Wynne, L. C. (2004). The emergence of "family integrity" in later life. *Family Process*, 43(1), 7–21.

Kleinman, A. (1988). *Illness narratives: Suffering, healing, and the human condition*. New York: Basic Books.

Kliman, G., Oklan, E., Wolfe, H., & Kliman, J. (2005). *My Hurricane Katrina story: A guided activity workbook*. San Francisco: Children's Psychological Health Center.

Knudsen-Martin, C., & Mahoney, A. R. (2005). Moving beyond gender: Processes that create relationship equity. *Journal of Marital and Family Therapy*, 31(2), 235–246.

Kobasa, S., Maddi, S., & Kahn, R. (1982). Hardiness and health: A prospective study. *Journal of Personality and Social Psychology*, 37, 1–11.

Koenig, H., McCullough, M. E., & Larson, D. (2001). *Handbook of religion and health*. New York: Oxford University Press.

Kotlowitz, A. (1991). *There are no children here*. New York: Doubleday.

Laird, J. (2003). Lesbian and gay families. In F. Walsh (Ed.), *Normal family processes* (3rd ed., pp. 176–209). New York: Guilford Press.

Laird, J., & Green, R.-J. (Eds.). (1996). *Lesbians and gays in families and family therapy.* San Francisco: Jossey-Bass.

Lamb, M. E. (Ed.). (2004). *The role of the father in child development* (4th ed.). New York: Wiley.

Landau, J. (2005). *Enhancing resilience: Families and communities as agents for change.* Manuscript submitted for publication.

Landau, J., & Saul, J. (2004). Family and community resilience in response to major disaster. In F. Walsh & M. McGoldrick (Eds.), *Living beyond loss: Death in the family* (2nd ed., 285–309). New York: Norton.

Lansford, J. E., Ceballo, R., Abby, A., & Stewart, A. J. (2001). Does family structure matter? A comparison of adoptive, two-parent biological, single-mother, stepfather, and stepmother households. *Journal of Marriage and the Family, 63,* 840–851.

Latimer, J., Dowden, C., & Muise, D. (2001). *The effectiveness of restorative justice practices: A meta-analysis.* Ottawa, Canada: Department of Justice.

Lattanzi-Licht, M., & Doka, K. (Eds.). (2003). *Living with grief: Coping with public tragedy.* Washington, DC: Hospice Foundation of America.

Lavee, Y., McCubbin, H. I., & Olson, D. H. (1987). The effect of stressful life events and transitions on family functioning and well-being. *Journal of Marriage and the Family, 49,* 857–873.

Lazarus, R., & Folkman, S. (1984). *Stress, appraisal, and coping.* New York: Springer.

Lebow, J. (1997). The integrative revolution in family therapy. *Family Process, 36(1),* 1–17.

Lee, S. (Director). (1994). *Crooklyn* [Motion picture]. New York: 40 acres and a mule.

Lefley, H. P. (1996). *Family caregiving in mental illness.* Thousand Oaks, CA: Sage.

Lev-Weisel, R., & Amir, M. (2001). Secondary traumatic stress, psychological distress, sharing of traumatic reminiscences, and marital quality among spouses of Holocaust child survivors. *Journal of Marital and Family Therapy, 27,* 433–444.

Lewis, J., Beavers, W. R., Gossett, J., & Phillips, V. (1976). *No single thread: Psychological health in family systems.* New York: Brunner/Mazel.

Liddle, H. A., Santisteban, D. A., Levant, R. F., & Bray, J. H. (Eds.). (2002). *Family psychology: Science-based interventions.* Washington, DC: American Psychological Association.

Lidz, T. (1963). *The family and human adaptation.* New York: International Universities Press.

Lifton, R. J. (1979). *The broken connection: On death and the continuity of life.* New York: Simon and Schuster.

Lifton, R. J. (1993). *The Protean self: Human resilience in an age of fragmentation.* New York: Basic Books.

Linley, P., & Joseph, S. (2004). Positive change following trauma and adversity: A review. *Journal of Traumatic Stress, 17,* 11–22.

Litz, B. (2004). *Early intervention for trauma and traumatic loss.* New York: Guilford Press.

Lopata, H. (1996). *Current widowhood: Myths and realities.* Thousand Oaks, CA: Sage.

Luthar, S. (Ed.). (2003). *Resilience and vulnerability: Adaptation in the context of childhood adversities.* New York: Cambridge University Press.

Luthar, S. S., Cicchetti, D., & Becker, B. (2000). The construct of resilience: A critical evaluation and guidelines for future work. *Child Development, 71,* 543–562.

Luthar, S. S., & Zigler, E. (1991). Vulnerability and competence: A review of research on resilience in childhood. *American Journal of Orthopsychiatry, 61,* 6–22.

Mackay, R. (2003). Family resilience and good child outcomes: An overview of the research literature. *Journal of New Zealand, 20,* 98–118.

Maddi, S. (2002). The story of hardiness: Twenty years of theorizing, research, and practice. *Consulting Psychology Journal, 54,* 173–185.

Madsen, W. C. (2003). *Collaborative therapy with multi-stressed families.* New York: Guilford Press. (Original edition published 1999)

Malkinson, R., Rubin, S., & Witztum, E. (2005). Terror, trauma, and bereavement: Implications for theory and therapy. In Y. Danieli, D. Brom, & J. Sills (Eds.), *The trauma of terrorism: Sharing knowledge and shared care: An international handbook* (pp. 467–481). New York: Haworth.

Markman, H., & Halford, W. K. (2005). International perspectives on couple relationship education. *Family Process, 44,* 139–146.

Markman, H., & Notarius, C. (1994). *We can work it out: Making sense of marital conflict.* San Francisco: Jossey-Bass.

Masten, A. S. (2001). Ordinary magic: Resilience processes in development. *American Psychologist, 56*(3), 227–238.

Masten, A. S., Best, K. M., & Garmezy, N. (1990). Resilience and development: Contributions from the study of children who overcome adversity. *Development and Psychopathology, 2,* 425–444.

Masten, A. S., & Coatsworth, J. D. (1998). The development of competence in favorable and unfavorable environments: Lessons from research on successful children. *American Psychologist, 53*(2), 205–220.

McAdoo, H. (Ed.). (1996). *Black families* (3rd ed.). Thousand Oaks, CA: Sage.

McCubbin, H., & Patterson, J. M. (1983). The family stress process: The Double ABCX model of adjustment and adaptation. *Marriage and Family Review, 6*(1–2), 7–37.

McCubbin, H., Thompson, E. A., Thompson, A. I., & Fromer, J. E. (Eds.). (1998a). *Resiliency in Native American and immigrant families.* Thousand Oaks, CA: Sage.

McCubbin, H., Thompson, E. A., Thompson, A. I., & Fromer, J. E. (Eds.). (1998b). *Stress, coping, and health in families: Sense of coherence and resiliency.* Thousand Oaks, CA: Sage

McCubbin, H., Thompson, E. A., Thompson, A. I., & Futrell, J. A. (Eds.). (1998). *Resiliency in African-American families.* Thousand Oaks, CA: Sage.

McDaniel, S., Campbell, T., Hepworth, J., & Lorenz, A. (2005). *Family-oriented primary care.* (2nd ed.). New York: Springer.

McDaniel, S., Hepworth, J., & Doherty, W. (Eds.). (1997). *The shared experience of illness: Stories of patients, families, and their therapists.* New York: Basic Books.

McFarlane, W. (Ed.). (2002). *Multifamily groups in the treatment of severe psychiatric disorders.* New York: Guilford Press.

McGoldrick, M. (1995). *You can go home again: Reconnecting with your family.* New York: Norton.

McGoldrick, M. (Ed.). (1998). *Re-visioning family therapy: Race, culture, and gender in clinical practice.* New York: Guilford Press.

McGoldrick, M., Anderson, C., & Walsh, F. (Eds.). (1989). *Women in families: A framework for family therapy.* New York: Norton.

McGoldrick, M., Gerson, R., & Shellenberger, S. (1999). *Genograms: Assessment and intervention* (2nd ed.). New York: Norton.

McGoldrick, M., Giordano, J., & Garcia-Preto, N. (Eds.). (2005). *Ethnicity and family therapy* (3rd ed.). New York: Guilford Press.

McGoldrick, M., Schlesinger, J. M., Lee, E., Hines, P., Chan, J., Almeida, R., et al. (2004). Mourning in different cultures. In F. Walsh & M. McGoldrick (Eds.), *Living beyond loss* (2nd. ed., pp. 119–160). New York: Norton.

McGoldrick, M., & Watson, M. (1999). Siblings through the life cycle. In B. Carter & M. McGoldrick (Eds.), *The expanded family life cycle* (3rd ed., pp. 153–168). Boston: Allyn & Bacon.

McHenry, P. C., & Price, S. J. (2005). *Families and change: Coping with stressful events and transitions* (3rd ed.). Thousand Oaks, CA: Sage.

McLanahan, S., Garfinkel, I., Reichman, N., Teitler, J., Carlson, M., & Audiger, C. N. (2003). *The Fragile Families and Child Well-being Study: Baseline national report*. Princeton, NJ: Center for Research on Child Well-being, Princeton University.

Mead, M. (1972). *Blackberry winter*. New York: Morrow.

Miklowitz, D., & Goldstein, M. (1997). *Bipolar disorder: A family-focused treatment approach*. New York: Guilford Press.

Miller, S., McDaniel, S., Rolland, J., & Feetham, S. (2006). *Individuals, families and the new era of genetics: Biopsychosocial perspectives*. New York: Norton.

Minkler, M., & Roe, J. (1993). *Grandparents as caregivers*. Newbury Park, CA: Sage.

Minuchin, P., Colapinto, J., & Minuchin, S. (1998). *Working with families of the poor*. New York: Guilford Press.

Minuchin, S. (1974). *Families and family therapy*. Cambridge, MA: Harvard University Press.

Minuchin, S., & Nichols, M. (1993). *Family healing: Tales of hope and renewal from family therapy*. New York: Free Press.

Mock, M. (1998). Clinical reflections on refugee families: Transforming crises into opportunities. In M. McGoldrick (Ed.), *Re-visioning family therapy*. New York: Guilford Press.

Mollica, R. (2004). Surviving torture. *New England Journal of Medicine, 35*(1), 5–7.

Moore, K. A., Chalk, R., Scarpa, J., & Vandevere, S. (2002). *Family strengths: Often overlooked, but real*. [Child Trends research brief.] Washington, DC: Child Trends.

Murphy, L. (1987). Further reflections on resilience. In E. J. Anthony & B. Cohler (Eds.), *The invulnerable child*. New York: Guilford Press.

Nadeau, J. W. (2001). Family construction of meaning. In R. Neimeyer (Ed.), *Meaning reconstruction and the experience of loss* (pp. 95–111). Washington, DC: American Psychological Association.

National Network for Family Resiliency. (1996). *Understanding resiliency* [Online]. Available at http://www.agnr.umd.edu/users/nnfr/pub_under.html.

Neimeyer, R. A. (Ed.). (2001). *Meaning reconstruction and the experience of loss*. Washington, DC: American Psychological Association.

Neugarten, B. (1976). Adaptation and the life cycle. *Counseling Psychologist, 6,* 16–20.

Nichols, M., & Schwartz, R. (2005). *Family therapy: Concepts and methods* (7th ed.). Needham Heights, MA: Allyn & Bacon.

Norris, F. H. (2002). 60,000 disaster victims speak: Part 1. An empirical review of the empirical literature, 1981–2001. *Psychiatry: Interpersonal and Biological Processes, 65*(3), 207–239.

Norris, F. H., & Alegria, M. (2005). Mental health care for ethnic minority individuals and communities in the aftermath of disasters and mass violence. *CNS Spectrums, 10*(2), 132–140.

Oliver, L. (1999). Effects of a child's death on the marital relationship: A review. *Omega, 39*(3), 197–227.

Olkin, R. (1999). *What psychotherapists should know about disability.* New York: Guilford Press.

Olson, D. H., & Gorell, D. M. (2003). Circumplex model of marital and family systems. In F. Walsh (Ed.), *Normal family processes* (3rd ed., pp. 514–548). New York: Guilford Press.

Ooms, T., & Wilson, P. (2004). The challenges of offering relationship and marriage education to low-income populations. *Family Relations, 53*(5), 440–447.

Oswald, R. F. (2002). Resilience within the family networks of lesbians and gay men: Intentionality and redefinition. *Journal of Marriage and the Family, 64*(2), 374–383.

Parkes, C. M. (2001). *Bereavement: Studies of grief in adult life* (3rd ed.). Philadelphia: Taylor & Francis.

Parsons, T., & Bales, R. F. (1955). *Family, socialization, and interaction processes.* Glencoe, IL: Free Press.

Patterson, G. R. (1983). Stress: A change agent for family process. In N. Garmezy & M. Rutter (Eds.), *Stress, coping, and development in children.* New York: McGraw-Hill.

Patterson, J. M. (2002). Integrating family resilience and family stress theory. *Journal of Marriage and the Family, 64,* 349–360.

Patterson, J. M., & Garwick, A. W. (1994). Levels of family meaning in family stress theory. *Family Process, 33,* 287–304.

Penn, P. (1985). Feed forward: Future questions, future maps. *Family Process, 24,* 299–310.

Perry, A., & Rolland, J. (1999). Spirituality expressed in community action and social justice. In F. Walsh (Ed.), *Spiritual resources in family therapy* (pp. 272–292). New York: Guilford Press.

Pertman, A. (2000). *Adoption nation: How the adoption revolution is transforming America.* New York: Basic Books.

Pipher, M. (1997). *The shelter of each other: Rebuilding our families.* New York: Ballantine.

Rampage, C., Eovaldi, M., Ma, C., & Weigel-Foy, C. (2003). Adoptive families. In F. Walsh (Ed.), *Normal family processes* (3rd ed., pp. 210–232). New York: Guilford Press.

Rando, T. (1993). *Treatment of complicated mourning.* Champaign, IL: Research Press.

Reiss, D. (1981). *The family's construction of reality.* Cambridge, MA: Harvard University Press.

Reiss, D., Hetherington, M., Plomin, R., & Neiderhiser, J. (2000). *The relationship code: Deciphering genetic and social influences on adolescent development.* New York: Wiley.

Risman, B. (1999). *Gender vertigo: American families in transition.* New Haven, CT: Yale University Press.

Rolland, J. S. (1994). *Families, illness, and disability: An integrative treatment model.* New York: Basic Books.

Rolland, J. S. (2003). Mastering family challenges in serious illness and disability. In F. Walsh (Ed.), *Normal family processes* (3rd ed., pp. 460–489). New York: Guilford Press.

Rolland, J. S., & Walsh, F. (2005). Systemic training for healthcare professionals: The Chicago Center for Family Health approach. *Family Process, 44*(3), 283–301.

Rolland, J. S., & Weine, S. (2000). Kosovar Family Professional Educational Collaborative. *American Family Therapy Academy Newsletter, 79,* 34–35.

Rolland, J. S., & Williams, J. (2005). Toward a biopsychosocial model for 21st century genomics. *Family Process, 44*(1), 3–24.

Root, M. P. P. (2001). *Love's revolution: Racial intermarriage.* Philadelphia: Temple University Press.

Rosen, E. (1998). *Families facing death* (2nd ed.). San Francisco: Jossey-Bass.

Rubin, L. B. (1996). *The transcendent child: Tales of triumph over the past.* New York: Basic Books.

Rutter, M. (1985). Resilience in the face of adversity: Protective factors and resistance to psychiatric disorder. *British Journal of Psychiatry, 147,* 598–611.

Rutter, M. (1987). Psychosocial resilience and protective mechanisms. *American Journal of Orthopsychiatry, 57,* 316–331.

Rutter, M. (1999). Resilience concepts and findings: Implications for family therapy. *Journal of Family Therapy, 21*(2), 119–144.

Ryan, C., Epstein, N. B., Keitner, G., Miller, I. W., & Bishop, D. S. (2005). *Evaluating and treating families: The McMaster approach.* New York: Routledge.

Sanders, G., & Krall, I. T. (2000). Generating stories of resilience: Helping gay and lesbian youth and their families. *Journal of Marital and Family Therapy, 26*(4), 433–442.

Satir, V. (1988). *The new peoplemaking.* Palo Alto, CA: Science & Behavior Books.

Schumm, W. (1985). Beyond relationship characteristics of strong families: Constructing a model of family strengths. *Family Perspective, 19,* 1–9.

Schwartz, P. (1994). *Love between equals.* New York: Free Press.

Schwartz, R. (1997, March–April). Don't look back. *Family Therapy Networker,* 40–47.

Sciolino, E. (1996, Nov. 11). A painful road from Vietnam to forgiveness. *New York Times,* A1, A8.

Seccombe, K. (2002). "Beating the odds" versus "changing the odds": Poverty, resilience, and family policy. *Journal of Marriage and the Family, 64*(2), 384–394.

Seligman, M. E. P. (1990). *Learned optimism.* New York: Random House.

Seligman, M. E. P. (1995). *The optimistic child.* Boston: Houghton-Mifflin.

Seligman, M. E. P., & Csikszentmihalyi, M. (2000). Positive psychology. *American Psychologist, 55*(1), 55–70.

Sexton, T., & Alexander, J. (2003). Functional family therapy: A mature clinical model for working with at-risk adolescents and their families. In T. Sexton, G. Weeks, & M. Robbins (Eds.), *Handbook of family therapy* (pp. 323–363). New York: Brunner-Routledge.

Shange, N., & Shabalala, J. (1995). *Nomathemba.* Performance. Chicago: Steppenwolf Theatre.

Shefsky, J. (2000). *A justice that heals* [Documentary film]. Chicago: WTTW, Windows of the World Communications.

Sheinberg, M., & Fraenkel, P. (2001). *The relational trauma of incest: A family-based approach to treatment.* New York: Guilford Press.

Shibusawa, T. (2005). Japanese families. In M. McGoldrick, J. Giordano, & N. Garcia-Preto (Eds.), *Ethnicity and family therapy* (3rd ed., pp. 399–348). New York: Guilford Press.

Siegel, D. (1999) *The developing mind: Toward a neurobiology of interpersonal experience.* New York: Guilford Press.

Silverman, L., & Goodrich, T. J. (2003). *Feminist family therapy: Empowerment in social context.* Washington, DC: American Psychological Association.

Simon, R. (1997, March–April). Systems therapy NBA style. *Family Therapy Networker,* pp. 49–61.

Sitterle, K. A., & Gurwitch, R. H. (1999). The terrorist bombing in Oklahoma City. In E. S. Zinner & M. B. Williams (Eds.), *When a community weeps.* New York: Brunner-Mazel.

Skolnick, A., & Skolnick, J. (2001). *Family in transition* (9th ed.). Boston: Allyn & Bacon.

Sluzki, C. (1983). Process, structure, and worldviews in family therapy: Toward an integration of systemic models. *Family Process, 22,* 469–476.

Sluzki, C. (1998). Migration and the disruption of the social network. In M. McGoldrick (Ed.), *Re-visioning family therapy* (pp. 360–369). New York: Guilford Press.

Sluzki, C. E. (2003). The process toward reconciliation. In A. Chayes & M. Minow (Eds.), *Imagine coexistence: Restoring humanity after violent ethnic conflict* (pp. 21–30). San Francisco: Jossey-Bass.

Speck, R. (2003). Social network intervention. In G. P. Sholevar & L. D. Schwoeri (Eds.), *Textbook of family and couples therapy* (pp. 193–201). Washington, DC: American Psychiatric Press.

Sprenkle, D., & Piercy, F. (Eds.). (2005). *Research methods in family therapy.* New York: Guilford Press.

Stacey, J. (1990). *Brave new families: Stories of domestic upheaval in late twentieth century America.* New York: Basic Books.

Stacey, J. (1996). *In the name of the family: Rethinking family values in the postmodern age.* Boston: Beacon Press.

Stacey, J., & Biblarz, T. J. (2001). How does the sexual orientation of parents matter? *American Sociological Review, 66*(2), 159–183.

Stanley, S. M., Markman, H. J., & Jenkins, N. H. (2004). *Marriage education using PREP with low-income and diverse clients.* Denver, CO: PREP.

Stanley, S. M., Markman, H. J., Saiz, C. C., Schumm, W. R., Bloomstrom, G., & Bailey, A. E. (2003). *Building strong and ready families: Interim report.* Washington, DC: Science Applications International.

Statistical Abstract of the United States: 2004–2005. Washington, DC: U.S. Government Printing Office.

Steinberg, L., Lamborn, S. D., Dornbusch, S. M., & Darling, N. (1992). Impact of parenting practices on adolescent achievement: Authoritative parenting, school involvement, and encouragement to succeed. *Child Development, 63,* 1266–1281.

Steinglass, P. (1998). Multiple family discussion groups for patients with chronic medical illness. *Families, Systems, and Health, 16*(1–2), 55–71.

Stinnett, N., & DeFrain, J. (1985). *Secrets of strong families.* Boston: Little, Brown.

Stone, E., Gomez, E., Hotzoglou, D., & Lipnitsky, J. (2005). Transnationalism as a motif in family stories. *Family Process*, 44(4), 381–398.

Stroebe, M. S., & Schut, H. (2001). Meaning making in the dual process model of coping with bereavement. In R. Neimeyer (Ed.), *Meaning reconstruction in the experience of loss* (pp. 55–73). Washington, DC: American Psychological Association.

Swadener, B. B., & Lubeck, S. (Eds.). (1995). *Children and families "at promise": Deconstructing the discourse of risk*. Albany: State University of New York Press.

Taggart, S. (1994). *Living as if: Belief systems in mental health practice*. San Francisco: Jossey-Bass.

Taylor, S. (1989). *Positive illusions: Creative self-deception and the healthy mind*. New York: Basic Books.

Taylor, S., Kemeny, M., Reed, G., Bower, J., & Gruenwald, T. (2000). Psychological resources, positive illusions, and health. *American Psychologist*, 55(1), 99–109.

Tedeschi, R. G., & Calhoun, L. G. (1995). *Trauma and transformation: Growing in the aftermath of suffering*. Thousand Oaks, CA: Sage.

Tedeschi, R. G., Park, L. C., & Calhoun, L. G. (1996). The Posttraumatic Growth Inventory: Measuring the positive legacy of trauma. *Journal of Traumatic Stress*, 9, 455–471.

Terkel, S. (2000). *Will the circle be unbroken?* New York: Norton.

Terkel, S. (2002). *Hope dies last: Keeping the faith in troubled times*. New York: Norton.

Tienari, P. et al. (2004). Genotype–environment interaction in schizophrenia-spectrum disorders. *British Journal of Psychiatry*, 184, 216–222.

Torrey, E. F. (2001) *Surviving schizophrenia: A manual for families, consumers, and providers* (4th ed.). New York: HarperCollins.

Torrey, E. F. (2002). *Surviving manic depression: A manual on bipolar disorder*. New York: Basic Books.

Towers, H., Spotts, E., & Reiss, D. (2003). Unraveling the complexity of genetic and environmental influences on family relationships. In F. Walsh (Ed.), *Normal family processes* (3rd ed., pp. 608–631). New York: Guilford Press.

Trepper, T., & Barrett, M. J. (1989). *Systemic treatment of incest: A therapeutic handbook*. New York: Brunner/Mazel.

Ungar, M. (2004a). The importance of parents and other caregivers to the resilience of high-risk adolescents. *Family Process*, 43(1), 23–41.

Ungar, M. (2004b). *Nurturing hidden resilience in troubled youth*. Toronto, Canada: University of Toronto Press.

Ungar, M. (Ed.). (2005). *Handbook for working with children and youth: Pathways to resilience across cultures and contexts*. Thousand Oaks, CA: Sage.

Vaillant, G. (1995). *Adaptation to life* (rev. ed.). Cambridge, MA: Harvard University Press.

Vaillant, G. (2002). *Aging well*. Boston: Little Brown.

Van der Kolk, B. A., McFarlane, A. C., & Weisaeth, L. (Eds.). (1996). *Traumatic stress: The effects of overwhelming experience on mind, body, and society*. New York: Guilford Press.

Vanderpool, M. (2002). Resilience: A missing link in our understanding of survival. *Harvard Review of Psychiatry*, 10, 302–306.

Visher, E., Visher, J. S., & Pasley, K. (2003). Remarriage families and stepparenting. In F.

Walsh (Ed.), *Normal family processes* (3rd ed., pp. 153–175). New York: Guilford Press.

Walker, A. (1983). *The color purple.* New York: Washington Square Press.

Waller, M. (2001). Resilience in ecosystemic context: Evolution of the concept. *American Journal of Orthopsychiatry, 71*(3), 1–8.

Walsh, F. (1983). The timing of symptoms and critical events in the family life cycle. In H. Liddle (Ed.), *Clinical implications of the family life cycle* (pp. 120–133). Rockville, MD: Aspen.

Walsh, F. (1985). Social change, disequilibrium, and adaptation in developing countries: A Moroccan example. In J. Schwartzman (Ed.), *Families and other systems.* New York: Guilford Press.

Walsh, F. (1989). Reconsidering gender in the "marital quid pro quo." In M. McGoldrick, C. Anderson, & F. Walsh (Eds.), *Women in families: A framework for family therapy* (pp. 267–285). New York: Norton.

Walsh, F. (1996). The concept of family resilience: Crisis and challenge. *Family Process, 35,* 261–281.

Walsh, F. (1998). Beliefs, spirituality, and transcendence: Keys to family resilience. In M. McGoldrick (Ed.), *Re-visioning family therapy: Race, culture, and gender in clinical practice.* New York: Guilford Press.

Walsh, F. (1999a). Families in later life: Challenges and opportunities. In B. Carter & M. McGoldrick (Eds.), *The expanded family life cycle* (3rd ed., pp. 307–326). Needham Heights, MA: Allyn & Bacon.

Walsh, F. (Ed.). (1999b). *Spiritual resources in family therapy.* New York: Guilford Press.

Walsh, F. (2002a). A family resilience framework: Innovative practice applications. *Family Relations, 51*(2), 130–137.

Walsh, F. (2002b). Bouncing forward: Resilience in the aftermath of September 11, 2001. *Family Process, 41*(1), 34–36.

Walsh, F. (2003a). Changing families in a changing world: Reconstructing family normality. In F. Walsh (Ed.), *Normal family processes* (3rd ed., pp. 3–26). New York: Guilford Press.

Walsh, F. (2003b). Clinical views of family normality, health, and dysfunction: From deficit to strengths perspective. In F. Walsh (Ed.), *Normal family processes* (3rd ed., pp. 27–57). New York: Guilford Press.

Walsh, F. (2003c). Crisis, trauma, and challenge: A relational resilience approach for healing, transformation, and growth. *Smith College Studies in Social Work, 74*(1), 49–71.

Walsh, F. (2003d). Family resilience: A framework for clinical practice. *Family Process, 42*(1), 1–18.

Walsh, F. (2004). Spirituality, death, and loss. In F. Walsh & M. McGoldrick (Eds.), *Living beyond loss: Death in the family* (2nd ed.). New York: Norton.

Walsh, F. (2006). *Pets: The relational significance of companion animals.* Manuscript submitted for publication.

Walsh, F., & Anderson, C. M. (Eds.). (1988). *Chronic disorders and the family.* New York: Haworth Press

Walsh, F., Jacob, L., & Simons, V. (1995). Facilitating healthy divorce processes: Therapy and mediation approaches. In N. Jacobson & A. Gurman (Eds.), *Clinical handbook of couple therapy.* New York: Guilford Press.

Walsh, F., & McGoldrick, M. (2004). Loss and the family: A systemic perspective. In F.

Walsh & M. McGoldrick (Eds.), *Living beyond loss: Death in the family* (2nd ed., pp. 3–26). New York: Norton.

Waters, D., & Lawrence, E. (1993). *Competence, courage, and change.* New York: Norton.

Watzlawick, P., Beavin, J., & Jackson, D. (1967). *Pragmatics of human communication.* New York: Norton.

Webb, N. B. (2003). *Mass trauma and violence: Helping families and children cope.* New York: Guilford Press.

Weihs, K., Fisher, L., & Baird, M. (2001). Families, health, and behavior: A section of the commissioned report for the Institute of Medicine, National Academy of Sciences. *Families, Systems, and Health, 20*(1), 7–47.

Weil, A. (1994). *Spontaneous healing.* New York: Knopf.

Weine, S. (1999). *When history is a nightmare.* New Brunswick, NJ: Rutgers University Press.

Weine, S., et al. (2004). Family consequences of refugee trauma. *Family Process, 43*(2), 147–160.

Weine, S. (2006). *Testimony after catastrophe: Narrating the traumas of political violence.* Evanston, IL: Northwestern University Press.

Weingarten, K. (2003). *Common shock: Witnessing violence every day: How we are harmed, how we can heal.* New York: Dutton.

Weingarten, K. (2004). Witnessing the effects of political violence in families: Mechanisms of intergenerational transmission of trauma and clinical interventions. *Journal of Marital and Family Therapy, 30*(1), 45–59.

Werner, E. E. (1993). Risk, resilience, and recovery: Perspectives from the Kauai longitudinal study. *Development and Psychopathology, 5,* 503–515.

Werner, E. E., & Johnson, J. L. (1999). Can we apply resilience? In M. J. Glantz & J. L. Johnson (Eds.), *Resilience and development: Positive life adaptations* (pp. 259–268). New York: Kluwer Academic/Plenum.

Werner, E. E., & Smith, R. S. (1982). *Vulnerable but invincible: A study of resilient children.* New York: McGraw-Hill.

Werner, E. E., & Smith, R. S. (1992). *Overcoming the odds: High-risk children from birth to adulthood.* Ithaca, NY: Cornell University Press.

Werner, E. E., & Smith, R. S. (2001). *Journeys from childhood to midlife: Risk, resilience, and recovery.* Ithaca: Cornell University Press.

West, C. (1995). *Race matters.* Cambridge, MA: Harvard University Press.

Weston, K. (1991). *Families we choose: Lesbians, gays, and kinship.* New York: Columbia University Press.

Whitaker, C., & Keith, D. (1981). Symbolic–experiential family therapy. In A. Gurman & D. Kniskern (Eds.), *Handbook of family therapy.* New York: Brunner/Mazel.

White, M., & Epston, D. (1990). *Narrative means to therapeutic ends.* New York: Norton.

Wiesel, E. (1995). *All rivers run to the sea: Memoirs.* New York: Knopf.

Wilson, W. J. (1996). *When work disappears: The world of the urban poor.* New York: Random House.

Wolin, S., & Wolin, S. (1993). *The resilient self: How survivors of troubled families rise above adversity.* New York: Villard.

Wood, B. (1985). Proximity and hierarchy: Orthogonal dimensions of family interconnectedness. *Family Process, 24,* 487–507.

Worden, W. J. (1996). *Children and grief: When a parent dies.* New York: Guilford Press.

Worden, W. J. (2002). *Grief counseling and grief therapy* (3rd ed.). New York: Springer.
World Health Organization. (1972). *International statistical classification of diseases and related health problems* (10th ed.). Geneva, Switzerland: Author.
Worthington, E. L., Jr., & Scherer, M. (2004). Forgiveness is an emotion-focused coping strategy that can reduce health risks and promote health resilience: Theory, review, and hypotheses. *Psychology and Health, 19,* 385–406.
Wortman, C., & Silver, R. (1989). The myths of coping with loss. *Journal of Counseling and Clinical Psychology, 57,* 349–357.
Wright, L., Watson, W. L., & Bell, J. M. (1996). *Beliefs: The heart of healing in families and illness.* New York: Basic Books.
Wuerffel, J., DeFrain, J., & Stinnett, N. (1990). How strong families use humor. *Family Perspective, 24,* 129–142.
Wyman, E., Cowen, W., Work, W., & Parker, G. (1991). Developmental and milieu correlates of resilience in urban children who have experienced major life stress. *American Journal of Community Psychology, 19,* 405–426.
Wynne, L. C., McDaniel, S., & Weber, T. (Eds.). (1986). *Systems consultation: A new perspective for family therapy* (pp. 253–272). New York: Guilford Press.
Yang, O-K., & Choi, M-M. (2001). Koreans' Han and resilience: Application to mental health social work. *Mental Health and Social Work, 11*(6), 7–29.
Zinner, E. S., & Williams, M. B. (Eds.). (1999). *When a community weeps: Case studies in group survivorship.* New York: Brunner/Mazel.

Index